Supervision in Psychiatric Practice

Practical Approaches Across Venues and Providers

Supervision in Psychiatric Practice

Practical Approaches Across Venues and Providers

Edited by

Sallie G. De Golia, M.D., M.P.H.

Kathleen M. Corcoran, Ph.D.

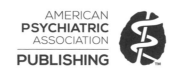

AMERICAN
PSYCHIATRIC
ASSOCIATION
PUBLISHING

If you wish to buy 50 or more copies of the same title, please go to www.appi.org/specialdiscounts for more information.

Copyright © 2019 American Psychiatric Association Publishing

ALL RIGHTS RESERVED

First Edition

Manufactured in the United States of America on acid-free paper
23 22 21 20 19   5 4 3 2 1

American Psychiatric Association Publishing
800 Maine Avenue SW
Suite 900
Washington, DC 20024-2812
www.appi.org

Library of Congress Cataloging-in-Publication Data
Names: De Golia, Sallie G., editor. | Corcoran, Kathleen M., editor. | American Psychiatric Association Publishing, issuing body.
Title: Supervision in psychiatric practice : practical approaches across venues and providers / edited by Sallie G. De Golia, Kathleen M. Corcoran.
Description: First edition. | Washington, D.C. : American Psychiatric Association Publishing, [2019] | Includes bibliographical references and index. |
Identifiers: LCCN 2019003832 (print) | LCCN 2019004876 (ebook) | ISBN 9781615372546 () | ISBN 9781615371648 (pbk. : alk. paper)
Subjects: | MESH: Psychiatry—organization & administration | Teaching | Professional Competence
Classification: LCC RC440.8 (ebook) | LCC RC440.8 (print) | NLM WM 100 | DDC 616.890068—dc23
LC record available at https://lccn.loc.gov/2019003832

British Library Cataloguing in Publication Data
A CIP record is available from the British Library.

Contents

Part 1

Introduction

Part 2

Supervision Formats

Part 3
Supervision Techniques

Part 4
Clinical Supervision Venues

Michelle Burke Parish, Ph.D., M.A.

Shannon Suo, M.D.

Rachel Robitz, M.D.

Jaesu Han, M.D.

Peter Yellowlees, M.B.B.S., M.D.

Ripal Shah, M.D., M.P.H.

Lawrence M. McGlynn, M.D., M.S.

Viet T. Nguyen, M.D., M.P.H.

Pragya Rimal, M.A.

Rebecca M. White, M.D.

Bibhav Acharya, M.D.

Part 5

Nonclinical Supervision Venues

Joshua Griffiths, M.D.

Joel Yager, M.D.

Ella M. Williams, M.D.

Adam M. Brenner, M.D.

Francesco N. Dandekar, M.D.

Belinda S. Bandstra, M.D., M.A.

Part 6

Special Issues in Supervision

Part 7

Legal and Ethical Issues

Part 8

Professional Development

Contributors

Bibhav Acharya, M.D.
UCSF Psychiatry HEAL Fellowship in Global Mental Health, Department of Psychiatry, University of California, San Francisco, California; Co-founder, Possible, a nonprofit organization, Kathmandu, Nepal

Esther Akinyemi, M.D.
Associate Training Director of Psychiatry, Henry Ford Hospital/Wayne State University, Detroit, Michigan

Melissa R. Arbuckle, M.D., Ph.D.
Professor of Psychiatry at CUIMC, Columbia University Irving Medical Center, New York, New York

Belinda S. Bandstra, M.D., M.A.
Clinical Associate Professor, Department of Psychiatry and Behavioral Sciences, Stanford University School of Medicine, Stanford, California

Jessica Bentzley, M.D.
Resident, Department of Psychiatry and Behavioral Sciences, Stanford University School of Medicine, Stanford, California

Joseph Biedrzycki, D.O.
Assistant Professor, Department of Psychiatry and Behavioral Sciences, SUNY Upstate Medical University, Syracuse, New York

Stephen T. Black, Ph.D.
Clinical Assistant Professor (Affiliated), Stanford University School of Medicine; Veterans Affairs Palo Alto Health Care System, Palo Alto, California

Adam M. Brenner, M.D.
Professor of Psychiatry, Distinguished Teaching Professor, Vice Chair of Education and Residency Training Director, University of Texas Southwestern, Dallas, Texas

Kim D. Bullock, M.D.
Clinical Associate Professor, Department of Psychiatry and Behavioral Sciences, Stanford University School of Medicine, Stanford, California

Michelle Burke Parish, Ph.D., M.A.
Researcher, University of California, Davis School of Medicine, Davis, California

Deborah L. Cabaniss, M.D.
Professor of Clinical Psychiatry and Associate Director of Residency Training, Columbia University Department of Psychiatry, New York, New York

Jennifer L. Callahan, Ph.D., ABPP
Professor of Psychology, University of North Texas, Denton, Texas

Randolph S. Charlton, M.D.
Adjunct Clinical Professor of Psychiatry, Stanford University School of Medicine, Stanford, California

Kathleen M. Corcoran, Ph.D.
Clinical Associate Professor and Training Director for the Clinical Psychology Postdoctoral Program (Adult), Department of Psychiatry and Behavioral Sciences, Stanford University, Stanford, California

Deborah Suzanne Cowley, M.D.
Professor and Vice Chair, Department of Psychiatry and Behavioral Sciences, University of Washington School of Medicine, Seattle, Washington

Francesco N. Dandekar, M.D.
College Mental Health Fellow, Department of Psychiatry and Behavioral Sciences, Stanford University School of Medicine, Stanford, California

Sallie G. De Golia, M.D., M.P.H.
Clinical Professor; Associate Chair, Clinician Educator Professional Development; and Associate Residency Director, Department of Psychiatry and Behavioral Sciences, Stanford University School of Medicine, Stanford, California

William O. Faustman, Ph.D.
Clinical Professor (Affiliated), Stanford University School of Medicine; Veterans Affairs Palo Alto Health Care System, Palo Alto, California

Amanda M. Franciscus, M.D.
Clinical Instructor (Affiliated), Department of Psychiatry and Behavioral Sciences, Stanford University Medical School, Stanford, California

G. Mark Freeman Jr., M.D., Ph.D.
Clinical Assistant Professor (Affiliated), Stanford University School of Medicine, Stanford, California

Elise Gibbs, Psy.D.
Clinical Instructor, Department of Psychiatry and Behavioral Sciences, Stanford University, Stanford, California

Jessica Gold, M.D., M.S.
Assistant Professor, Department of Psychiatry, Washington University in St. Louis School of Medicine, St. Louis, Missouri

Michelle Goldsmith, M.D.
Clinical Associate Professor, Department of Psychiatry and Behavioral Sciences, Stanford University School of Medicine, Stanford, California

Cheryl Yund Goodrich, Ph.D.
Private Practice of Psychoanalytic Psychotherapy and Mentalization Based Therapy, Los Altos, California; Adjunct Clinical Assistant Professor, Department of Psychiatry and Behavioral Sciences, Stanford University School of Medicine, Stanford, California

Carlos C. Greaves, M.D.
Adjunct Clinical Associate Professor, Department of Psychiatry and Behavioral Sciences, Stanford University School of Medicine, Stanford, California

John M. Greene, M.D.
Adjunct Clinical Assistant Professor, Department of Psychiatry and Behavioral Sciences, Stanford University School of Medicine, Stanford, California

Joshua Griffiths, M.D.
Fellow in Forensic Psychiatry, Department of Psychiatry, University of Colorado School of Medicine, Aurora, Colorado

Jaesu Han, M.D.
Clinical Professor, Department of Psychiatry & Human Behavior, University of California, Irvine School of Medicine, Irvine, California

Joshua J. Hubregsen, M.D.
Assistant Professor of Psychiatry, University of Texas at Southwestern Medical Center, Dallas, Texas

Shani Isaac, M.D.
Staff Psychiatrist, Momentum for Mental Health, Palo Alto, California

Joanna Jarecki, M.D.
Assistant Professor, Department of Psychiatry and Behavioural Sciences, McMaster University, Hamilton, Ontario, Canada

Agnes Kalinowski, M.D., Ph.D.
Clinical Instructor and Research Fellow, Department of Psychiatry and Behavioral Sciences, Stanford University School of Medicine, Stanford, California

Anita R. Kishore, M.D.
Clinical Associate Professor of Psychiatry, Stanford University School of Medicine, Stanford, California

Malathy Kuppuswamy, M.D.
Clinical Associate Professor (Affiliated), Stanford University School of Medicine; Site Director for Residency Training Program in Psychiatry, Veterans Affairs Palo Alto Health Care System, Palo Alto, California

Sheila Lahijani, M.D.
Clinical Assistant Professor, Department of Psychiatry and Behavioral Sciences, Stanford University School of Medicine, Stanford, California

Angela Lee, A.B.
Third-Year Medical Student, Stanford University School of Medicine, Stanford, California

Hanna Levenson, Ph.D.
Professor, Wright Institute, Berkeley, California; Private Practice, Oakland, California

Kristine H. Luce, Ph.D.
Clinical Associate Professor, Department of Psychiatry and Behavioral Sciences, Stanford University School of Medicine, Stanford, California

Lisa MacLean, M.D.
Clerkship Director, Henry Ford Health System, Detroit, Michigan

Jan Malat, M.D.
Assistant Professor, Department of Psychiatry, University of Toronto, Toronto, Canada

John M. Manring, M.D.
Professor, Department of Psychiatry and Behavioral Sciences, SUNY Upstate Medical University, Syracuse, New York

Jesse David Markman, M.D., M.B.A.
Assistant Professor and Associate Training Director, Department of Psychiatry and Behavioral Sciences, University of Washington School of Medicine, Seattle, Washington

Margaret May, M.D.
Clinical Instructor (affiliated), Palo Alto VAHCS and Stanford University School of Medicine, Palo Alto, California

Robert M. McCarron, D.O.
Professor and Vice Chair of Education and Integrated Care, Residency Training Director, and Co-Director, UCI/UC Davis Train New Trainers Primary Care Psychiatry Fellowship, Department of Psychiatry & Human Behavior, University of California, Irvine School of Medicine, Irvine, California

Lawrence M. McGlynn, M.D., M.S.
Clinical Professor, Department of Psychiatry and Behavioral Sciences, Stanford University School of Medicine, Stanford, California

Susan McNair, M.D.
Assistant Professor, Department of Psychiatry and Behavioural Sciences, McMaster University, Hamilton, Ontario, Canada

Zsuzsa Szombathyne Meszaros, M.D., Ph.D.
Associate Professor, Department of Psychiatry and Behavioral Sciences, SUNY Upstate Medical University, Syracuse, New York

Viet T. Nguyen, M.D., M.P.H.
UCSF Psychiatry HEAL Fellow in Global Mental Health, University of California, San Francisco—HEAL Initiative, San Francisco, California

Natalie Pon, M.D.
Child and Adolescent Psychiatrist, Children's Health Council, Palo Alto, California

Deepak Prabhakar, M.D., M.P.H.
Clinical Associate Professor and Director of Psychiatric Education, Henry Ford Health System; Training Director, Psychiatry Residency Program, Henry Ford Hospital/ Wayne State University, Detroit, Michigan

Douglas S. Rait, Ph.D.
Clinical Professor and Chief, Couples and Family Therapy Clinic, Department of Psychiatry and Behavioral Sciences, Stanford University School of Medicine, Stanford, California

Kristin S. Raj, M.D.
Clinical Assistant Professor, Department of Psychiatry and Behavioral Sciences, Stanford University School of Medicine, Stanford, California

Anna Ratzliff, M.D., Ph.D.
Associate Professor, Depression Therapy Research Endowed Professorship, and Associate Director for Education, AIMS Center; Director, University of Washington Integrated Care Training Program, Seattle, Washington

Divy Ravindranath, M.D.
Clinical Assistant Professor (affiliated), Palo Alto VAHCS and Stanford University School of Medicine, Palo Alto, California

Matthew Reed, M.D., M.S.P.H.
Assistant Professor of Clinical Psychiatry, Associate Residency Training Director, Director of Consultation and Liaison Psychiatry, and Director of Education, Train New Trainers Primary Care Psychiatry Fellowship, Department of Psychiatry & Human Behavior, and Assistant Dean for Student Affairs, University of California, Irvine School of Medicine, Irvine, California

Pragya Rimal, M.A.
Mental Health Research Manager, UCSF Psychiatry HEAL Fellow in Global Mental Health, University of California, San Francisco—HEAL Initiative, San Francisco, California; Mental Health Research Manager, Possible, a nonprofit organization, Kathmandu, Nepal

Thalia Robakis, M.D., Ph.D.
Clinical Assistant Professor, Department of Psychiatry and Behavioral Sciences, Stanford University School of Medicine, Stanford, California

Rachel Robitz, M.D.
Assistant Clinical Professor, Department of Psychiatry and Behavioral Sciences, University of California, Davis School of Medicine, Davis, California

Tony Rousmaniere, Psy.D.
Clinical Faculty, University of Washington, Seattle, Washington

Marie E. Rueve, M.D.
Assistant Clinical Professor, Department of Psychiatry and Behavioral Neuroscience, University of Cincinnati, Lindner Center of HOPE, Cincinnati, Ohio

Jennifer Ruzhynsky, M.D., M.A.
Assistant Professor, Department of Psychiatry and Behavioural Sciences, McMaster University, Hamilton, Ontario, Canada

Debra L. Safer, M.D.
Associate Professor and Co-director, Eating Disorders Clinic, Stanford University
School of Medicine, Stanford, California

Ann C. Schwartz, M.D.
Professor and Director of Psychiatry Residency Education, Department of Psychiatry
and Behavioral Sciences, Emory University School of Medicine, Atlanta, Georgia

Ripal Shah, M.D., M.P.H.
Clinical Instructor, Department of Psychiatry and Behavioral Sciences, Stanford University School of Medicine, Stanford, California

Dorothy E. Stubbe, M.D.
Associate Professor of Psychiatry, Program Director, Yale University School of Medicine
Child Study Center, Yale University School of Medicine, New Haven, Connecticut

Donna M. Sudak, M.D.
Professor of Psychiatry, Drexel University, Philadelphia, Pennsylvania

Shannon Suo, M.D.
Associate Professor, Residency Program Director, Family Medicine Psychiatry, and
Co-Director, UCI/UC Davis Train New Trainers Primary Care Psychiatry Fellowship,
Department of Psychiatry & Behavioral Sciences, University of California, Davis
School of Medicine, Davis, California

Megan Tan, M.D., M.S.
Resident in Psychiatry, Department of Psychiatry and Behavioral Sciences, Stanford
University School of Medicine, Stanford, California

Camilla N. Van Voorhees, M.D.
Faculty, San Francisco Center for Psychoanalysis, San Francisco, California

Katherine Walia Cerio, M.D.
Clinical Assistant Professor, Department of Psychiatry and Behavioral Sciences,
SUNY Upstate Medical University and Syracuse Veterans Administration Hospital,
Syracuse, New York

S. Dina Wang-Kraus, M.D.
Resident, Department of Psychiatry and Behavioral Sciences, Stanford University
School of Medicine, Stanford, California

C. Edward Watkins Jr., Ph.D.
Professor of Psychology, University of North Texas, Denton, Texas

Priyanthy Weerasekera, M.D., M.Ed.
Professor, Department of Psychiatry and Behavioural Sciences, McMaster University,
Hamilton, Ontario, Canada

Randon S. Welton, M.D.
Associate Professor and Director of Residency Training, Department of Psychiatry,
Wright State University, Dayton, Ohio

Rebecca M. White, M.D.
UCSF Psychiatry HEAL Fellow in Global Mental Health, University of California,
San Francisco—HEAL Initiative, San Francisco, California

Dana Wideman, Ph.D.
Adjunct Clinical Assistant Professor, Stanford University School of Medicine, Stanford, California

Ella M. Williams, M.D.
Assistant Professor of Psychiatry, University of Texas Southwestern, Dallas, Texas

Katherine E. Williams, M.D.
Clinical Professor and Director of the Women's Wellness Clinic, Stanford University School of Medicine, Stanford, California

Joel Yager, M.D.
Professor, Department of Psychiatry, University of Colorado School of Medicine, Aurora, Colorado

Peter Yellowlees, M.B.B.S., M.D.
Professor of Psychiatry and Vice Chair for Faculty Development, Department of Psychiatry and Behavioral Sciences, University of California, Davis, Sacramento, California

Disclosure of Competing Interests

The following contributors to this book have indicated a financial interest in or other affiliation with a commercial supporter, a manufacturer of a commercial product, a provider of a commercial service, a nongovernmental organization, and/or a government agency, as listed below:

Susan McNair, M.D.—*Royalties:* Psychotherapy Training e-Resources (PTeR)

Jennifer Ruzhynsky, M.D., M.A.—*Royalties:* Psychotherapy Training e-Resources (PTeR)

Donna M. Sudak, M.D.—*Book royalties:* John Wiley & Sons, Lippincott Williams & Wilkins

Priyanthy Weerasekera, M.D., M.Ed.—*Royalties:* Psychotherapy Training e-Resources (PTeR)

The following contributors have indicated that they have no financial interests or other affiliations that represent or could appear to represent a competing interest with the contributions to this book:

Bibhav Acharya, M.D.
Esther Akinyemi, M.D.
Melissa R. Arbuckle, M.D., Ph.D.
Belinda S. Bandstra, M.D., M.A.
Jessica Bentzley, M.D.
Joseph Biedrzycki, D.O.
Stephen T. Black, Ph.D.
Adam M. Brenner, M.D.
Kim D. Bullock, M.D.
Michelle Burke Parish, Ph.D., M.A.

Kristine H. Luce, Ph.D.
Lisa MacLean, M.D.
Jan Malat, M.D.
John M. Manring, M.D.
Jesse David Markman, M.D., M.B.A.
Margaret May, M.D.
Robert M. McCarron, D.O.
Lawrence M. McGlynn, M.D., M.S.
Zsuzsa Szombathyne Meszaros, M.D., Ph.D.
Viet T. Nguyen, M.D., M.P.H.

Deborah L. Cabaniss, M.D.

Jennifer L. Callahan, Ph.D., ABPP

Randolph S. Charlton, M.D.

Kathleen M. Corcoran, Ph.D.

Deborah Suzanne Cowley, M.D.

Francesco N. Dandekar, M.D.

Sallie G. De Golia, M.D., M.P.H.

William O. Faustman, Ph.D.

Amanda M. Franciscus, M.D.

G. Mark Freeman Jr., M.D., Ph.D.

Elise Gibbs, Psy.D.

Jessica Gold, M.D., M.S.

Michelle Goldsmith, M.D.

Cheryl Yund Goodrich, Ph.D.

Carlos C. Greaves, M.D.

John M. Greene, M.D.

Joshua Griffiths, M.D.

Jaesu Han, M.D.

Joshua J. Hubregsen, M.D.

Shani Isaac, M.D.

Joanna Jarecki, M.D.

Agnes Kalinowski, M.D., Ph.D.

Anita R. Kishore, M.D.

Malathy Kuppuswamy, M.D.

Sheila Lahijani, M.D.

Angela Lee, A.B.

Hanna Levenson, Ph.D.

Deepak Prabhakar, M.D., M.P.H.

Douglas S. Rait, Ph.D.

Kristin S. Raj, M.D.

Divy Ravindranath, M.D.

Matthew Reed, M.D., M.S.P.H.

Pragya Rimal, M.A.

Thalia Robakis, M.D., Ph.D.

Rachel Robitz, M.D.

Tony Rousmaniere, Psy.D.

Marie E. Rueve, M.D.

Debra L. Safer, M.D.

Ann C. Schwartz, M.D.

Ripal Shah, M.D., M.P.H.

Dorothy E. Stubbe, M.D.

Shannon Suo, M.D.

Megan Tan, M.D., M.S.

Camilla N. Van Voorhees, M.D.

Katherine Walia Cerio, M.D.

S. Dina Wang-Kraus, M.D.

C. Edward Watkins Jr., Ph.D.

Randon S. Welton, M.D.

Rebecca M. White, M.D.

Dana Wideman, Ph.D.

Ella M. Williams, M.D.

Katherine E. Williams, M.D.

Joel Yager, M.D.

Peter Yellowlees, M.B.B.S., M.D.

Acknowledgments

We are most grateful to the dozens of authors who graciously agreed to submit manuscripts to our publication and tolerated our, sometimes excessive, editorial comments. Without their wise insight and experience, this book would never have taken shape. We would also like to thank our Chair, Dr. Laura Roberts, for providing us the exceptional opportunity to take on this challenge, as well as our colleagues who helped by reading our drafts and supporting this book, including Bruce Arnow, Chris Hayward, Kathryn DeWitt, and Katherine Williams.

We are also grateful to our own supervisors from the past who helped shape our passion for this work, and to our trainees, who are a source of constant inspiration.

And finally, this effort would not have happened without the enduring support and love of our families. We cannot thank you all enough.

Part 1 Introduction

Chapter 1   Elements of Supervision

Sallie G. De Golia, M.D., M.P.H.

Supervision is central to the field of psychiatry. It is how we learn, it is how we prepare for unsupervised practice, it is how we develop into who we are as professionals. It is also what many of us do as part of our jobs as psychiatrists, psychologists, or other mental health professionals—from supervising psychotherapy to supervising a team of mental health care providers. And, as supervisees, it is what many of us continue to engage in well into our careers (Grant et al. 2012; Psychology Board of Australia 2018). In short, it represents a dominant feature of our professional development and professional activities. Yet, most mental health supervisors, particularly psychiatrists, receive little or no training in how to supervise (Reiss and Fishel 2000; Rodenhauser 1992). And despite supervision's central place in psychiatry's professional training and work, supervision is the least developed and researched aspect of clinical teaching (Kilminster et al. 2007).

In fact, even agreement on how to define supervision across mental health disciplines and venues remains controversial. For the purposes of this book, Milne's definition of supervision is appropriate (though originally developed in the context of clinical psychotherapy supervision): "the formal provision, by approved supervisors, of a relationship-based education and training that is work focused and which manages, supports, develops and evaluates the work of colleagues" (Milne 2009, p. 15). Using this definition, this book seeks to provide practical insights into a variety of aspects of supervision within both clinical and nonclinical venues. It explores a variety of supervisory techniques and issues related to specific supervisory topics in addition to reviewing legal issues associated with supervision and the current state of professional development.

3

Within the past couple of decades significant progress in understanding clinical supervision has occurred, particularly through the supervision competency movement (Falender and Shafranske 2004; Psychology Board of Australia 2018; UCL Psychology and Language Sciences 2018) and identification of evidence-based practices in supervision. As Borders (2014) describes, effective supervision needs both competencies and best practices to offer critical supervisory guidelines. Though immensely valuable, the current clinical competency frameworks are based on expert consensus and do not as of this writing have empirical support; nor do they have demonstrated predictive or construct validity (Gonsalvez et al. 2013). Furthermore, the lack of guidance on supervision from psychiatry's main accrediting institution for residency and fellowship training, the Accreditation Council for Graduate Education (ACGME), underscores the absence of evidence-based guidelines. The ACGME offers only nonspecific guidelines: "faculty must devote sufficient time to the educational program to fulfill their supervisory and teaching responsibilities...." (Accreditation Council for Graduate Medical Education 2017). Accordingly, each residency and fellowship program must independently determine the behaviors and logistics associated with supervision, and ultimately how supervision competency is evaluated and tracked within the program.

This chapter serves as a basic roadmap for supervision; it covers the core elements of supervision within psychiatry, irrespective of discipline, venue, or format. These core elements are relevant when supervising a variety of mental health professionals as well as physicians from other disciplines and auxiliary health care professionals and administrators; when supervising within a variety of settings, from inpatient to community-based settings or diverse administrative to scholarly environments; when supervising an individual, group, or team; and/or when supervising live or through virtual means. The core elements presented in this chapter are relevant to all supervisory situations, yet they are *not* prescriptive in nature.

Phases of Supervision

There are multiple ways to examine supervision. One way is to break down supervision into four phases (Figure 1–1). The *preparatory phase* involves aspects the supervisor might consider *before* initiating a supervisory relationship, while the *introductory phase* explores what happens within the initial meetings with a supervisee. The *working phase* of supervision is where the bulk of learning and skill development occurs, while the *termination phase* focuses on transitioning the supervisee(s) to future supervision, unsupervised practice, or work with a consultant and may include a final assessment.

Preparatory Phase

Before meeting with supervisees, supervisors might familiarize themselves with adult learning theory principles to orient around a framework for teaching. It is also critical to understand the context in which one is asked to supervise. With an understanding of the context, supervisors must prepare for the many roles they may need to assume, taking into account supervisee needs, the system in which supervision occurs, and the supervisor's own limitations.

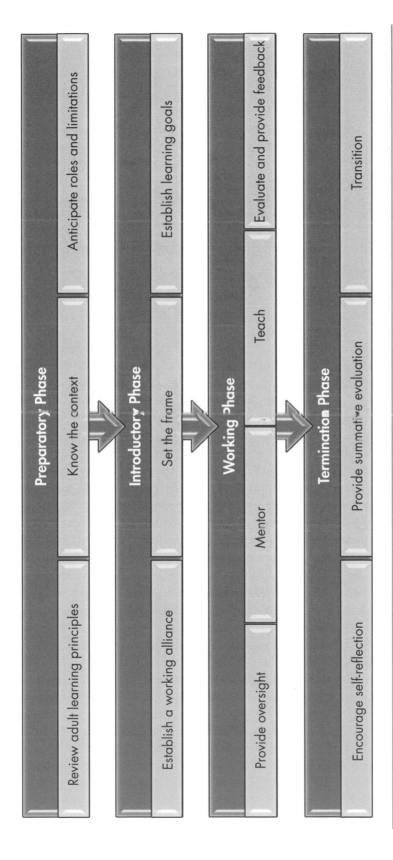

FIGURE 1–1. Four phases of supervision.

Key Points

- Review adult learning principles.
    - Adult learners are self-directed and motivated, seek participation in the learning process, and focus on meaning and application.
- Know the context.
    - Know the environment in which you supervise (resources and limitations), supervisor requirements and expectations, and how the supervisor will be evaluated.
- Anticipate supervisor roles and limitations.
    - Many supervisory roles occur concurrently and are seemingly conflictual.
    - Be cognizant of the power differentials, culture, and privilege issues.
    - Avoid dual relationships and balance support and self-disclosure while maintaining clear boundaries.

Review Adult Learning Principles

In recent years, medical and mental health education has integrated more intentional, interactive and explicit learning processes into the practice of supervision. This represents movement beyond the more traditional apprenticeship model of learning. Research has shown that learning improves when educators are able to implement principles from learning theories (Bergman et al. 2013). Although an exhaustive discussion of learning theories is beyond the scope of this chapter, *andragogy*, or principles used in adult learning, offers a description of the adult learner and his or her needs which is relevant to the supervisory situation (Knowles 1984). Supervisees (and supervisors) are adult learners. Knowles (1984) characterizes adult learners as being self-directed and motivated. They seek active participation in the learning process in order to accept and integrate new information in a meaningful way.

To achieve meaningful or deep learning, adult learners focus on understanding. They strive to understand the new knowledge as a coherent whole, rather than as a set of disparate facts. According to the theory, it is important to actively involve the learner in constructing meaning for the supervision. Learners want evidence to explain how learning a given content will contribute to their professional understanding. Once relevance is established, adult learners want to know how they might apply the content in the future. This will help motivate the supervisee to attend to the content, absorb the material, and, in turn, retain it.

Adult learners also rely on their prior experience to enhance their learning. To integrate new knowledge into the learner's awareness as a meaningful whole, learners must relate new information provided by the supervisor to what they already know or perceive. If the preexisting knowledge has been activated and is closely related to the new incoming material, this new information will be more readily received by the long-term memory.

And, finally, adult learners want to apply their new knowledge immediately in solving problems and receive feedback with regard to their progress. Because psychiatric supervision is so inextricably linked to the workplace through its role in overseeing clinical and academic activities, it represents the ideal context for fostering experiential learning.

All learning starts with participation in work-related tasks of the day-to-day activities in which a wide variety of medical and cultural content is embedded (Teunissen et al. 2007). Through interpreting and constructing meaning from their work activities, whether clinical, administrative, or scholarly, supervisees transform the essence of these activities into personal knowledge. Supervisors guide this learning through modeling, guided reflection, feedback, and mentorship.

Supervisors need to reflect on their own competencies and teaching methods in an attempt to more closely align their approaches to best meet the needs of an adult learner. They might also seek didactic or experiential training in supervision and/or teaching to enhance their supervisory skills.

Know the Context

The context in which one supervises involves not only the immediate setting of the supervision (e.g., inpatient ward with trainees vs. managing other clinic providers) but also the broader environment. Does the environment allow for enough time for knowledge acquisition or adequate case assessment? Does it support resources needed to help supervisees (e.g., technology, office space)? Does it value, prioritize, or incentivize teaching (e.g., protected time)? Furthermore, supervisory activities may not always be driven by education or patient safety considerations; they may also be driven by rules and regulations not clearly specified. For example, Medicare rules and insurance guidelines often dictate what and how supervision will be conducted with trainees in order to receive reimbursement for services provided instead of supervision being based on oversight or teaching needs (Kuttner 1999; Stern 2002).

It is important to understand the site of initiation of the supervision. If the supervisee is unaffiliated, the supervisor will want to understand the supervisee's specific needs and whether there are any legal or evaluative requirements. If supervision is requested by a program or organization, the supervisor will need to know who ultimately is overseeing the supervision and to whom he or she would report in case of questions, resource needs, or supervisee performance concerns. It is also important to clarify the format of supervision (individual or group; live or virtual), specific logistical considerations (meeting place, frequency, duration), and/or expected supervisory methods (videotaping, one-way mirror, deliberate practice). What would be expected if a meeting were cancelled or a supervisee missed a session? Who would cover if the supervisor (or supervisee) is on vacation? If remediation is required, what role might the supervisor play?

Clarifying the conceptual framework used for evaluating supervisees is important: these may include measures such as ACGME competencies and milestones, Entrustable Professional Activities (EPAs), established supervisory guidelines (e.g., Psychology Board of Australia 2018), or other approaches derived from frameworks such as psychotherapy-based (e.g., CBT or psychodynamic) or supervision-based psychotherapy models (e.g., developmental or integrative). Which supervisee competencies are expected to be accomplished within a given supervisory time period? If there are no internal competency guidelines, guidelines from national organizations (e.g., ACGME) may be helpful. Another approach to determine supervision expectations is to review evaluation forms, though not all evaluative tools fully reflect an organization's expectations, particularly by supervisee level.

Conversely, it is also important to determine how the supervisor will be evaluated within the system. The program director or workplace manager should be able to clarify the process. If a supervisor evaluation form exists, it would be useful to review it prior to starting supervision.

Optimally, all these issues would be clarified and understood in advance, but unfortunately much of this information is not always explicitly described or available. The clearer the structural issues of supervision, the more transparent and tension-free the relationship, both with the system and with the supervisee, may be.

Anticipate Supervisor Roles and Limitations

Supervisory roles can range from managerial to educational to service to support. Responsibilities will vary according to the context, and, often, many of these roles exist concurrently. For example, managerial roles encompass a broad array of responsibilities, including modeling and maintaining effective communication, creating and maintaining an effective team, distributing workloads, setting deadlines, establishing and maintaining clear boundaries, protecting and maintaining resources, establishing and clarifying staff roles, establishing and/or enforcing policies and procedures, observing societal laws, disciplining, and remediating and resolving conflict. The educator role involves engaging in a host of teaching techniques and methods, including evaluating, providing feedback, and fostering self-directed (lifelong) learning. As a clinical provider, the supervisor has responsibility for maintaining patient safety, and, at times, he or she may need to provide direct service. And mentoring involves coaching, supporting, and nurturing behaviors to enhance learner or professional development. Sometimes these roles may be seemingly in opposition to one another, leading to inherent tension within the supervisory relationship, and highlighting the complex skills required and challenges of the supervisory function.

When one is preparing for supervision, it is important to be aware of the potential power differential between the supervisor and supervisee. The supervisee may be fearful of being open and honest with the supervisor for fear of criticism or a poor evaluation. In addition to power, the supervisor should be self-reflective around cultural and privilege issues (see Chapter 35, "Cultural Issues Within the Supervisory Relationship"). Another complicating factor involves the multiple roles a supervisor might have within an organization, which may lead to dual relationships with the supervisee. Supervisors are often engaged with learners in a variety of contexts: as didactic teachers, ward supervisors, coauthors on publications, members of committees, colleagues in national organizations, and friends. As a supervisor, it is advisable to avoid dual relationships, though occasionally this may not be possible. A related issue to consider is the maintenance of boundaries (see Chapter 38, "Boundaries: Management of Supervisory Roles and Behaviors"). Supervision is not mentorship, and it is not therapy. It has an evaluative function. However, it may embody aspects of both mentorship and therapy. The supervisor must balance allowing the supervisee to explore internal feelings and reactions with avoiding too much disclosure (Sarnat 2010). On the other hand, self-disclosure by a supervisor may be quite useful and appropriate, particularly as it relates to supervisees presenting concerns (Ladany et al. 2013), whereas this would be more carefully restricted within a therapy context. Furthermore, though a sound working alliance is critical, the supervisory relationship must tolerate the fact it is not entirely confidential. In the context of a training program, supervisors are mandated to evaluate trainees and, at times, may need to inform the program of serious concerns they have with a supervisee. As problems arise, the supervisor needs to be prepared to address them.

Introductory Phase

Supervision is a proactive, planned, purposeful, goal-oriented, and intentional activity (Borders and Brown 2005). As such, the first sessions will be predominantly associated with developing a working alliance, setting the supervisory frame, and establishing learning goals.

Key Points

- Establish a working alliance.
  - Invest time in getting to know the supervisee.
  - Supervisees value being empowered through encouragement of autonomy and sharing ideas.
  - Keep lines of communication open: consider addressing power dynamics, diversity and cultural issues, and dual relationships and how to manage potential ruptures.
- Set the frame.
  - Explain supervisory benefits and relevance to supervisee.
  - Review issues and limitations of confidentiality within supervision.
  - Review terms, framework, and expectations of supervision.
- Establish learning objectives.
  - Assess the supervisee's level of competence and areas for improvement.
  - Collaboratively develop clear goals and objectives.
  - Identify educational activities based on goals.

Establish a Working Alliance

Prior to jumping into the content or "work" of supervision, the supervisor needs to know and understand the supervisee. By investing in the development of a safe, comfortable, and respectful relationship, the supervisee will be more able to express concerns, vulnerabilities, fears, mistakes, and therapeutic blunders without experiencing excessive shame or anxiety. However, supervisee anxiety and resistance are normal, particularly with less experienced supervisees. A strong supervisory working alliance sets the stage for effective learning, much like a therapeutic alliance with a patient. Active listening, reflection of feelings, and empathy all facilitate this bond and allow for a more trusting and effective working alliance (Bernard and Goodyear 2009; Shanfield et al. 1992); improve motivation (Orsini et al. 2018), self-confidence, and overall morale (van der Wal et al. 2016); and may have an impact on academic achievement (Lucas et al. 1993) and contribute to burnout (Edwards et al. 2006) and medical errors (Chang and Mark 2011). Supervisees value being empowered by supervisors who encourage autonomy and facilitate openness to their ideas (Ladany et al. 2013). A strong supervisory working alliance encourages a supervisee to feel more comfortable seeking help, receiving feedback, and incorporating changes (Kaufman and Schwartz 2004). A weaker supervisory working alliance has been associated with supervisor ethical infractions; limited supervisor multicultural competence, as well as supervisee nondisclosure, role conflict, and role ambiguity (Ladany 2004); poor coping skills, with adverse client-related events (Kozlowska et al. 1997b); and high levels of supervisee despair and psychological difficulties (Kozlowska et al. 1997a).

Supervisors are encouraged to learn about their supervisees' past experiences and knowledge base. What are the challenges they face, and the relevant issues they may have personally and professionally? Understanding their context fosters an authentic, caring environment where commitment to education and development is demonstrated.

Diversity and cultural issues and the implicit power differential within the supervisory relationship are important to address because this may lead to deeper understanding between participants. Being explicit about the nature of the dynamic in the relationship will help keep lines of communication open. Furthermore, it is important to avoid, or at least to be explicit about, existing dual relationships within the supervisory relationship and how they might affect this relationship. By being clear about these issues and how to handle them, supervisors help minimize potential barriers to communication and learning.

At the outset of supervision, the supervisor might articulate a commitment to explore and work through any ruptures or difficulties in the supervisory relationship (see Chapter 36, "Ruptures in the Supervisory Alliance"). By encouraging honesty and openness in the process of supervision, particularly around potential conflicts, the supervisor may help the supervisee to feel more comfortable bringing up such issues to explore. If difficulties arise, it is important for supervisors to find ways to manage tensions productively and be aware of their own role in creating tension, whether based on supervisor interpersonal style, diverging values and beliefs, or unwanted supervisor requests. By modeling how to manage conflicts, the supervisor can provide valuable learning opportunities for the supervisee around core professionalism values. Such modeling helps inform the learner how to acknowledge uncertainty, take personal responsibility, and admit limitations (Ramani and Orlander 2013).

Set the Frame

Many junior supervisees do not know what to expect from supervision. It is helpful to explain supervisory benefits and their relevance to supervisees. Once the utility and purpose of supervision are accepted, the terms of the supervisory relationship can be defined: how often to meet, when, where, what the expectations are, how to contact each other (particularly in the case of a crisis), and how to manage absences. The supervisor will also want to review his or her legal obligations vis-à-vis the patient and/or program.

Discussing explicitly the limits of confidentiality at the outset of supervision is advisable. The supervisee needs to understand those issues or behaviors that will require supervisors to break confidentiality by informing the appropriate program leadership who oversee the supervisory program. Issues of concern may range from excessive absences in supervision, inadequate work that has been refractory to feedback, unethical behavior, or mental health issues such as suicidality or cognitive impairment. The program may provide guidance about those behaviors that warrant breaking of confidentiality and what procedures to follow. Any of these issues require thoughtful, sensitive discussion with the supervisee.

Finally, it is advised to make the framework (e.g., competency, milestone, EPA) on which supervision will be based and methods of evaluation explicit to the supervisee.

The supervisor might also explore what types of oversight and learning approaches tend to work best for the supervisee. Ideally, there would be a clear agreement about the expected approach to each session, the method of content presentation, and the ways the supervisee might utilize the new material after supervision. For example, the supervisee might be encouraged to come prepared to supervision with questions, an agenda, and/or a video. The supervisee might be expected to complete homework or to practice a skill discussed before the next session.

Establish Learning Objectives

Goals drive learning by providing learners with a guide for what is expected. Goals are at the core of the supervisory process. Trainees are often unclear what they are supposed to be learning (Rojas et al. 2010). However, learners find goals and objectives useful in self-monitoring to gauge and inform their progress. This is helpful in guiding and stimulating deeper reflection on clinical performance as well as encouraging self-directed learning (Sargeant et al. 2011).

Knowing a supervisee's level of competence is important not only for developing and/or collaborating on appropriate learning goals but also to avoid compromising supervisee and patient safety. However, getting a handle on a supervisee's level of competence at the outset of supervision is not always easy. What exposure has the supervisee had to relevant didactics or educational and/or past clinical or work-associated experiences germane to the supervision? What has he or she been able to master? What are his or her struggles and/or vulnerabilities? Be mindful that some supervisees may not be able to articulate these gaps or be aware of their own deficiencies. Supervisees' level of competence will become clearer as supervisors directly observe their work. Furthermore, a supervisor might ask other staff or prior supervisors about their perceptions of the supervisee's level of competence and areas for improvement.

What are the supervisees' specific interests and goals in supervision? By collaborating with supervisees in creating clear goals regarding not only knowledge but also skills and attitudes, supervisees own their learning and have their intrinsic motivation reinforced. Focusing only on program or supervisor goals leads supervisees to perceive goals as external criteria on which they will be judged, leading to extrinsic motivation. By collaborating on goals, learners tend to perform better and have higher self-efficacy than those who do not collaborate on goals (Latham et al. 1994). The ideal would be to align personal and program goals with supervisee needs to ensure relevance and enhance motivation, ownership, and responsibility.

Developing clear and useful goals is a collaborative learning process and skill in and of itself. The SMART goal format (Specific, Measurable, Achievable, Realistic, Time-phased) is a useful tool for developing sound and effective goals to ensure clarity of expectations toward achievement success (Doran 1981). The goals should match the supervisee's developmental level and be within the supervisor's area of competence.

The next step is to identify educational activities to ensure that supervisee goals will be attained. Activities might involve assigning readings, participating in role-plays, reviewing video, responding to questions, encouraging time for reflection, requesting narrative writings or an annotated transcript, and/or encouraging conference attendance. The goals and context will guide the selection of and approach to educational activities.

Writing down the mutually accepted goals and educational activities will allow both supervisor and supervisee to review and track goals regularly as supervision proceeds. This will also allow the supervisor to intentionally evaluate and provide feedback to the supervisee on each of the established goals. A supervision contract or supervision log might be helpful and creates a clear understanding between partners (see "Additional Resources" at the end of this chapter for more information on supervision contracts, and Figure 1–2 for a sample supervision log). Goals will need to be modified as the supervision proceeds based on increased learner experience, evaluation, and feedback, leading to a recognition of new needs and skills to be mastered.

Working Phase

The working phase involves four major supervisory domains: oversight, mentorship, teaching, and evaluation and feedback activities. These functions often overlap in a fluid manner. A supervisor develops, on the basis of learner goals, a plan of how to fill the perceived gaps. Ideally, the supervisor has the ability to respond flexibly, taking into account the supervisee's developmental stage and particular needs, abilities, and deficiencies.

Before describing each of these domains, supervisors might consider how to manage a supervisory session. A supervisory agenda is often generated in an impromptu manner, but this approach may leave a lot of learning to chance. Prior to meetings, it is valuable to review a supervisee's learning goals, developmental needs, learning style, cultural characteristics, and responsiveness to previous sessions. It is important to keep track of what has (or has not) worked within supervisory sessions, supervisee strengths and areas of deficiency, and whether the supervisee, patient, and project are progressing. A planned, preset agenda may be helpful before each session is begun in order to gain the most from the experience. It may also be helpful to keep a written record of sessions in order to track these parameters (see Figure 1–2).

Key Points

- Provide oversight.
  - Ensure patient care and safety, research and scholarship progress, and leadership successes.
  - Monitor performance.
  - Ensure adherence to rules, regulations, procedures, and laws.
- Mentor.
  - Support, coach, advocate, and model professionalism and self-care.
  - Help socialize supervisee to profession.
  - Unlike mentors, supervisors evaluate supervisees.
- Teach.
  - Seek a more learner-centered and collaborative teaching approach targeting the level of the supervisee.
  - Align teaching methods with learner goals, interests, and the context.
  - Try to use more than one teaching modality to enhance learning.
- Evaluate and provide feedback.
  - Seek to evaluate carefully through direct observation and questioning.
  - Engage in interactive feedback.

Clinical Supervision Log

Supervisee: _____ Contact: _____ Supervision time: _____

GOAL SETTING   Date discussed: _____

Supervisee's Goals   Supervisor's Goals

1.   1.

2.   2.

3.   3.

Midterm Feedback About Supervision _____   Completed Y/N
                                        date

Date	Supervision question	Discussion	Reflection: What seemed to work in supervision	Supervisee/ supervisor action plan

FIGURE 1–2. Sample supervision log.

Provide Oversight

Managing the competing needs of guiding supervisee learning while monitoring the health care needs of patients, supervisee research needs, or administrative dilemmas in the context of maintaining quality standards and adherence to policies makes supervisory oversight a complicated process.

Within the context of patient care, Kilminster et al. (2007) describe the object of supervision as "to provide the patient with the best possible quality service under the prevailing circumstances and to provide the community from which that patient comes with the quality of service which meets its needs" (p. 3). The clinical supervisor must ensure that the supervisee is competent and performing only at his or her appropriate level. This is not always easy to determine and may require direct observation or feedback from other staff. Supervisors make decisions on how much to trust a supervisee to independently carry out a patient care activity based on supervisee factors, including developmental level, work context or circumstances, tasks or activities involved, and the supervisee/supervisor relationship (Ten Cate et al. 2016). While ensuring quality care, supervisors often allow supervisees to experience some level of autonomy (Babbott 2010). However, as learners seek to perform tasks in the service of learning and identity formation, they are at risk of performing an unsafe act (de Feijter et al. 2011). This underscores how critical effective supervision is, particularly while supervisees are acquiring new skills. Inadequate supervision can compromise patient safety and supervisee learning (Baldwin et al. 2010; Ten Cate et al. 2016).

Kennedy et al. (2007) have developed a topography of four oversight activities in an attempt to operationalize clinical oversight, starting with the least intensive form of supervisory involvement to the most. These activities include routine oversight (carries out activities planned in advance; e.g., daily rounds or prearranged case discussions), responsive oversight (responds to supervisee regarding patient-specific issues; e.g., discrepancies in clinical information or changed condition of severely ill patient that triggers supervisor to examine patient), direct patient care (actively cares for patient as beyond supervisee's competence level), or backstage oversight (occurs outside the supervisee's awareness either routinely or in response to trigger; e.g., lab review or patient exam). Though these activities were described within the clinical context, they could apply to other supervisory venues as well.

Mentor

Supervision involves many aspects of mentorship, and yet it is distinctly different. Similar to mentors, supervisors are supportive and reflective and ask reflective questions associated with career and personal development. They coach supervisees to develop skills in specific areas, including management, organizational, and leadership skills. They may advocate for learning resources and adequate time for supervision and/or ensure that learning needs are met. They model professionalism and help supervisees socialize to the professional culture. As in mentorship, these tasks are accomplished through using active listening, role modeling, and empathic and analytical skills and providing honest and specific feedback while maintaining clear boundaries. Supervisors also model recognizing their own limitations.

Another important role of the supervisor-mentor is to model self-care. Burnout and stress among mental health workers are well documented, as is their impact on health, job satisfaction, retention, quality care, patient outcomes, and systemic cost (Morse et al. 2012). The supervisor needs to attend to a supervisee's levels of stress and well-being through listening, supporting, and helping supervisees to improve their capacity to cope. When supervisees are helped to process their workplace experience, then burnout, stress levels, and compassion fatigue can be reduced and supervisees can be more effective in the workplace (Wallbank and Robertson 2008). The supervisor may need to recommend resources to help supervisees or, in extreme cases, inform the program leadership of the supervisee's areas of struggle.

But, unlike the mentor, the supervisor-mentor is in a position to assess and provide feedback on performance to a program or institution. Supervisors are also responsible for outcomes in patient care and may be associated, if not responsible, for supervisee research and/or administrative performance. They are required to provide final assessments in an attempt to maintain professional standards.

Teach

Supervision and education are tightly entwined. Better supervisory teaching within the clinical setting has been shown to have a direct effect on trainee clinical competence (Wimmers et al. 2006). However, supervisees' ability to learn is negatively impacted if their work pressure or workload exceeds a certain level (Dornan 2012).

Though modeling remains a powerful learning modality, teaching within supervision has progressed over the years from teacher-centered approaches emphasizing information transfer to more learner-centered approaches with a collaborative focus. However, clinical supervisors still report deficiencies in teaching strategies, feedback skills, and ways to promote learner reflection and insight, suggesting that they remain less comfortable with learner-centered teaching strategies (Bearman et al. 2018).

Supervisors might start with reviewing the goals constructed early in supervision, which serve as a roadmap for teaching and evaluation. It is important to select teaching methods that align with supervisees' goals and interests and the context. It is valuable to be clear and intentional about one's teaching approach, yet flexible enough to accommodate supervisees' preferred learning style and needs, the content, and any unexpected circumstances that may arise. Also, targeting the teaching at the level of a supervisee will help avoid missed learning opportunities (Newman et al. 2016). In general, less-experienced supervisees tend to appreciate clear structure and concrete instructions.

Research has demonstrated that the use of more than one teaching modality improves retention (Dwyer 1978). This can be achieved by incorporating a range of educational modalities targeting aural (e.g., guided discussions of readings, podcasts, videos, lectures), visual (e.g., assigned readings, particularly with diagrams; PowerPoint presentations), and kinesthetic (e.g., role-plays for practice, transcript annotation, note taking) modalities that are relevant to the intended learning outcomes and appropriate for the content. Understanding and retention can be further promoted by presenting well-organized material, explaining relationships in the material, responding adequately to learner's questions, and asking a supervisee to reformulate the information and prioritize it with their existing knowledge—all approaches that can lead to a deeper processing of the material. Newly learned information can be reinforced by encouraging its incorporation into the task at hand or role-play. Knowledge that is not used or not useful will most likely not be retained. Modeling is another powerful method of teaching: role-modeling good clinical practice, leadership, time management, effective and open communication, teamwork, ability to critically self-evaluate, and self-care, as appropriate. If supervision parallels didactic courses, incorporating what has been learned within the classroom can reinforce concepts (Cabaniss and Arbuckle 2011). (See Part 3: "Supervision Techniques," for examples of how to integrate different teaching modalities into supervision.)

Evaluate and Provide Feedback

Evaluation is the process of making a judgment or assessment of a learner based on his or her knowledge, skills, and attitudes associated with learning goals developed throughout the supervisory process. Supervisees often do not know how they will be evaluated (Rojas et al. 2010), and certainly not what criteria they will be judged on. Both the supervisee and the supervisor should be the target of evaluation.

There are different ways to evaluate. One obvious way is through direct observation. Direct observation of a supervisee, whether he or she is engaged in clinical care or project management, is a valid and reliable approach to predicting competence (Hasnain et al. 2004). Thanks to developing technology, it is much easier to video-record patient sessions, teaching performances, and even supervisory sessions, and the supervisor can then evaluate these and provide feedback (see Chapter 9, "Video Recordings: Learning Through Facilitated Observation and Feedback"). Feedback based on direct observation is more likely to result in behavioral change (Watling et al. 2008). In addition to observing the supervisee in relation to others (e.g., patients, colleagues), supervisors observe supervisees within supervision as a proxy for how they engage with others or understand the task at hand. Supervisors may be able to determine if supervisees are self-reflective, defensive, and able to manage anxiety and whether they present themselves in a professional and/or ethical manner.

Another way of evaluating supervisees is by asking questions, both open- and closed-ended. Questions may be categorized into two types: fundamental (associated with principles) and applied (associated with a case, project or situation). A question can be formulated at different levels to elicit a response based on memory (recall) or require the learner to analyze and synthesize information. By utilizing different types and levels of questions, the supervisor has the opportunity to deepen his or her understanding of a supervisee's capacities.

By asking the supervisee to self-reflect and self-evaluate based on learning goals, the supervisor is able to evaluate how a learner understands one's self and one's knowledge and skills. It allows the supervisee to reveal those behaviors of which he or she may not be consciously aware. In addition, the supervisor can plan how best to deliver feedback-based on the supervisee's self-assessment.

Finally, one area of active research involves developing empirically validated assessment tools that could be utilized within the supervisory context (see Chapter 42, "Integrating Measurement-Based Care Into Supervision"). Some examples of reliable and validated assessment tools include Clinical Skills Verification forms to evaluate inpatient or outpatient clinical skills of residents or fellows (Dalack and Jibson 2012), a teaching skills tool for supervisors of clinician educators (Ricciotti et al. 2017), or various tools utilized within psychotherapy supervision, such as the Cognitive Therapy Scale (Vallis et al. 1986). These tools can be shared with supervisees prior to their use, and each of them allows for evaluation and can serve as a basis for rich feedback.

Effective feedback is essential for promoting learning and achieving defined goals (Bing-You and Trowbridge 2009). It is the "specific information about the comparison between a trainee's observed performance and a standard, given with the intent to improve the trainee's performance" (van de Ridder et al. 2008, p. 193). *Formative feedback* serves the purpose of improving or modifying a supervisee's behavior and is given regularly and ongoing, whereas *summative feedback* is a judgment made about a supervisee's performance at the end of a supervisory relationship. This summative feedback is based on overall performance and is given with the intent to document achievement, assess competence, or compare actual performance with standards. Without feedback, learners feel isolated, uncertain, and concerned about the potential inadequacy of their performance (Sargeant et al. 2010). Feedback is also important in helping inform and enhance the accuracy of a supervisees' self-assessment (Sargeant et al. 2011). Furthermore, it is important to encourage and support supervisees not only to be proactive regarding asking for feedback from the supervisor but also to be alert to feedback from patients and colleagues.

Feedback is no easy task. Despite a body of literature describing a variety of techniques and methods by which to provide effective feedback (Bienstock et al. 2007; Ende 1983; French et al. 2015; Hewson and Little 1998; Sargeant et al. 2015), trainees have been dissatisfied by the quantity and quality of feedback received (Bing-You and Trowbridge 2009; Jensen et al. 2012; Sargeant et al. 2011), and faculty have described feeling uncomfortable and inadequately prepared to give feedback (Bearman et al. 2018). The failure to provide effective feedback has been linked to the supervisor's desire to preserve the learner's self-confidence and self-esteem, protect a collegial relationship, preserve a commitment to active learning, enhance and maintain a learner's sense of agency, and avoid a supervisee's emotional response (Ende et al. 1995; Kogan et al. 2012). Also, fear of retaliation, feeling that behaviors will not change (Thomas and Arnold 2011), and a supervisor's lack of time or understanding of the importance of feedback (Bing-You and Trowbridge 2009) can also lead to inadequate feedback. Supervisees need to understand that the purpose of feedback is to help them improve their performance.

Effective feedback is based on several characteristics, including a sound learning climate. Feedback will be easier to accept and incorporate if the supervisory relationship involves mutual trust and respect (Sargeant et al. 2010). A strong supervisory relationship enables the delivery of more specific feedback that provides more precise guidance for the supervisee's development (Watling et al. 2012). Other characteristics of effective feedback include having clearly defined (and mutually understood) goals, evaluating the supervisee thoroughly, providing specific and behaviorally based statements involving both positive and corrective comments, delivering feedback in a timely manner (as close to the event as possible), assessing the learner's reaction, and developing an action plan for improvement. The supervisor should avoid feedback based on assumptions, intentions, or personality aspects. He or she should also consider giving feedback at each supervisory session: feedback should not be left to a midterm or final supervision session. Delayed feedback may lead to a decreased learning opportunity.

There are several feedback models described in the literature, including the feedback sandwich (Dohrenwend 2002), Ask-Tell-Ask (French et al. 2015), and the Facilitated Feedback Model, or R2C2 (Sargeant et al. 2015). In the past few years, feedback research has demonstrated that a more interactive, learner-centered approach of giving feedback is preferable to the conventional unilateral provision of information (such as the feedback sandwich) and helps integrate external feedback with the learner's self-perceptions of performance (Sargeant et al. 2011; Telio et al. 2015; Watling et al. 2008). In these interactive and learner-centered approaches, the supervisor guides the supervisee in a reflective, intentional dialogue about the performance to ensure that the supervisee understands both the performance and the feedback, as well as to develop strategies for improving performance. Reflection and clarification of the feedback can be beneficial and empowering and can lead to performance ownership (Sargeant et al. 2015), as well as enable acceptance and use of the feedback (Sargeant et al. 2011). It is important to try to clarify the supervisee's understanding of the feedback and whether any part of the feedback remains unclear; this will ensure that the supervisee perceives the strengths as well as deficits, and opportunities for change. The supervisor can problem-solve with the supervisee to develop specific strategies for improvement based on the feedback. This can help the supervisee incorporate the feedback and make use of it for real change (Sargeant et al. 2015). An interactive feedback approach such as Ask-Tell-Ask can be executed as follows:

Ask supervisee to self-assess. Self-assessment allows the learner to identify strengths as well as areas for improvement. Supervisors can assess how learners understand their performance without making assumptions. To encourage self-reflection, the supervisor might ask a supervisee in a nonjudgmental manner to reflect back on an experience he or she had: What transpired? Why did you act in a particular way? Did anything surprise you about the situation? Did you have the information or skills needed to deal with the situation, and if not, why was that? Was there a reason a given situation wasn't resolved?

The supervisor can then help the supervisee process the feelings, thoughts and experiences. Making sense of an experience can be associated with strong emotions (Boud et al. 1985), and supervisees may unconsciously (or consciously) block awareness of an experience and/or be reluctant to discuss it. The self-assessment gives the supervisor insight into those weaknesses the supervisee is aware of and those that remain outside consciousness. This reflection facilitates deeper learning, allowing new learning to be integrated into existing knowledge and skills (Mann et al. 2009). The supervisee's ability to self-assess and reflect on, translate, interpret, and assimilate information enhances his or her ability to take in feedback (Bing-You and Trowbridge 2009).

Unfortunately, research has shown that physicians, particularly those with the most deficient performances, tend to be poor self-assessors (Davis et al. 2006). As learners move beyond the training context, self-assessment, particularly in psychiatry, becomes a critical skill and is important to lifelong learning. By receiving accurate feedback, the supervisee has a better chance of developing a more accurate self-assessment and, therefore, will have more sound information to rely on to modify behaviors in the future.

Provide specific, behaviorally based feedback (tell). Feedback should be based preferably on direct observations, with care taken not to shame or undercut the supervisee. Feedback without observation is much less useful and undermines supervisor credibility (Sargeant et al. 2011; Telio et al. 2015). The supervisor should not use evaluative language, because the purpose of formative feedback is to improve performance, not to judge. Furthermore, the supervisor should avoid generalizations, personality-focused feedback, assumptions, and over-interpretation and limit the amount of feedback. Too many comments risk the chance of the supervisee forgetting what was discussed or being overwhelmed.

Both relevant, positive comments—to highlight strengths and reinforce desirable behaviors—and corrective feedback should be provided. Corrective feedback is the most challenging type to give. The supervisor should avoid being an adversary; instead, he or she should take the position of an ally. It may be no surprise that feedback that affirms the supervisee's self-perceptions tends to be more readily accepted, whereas that which disconfirms his or her self-perception tends to result in a strong emotional reaction and may result in it being more difficult for the supervisee to accept (Sargeant et al. 2010). Although learners may tend to be more satisfied with compliments, corrective feedback results in more significant performance improvement (Boehler et al. 2006).

Ask supervisee to summarize feedback session. Asking the supervisee to summarize the feedback session allows the supervisor to feel satisfied that the supervisee understood what the issues are and how the supervisee plans to go about modifying them, in what time frame, and how progress will be assessed moving forward. The content of the session needs to be documented as a reminder of added goals and action plans.

If a supervisee fails to reach the agreed-on goals during the supervision or performs poorly despite several attempts at appropriate feedback, the supervisor should thoughtfully discuss the issues with the supervisee well in advance of termination of supervision. Identifying the reason for delayed or stymied progress is essential. Even after identifying reasons for inadequate progress, the supervisor may need to alert the program overseeing supervision if the situation cannot be rectified within the current supervision. The supervisee also must be informed of the need to discuss the deficient performance with the administration *prior* to the supervisor's doing so. Even though limits of confidentiality may have been discussed during the introductory phase of supervision, the supervisor must guard against blindsiding, betraying, or shaming the supervisee by disclosure. Depending on the context, it may be the responsibility of the supervisor to develop a remediation plan with clear objectives and a timeline (see Chapter 39, "Unprofessional Behavior: Identification and Remediation in Supervision").

To enhance the working alliance, resolve any ruptures within the relationship, and improve supervisory skills, supervisors are advised to seek feedback from supervisees. What did the supervisee find helpful and not helpful? Modeling an open and receptive stance is an important learning opportunity for the supervisee and may increase the amount of information the supervisee is willing to provide. Another way to receive supervisor-targeted feedback is to request peer evaluation from a trusted colleague. Having a colleague sit in on a supervisory session or asking an expert educator to review a video-recorded supervisory session can lead to important insights for the supervisor.

In sum, feedback is *not* an easy skill to master, and providing feedback takes a significant amount of practice. It will be important for supervisors to work on this skill and, if possible, receive training.

Termination Phase

Little has been written about the termination phase of supervision. Termination occurs when the supervisory relationship reaches an endpoint based on a program-dictated timeframe or the achievement of agreed-on goals, the supervisee leaves an organization, or the supervisee is promoted or obtains licensure.

Key Points

- Encourage self-reflection.
  - Guide the supervisee in self-reflection and encourage transfer to next supervisor.
- Provide summative evaluation.
  - Review progress on all goals, and identify areas for continued improvement prior to supervisee's receipt of written summary report.
  - Complete all documentation by the end of the supervision.
- Help ensure a smooth transition.

- Encourage the supervisor to share strengths and areas of improvement with the new supervisor.

- Consider creating an ongoing action plan to be shared with the new supervisor.

- Consider contacting the new supervisor to provide "handoff."

Encourage Self-Reflection

It is important to guide the supervisee in self-reflection: What has been useful in the supervisory experience? How has the experience affected you from the standpoint of knowledge, skills, and attitudes? How have you grown and developed, and what are the ongoing opportunities for growth? It is valuable to discuss with the supervisee how to take these considerations into the next supervisory experience, whether with a supervisor or a consultant, and explore the supervisee's future challenges and resources (see Chapter 47, "Clinical Consultation: How Consulting Differs From Supervision").

Provide Summative Evaluation

The summative evaluation is often a requirement of the institution or program. It is not too difficult to create if ongoing evaluation and feedback have been taking place throughout the process of working with the supervisee. The supervisor might reflect on all goals developed throughout the supervisory experience and provide clear and specific feedback on each one. Such feedback typically will be in written form, and it is important to discuss the content of the feedback with the supervisee before supervision terminates and the supervisee receives the written report. Receipt of a written summary feedback report without prior discussion can be confusing and, at times, upsetting to a supervisee if it contains information that the supervisee is not aware of in advance.

It is important to complete all documentation by the end of supervision—whether it is signing off on patient notes or completing final evaluations of the supervisee. Failure to complete final evaluations in a timely manner may undermine the credibility of the feedback provided and diminish the value of the final assessment report (Watling et al. 2008).

Help Ensure a Smooth Transition

If the supervisor is leaving the supervisory relationship and a new supervisor will be taking over, supervisors might help ensure a smooth transition. A supervisee might be encouraged to inform the subsequent supervisor of areas for improvement. In the spirit of a longitudinal assessment, the current supervisor could also contact the future supervisor to share information about the supervisee's development and create an ongoing, meaningful action plan that may help with the transition. However, some supervisors and/or program leadership are not comfortable with possible "biasing" of the new supervisor (see Chapter 40, "Termination: Supervising a 'Good Goodbye'").

Conclusion

Supervisors prepare trainees for unsupervised practice, help deepen and enrich the future work of post-trainees, and contribute to supervisees' career development. The process involves a complex set of competencies and approaches that may vary depending on the setting and format of supervision. The core elements of supervision presented in this chapter serve as a basis for approaching this complex process, which is revealed in greater depth in future sections of this book.

By setting up the core elements and evidence behind supervision (Chapter 2, "Psychotherapy Supervision Research: A Status Report and Proposed Model"), we encourage readers to make use of this compendium by referring to those sections that may have greatest significance to them—whether it be understanding different formats and delivery systems of supervision (Part 2: "Supervisory Formats") or learning particular supervisory techniques (Part 3: "Supervision Techniques"). Both clinical (Part 4: "Clinical Supervision Venues") and nonclinical (Part 5: "Nonclinical Supervision Venues") supervision venues present more in-depth descriptions of supervision within each particular environment. Part 6 ("Special Issues in Supervision") explores a variety of special issues in supervision, including selecting a supervisor, supervising issues of termination, integrating neuroscience within supervision, and so forth. Part 7 ("Legal and Ethical Issues") explores the legal aspects and ethical codes within supervision, while Part 8 ("Professional Development") outlines the current state of professional development related to supervision and how to develop a supervisor training program.

Whether you are a novice or an expert supervisor (or supervisee), we hope this book provides an effective resource by clarifying an often-convoluted process while providing concrete approaches to improving the process, as well as inspiring future research and educational development and leadership.

Additional Resources

Adult Learning Theory

Teaching Excellence in Adult Literacy Center: Adult Learning Theories. TEAL Center Fact Sheet No 11. Washington, DC, American Institutes for Research, 2011. Available at: https://lincs.ed.gov/sites/default/files/11_%20TEAL_Adult_Learning_Theory.pdf.

Supervision Contracts

American Psychological Association: Summary of Supervisory Contract. Available at: http://supp.apa.org/books/Essential-Ethics-for-Psychologists/summary.pdf.

Milne DL, Reiser RP: A Manual for Evidence-Based Supervision. Hoboken, NJ, Wiley, 2017

Sudak DM, Codd RT III, Ludgate J, et al: Teaching and Supervising Cognitive Behavioral Therapy. Hoboken, NJ, Wiley, 2016

Learning Goals

Doran GT: There's a S.M.A.R.T. way to write management's goals and objectives. Management Review (AMA Forum) 70(11):35–36, 1981

Mentorship

Clinical and Translational Science Institute, University of Minnesota: Free web-based interactive modules: https://www.ctsi.umn.edu/education-and-training/mentoring/mentor-training

Johnson WB: On Being a Mentor: A Guide for Higher Education Faculty, 2nd Edition. New York, Routledge, 2016

Feedback

French J, Colbert C, Pien L, et al: Targeted feedback in the milestones era: utilization of the ask-tell-ask feedback model to promote reflection and self-assessment. J Surg Educ 72(6):e274–e279, 2015

References

Accreditation Council for Graduate Medical Education: Program requirements. July 1, 2017. Section 11.B.1.a. Available at: http://acgme.org/Specialties/Program-Requirements-and-FAQs-and-Applications/pfcatid/21/Psychiatry. Accessed August 6, 2018.

Babbott S: Commentary: watching closely at a distance: key tensions in supervising resident physicians. Acad Med 85(9):1399–1400, 2010 20736665

Baldwin DC Jr, Daugherty SR, Ryan PM: How residents view their clinical supervision: a reanalysis of classic national survey data. J Grad Med Educ 2(1):37–45, 2010 21975882

Bearman M, Tai J, Kent F, et al: What should we teach the teachers? Identifying the learning priorities of clinical supervisors. Adv Health Sci Educ Theory Pract 23(1):29–41, 2018 28315114

Bernard JM, Goodyear RK: Fundamentals of Clinical Supervision, 4th Edition. Upper Saddle River, NJ, Pearson Education, 2009

Bergman EM, Sieben JM, Smailbegovic I, et al: Constructive, collaborative, contextual, and self-directed learning in surface anatomy education. Anat Sci Educ 6(2):114–124, 2013 22899567

Bienstock JL, Katz NT, Cox SM, et al; Association of Professors of Gynecology and Obstetrics Undergraduate Medical Education Committee: To the point: medical education reviews—providing feedback. Am J Obstet Gynecol 196(6):508–513, 2007 17547874

Bing-You RG, Trowbridge RL: Why medical educators may be failing at feedback. JAMA 302(12):1330–1331, 2009 19773569

Boehler ML, Rogers DA, Schwind CJ, et al: An investigation of medical student reactions to feedback: a randomized controlled trial. Med Educ 40(8):746–749, 2006 16869919

Borders LD: Best practices in clinical supervision: another step in delineating effective supervision practice. Am J Psychother 68(2):151–162, 2014 25122982

Borders LD, Brown LL: The New Handbook of Counseling Supervision. Mahwah, NJ, Lahaska/Lawrence Erlbaum, 2005

Boud D, Keogh R, Walker D: Reflection: Turning Experience into Learning. London, Kogan, 1985

Cabaniss D, Arbuckle M: Course ad lab: a new model for supervision. Acad Psych 35:4, 2011

Chang Y, Mark B: Effects of learning climate and registered nurse staffing on medication errors. Nurs Res 60(1):32–39, 2011 21127452

Dalack GW, Jibson MD: Clinical skills verification, formative feedback, and psychiatry residency trainees. Acad Psychiatry 36(2):122–125, 2012 22532202

Davis DA, Mazmanian PE, Fordis M, et al: Accuracy of physician self-assessment compared with observed measures of competence: a systematic review. JAMA 296(9):1094–1102, 2006 16954489

de Feijter JM, de Grave WS, Dornan T, et al: Students' perceptions of patient safety during the transition from undergraduate to postgraduate training: an activity theory analysis. Adv Health Sci Educ Theory Pract 16(3):347–358, 2011 21132361

Dohrenwend A: Serving up the feedback sandwich. Fam Pract Manag 9(10):43–46, 2002 12469676

Doran GT: There's a s.m.a.r.t. way to write management's goals and objectives. Management Review. AMA Forum 70(11):35–36, 1981

Dornan T: Workplace learning. Perspect Med Educ 1(1):15–23, 2012 23316455

Dwyer FM: Strategies for Improving Visual Learning: A Handbook for the Effective Selection, Design, and Use of Visualized Materials. State College, PA, Learning Services, 1978, pp 1–20

Edwards D, Burnard P, Hannigan B, et al: Clinical supervision and burnout: the influence of clinical supervision for community mental health nurses. J Clin Nurs 15(8):1007–1015, 2006 16879545

Ende J: Feedback in clinical medical education. JAMA 250(6):777–781, 1983 6876333

Ende J, Pomerantz A, Erickson F: Preceptors' strategies for correcting residents in an ambulatory care medicine setting: a qualitative analysis. Acad Med 70(3):224–229, 1995 7873011

Falender CA, Shafranske EP: Clinical Supervision: A Competency Based Approach. Washington, DC, American Psychological Association, 2004

French J, Colbert C, Pien L, et al: Targeted feedback in the milestones era: utilization of the ask-tell-ask feedback model to promote reflection and self-assessment. J Surg Educ 72(6):e274–e279, 2015 26123726

Gonsalvez CJ, Bushnell J, Blackman R, et al: Assessment of psychology competencies in field placements: standardized vignettes reduce rater bias. Train Educ Prof Psychol 7(2):99–111, 2013

Grant J, Schofield MJ, Crawford S: Managing difficulties in supervision: supervisors' perspectives. J Couns Psychol 59(4):528–541, 2012 23088684

Hasnain M, Connell KJ, Downing SM, et al: Toward meaningful evaluation of clinical competence: the role of direct observation in clerkship ratings. Acad Med 79(10)(Suppl):S21–S24, 2004 15383380

Hewson MG, Little ML: Giving feedback in medical education: verification of recommended techniques. J Gen Intern Med 13(2):111–116, 1998 9502371

Jensen AR, Wright AS, Kim S, et al: Educational feedback in the operating room: a gap between resident and faculty perceptions. Am J Surg 204(2):248–255, 2012 22537472

Kaufman J, Schwartz T: Models of supervision. Clin Supervisor 22(1):143–158, 2004

Kennedy TJ, Lingard L, Baker GR, et al: Clinical oversight: conceptualizing the relationship between supervision and safety. J Gen Intern Med 22(8):1080–1085, 2007 17557190

Kilminster S, Cottrell D, Grant J, et al: AMEE Guide No. 27: Effective educational and clinical supervision. Med Teach 29(1):2–19, 2007 17538823

Knowles MS: The Adult Learner: A Neglected Species, 3rd Edition. Houston, TX, Gulf Publishing, 1984

Kogan JR, Conforti LN, Bernabeo EC, et al: Faculty staff perceptions of feedback to residents after direct observation of clinical skills. Med Educ 46(2):201–215, 2012 22239334

Kozlowska K, Nunn K, Cousens P: Adverse experiences in psychiatric training. Part 2. Aust N Z J Psychiatry 31(5):641–652, discussion 653–654, 1997a 9400870

Kozlowska K, Nunn K, Cousens P: Training in psychiatry: an examination of trainee perceptions. Part 1. Aust N Z J Psychiatry 31(5):628–640, discussion 653–654, 1997b 9400869

Kuttner R: Managed care and medical education. N Engl J Med 341(14):1092–1096, 1999 10502601

Ladany N: Psychotherapy supervision: what lies beneath. Psychother Res 14(1):1–19, 2004 22011114

Ladany N, Mori Y, Mehr K: Effective and ineffective supervision. Couns Psychol 41:28–47, 2013

Latham GP, Winters D, Locke E: Cognitive and motivational effects of participation: a mediator study. J Organ Behav 15:49–63, 1994

Lucas CA, Benedek D, Pangaro L: Learning climate and students' achievement in a medicine clerkship. Acad Med 68(10):811–812, 1993 8397620

Mann K, Gordon J, Macleod A: Reflection and reflective practice in health professions education: a systematic review. Adv Health Sci Educ 14(4):595–621, 2009 18034364

Milne DL: Evidence-Based Clinical Supervision: Principles and Practice. Malden, MA, BPS/Blackwell, 2009

Morse G, Salyers MP, Rollins AL, et al: Burnout in mental health services: a review of the problem and its remediation. Adm Policy Ment Health 39(5):341–352, 2012 21533847

Newman M, Ravindranath D, Figueroa S, et al: Perceptions of supervision in an outpatient psychiatry clinic. Acad Psychiatry 40(1):153–156, 2016 25085500

Orsini C, Binnie V, Wilson S, et al: Learning climate and feedback as predictors of dental students' self-determined motivation: the mediating role of basic psychological needs and satisfaction. Eur J Dent Educ 22(2):e228–e236, 2018 28643884

Psychology Board of Australia: Guidelines for supervisors and supervisor training providers. January 8, 2018. Available at: http://www.psychologyboard.gov.au/Standards-and-Guidelines/ Codes-Guidelines-Policies.aspx. Accessed Aguust 6, 2018.

Ramani S, Orlander JD: Human dimensions in bedside teaching: focus group discussions of teachers and learners. Teach Learn Med 25(4):312–318, 2013 24112200

Reiss H, Fishel AK: The necessity of continuing education for psychotherapy supervisors. Acad Psychiatry 24:147–155, 2000

Ricciotti HA, Freret TS, Aluko A, et al: Effects of a short video-based resident-as-teacher training toolkit on resident teaching. Obstet Gynecol 130(1)(Suppl 1):36S–41S, 2017 28937517

Rodenhauser P: Psychiatry residency programs: trends in psychotherapy supervision. Am J Psychother 46(2):240–249, 1992 1605331

Rojas A, Arbuckle M, Cabaniss D: Don't leave teaching to chance: learning objectives for psychodynamic psychotherapy supervision. Acad Psychiatry 34(1):46–49, 2010 20071725

Sargeant J, Armson H, Chesluk B, et al: The processes and dimensions of informed self-assessment: a conceptual model. Acad Med 85(7):1212–1220, 2010 20375832

Sargeant J, Eva KW, Armson H, et al: Features of assessment learners use to make informed self-assessments of clinical performance. Med Educ 45(6):636–647, 2011 21564201

Sargeant J, Lockyer J, Mann K, et al: Facilitated reflective performance feedback: developing an evidence- and theory-based model that builds relationship, explores reactions and content, and coaches for performance change (R2C2). Acad Med 90(12):1698–1706, 2015 26200584

Sarnat J: Key competencies of the psychodynamic psychotherapist and how to teach them in supervision. Psychotherapy (Chic) 47(1):20–27, 2010 22401997

Shanfield SB, Mohl PC, Matthews KL, et al: Quantitative assessment of the behavior of psychotherapy supervisors. Am J Psychiatry 149(3):352–357, 1992 1536274

Stern RS: Medicare reimbursement policy and teaching physicians' behavior in hospital clinics: the changes of 1996. Acad Med 77(1):65–71, 2002 11788328

Telio S, Ajjawi R, Regehr G: The "educational alliance" as a framework for reconceptualizing feedback in medical education. Acad Med 90(5):609–614, 2015 25406607

Ten Cate O, Hart D, Ankel F, et al; International Competency-Based Medical Education Collaborators: Entrustment decision making in clinical training. Acad Med 91(2):191–198, 2016 26630606

Teunissen P, Scheele F, Scherpbier A, et al: How residents learn: qualitative evidence for the pivotal role of clinical activities. Med Educ 41(8):763–770, 2007 17661884

Thomas JD, Arnold RM: Giving feedback. J Palliat Med 14(2):233–239, 2011 21314576

UCL Psychology and Language Sciences: Competence frameworks. 2018. Available at: http:// www.ucl.ac.uk/pals/research/cehp/research-groups/core/competence-frameworks. Accessed August 6, 2018.

Vallis TM, Shaw BF, Dobson KS: The Cognitive Therapy Scale: psychometric properties. J Consult Clin Psychol 54(3):381–385, 1986 3722567

van de Ridder JM, Stokking KM, McGaghie WC, et al: What is feedback in clinical education? Med Educ 42(2):189–197, 2008 18230092

van der Wal M, Schonrock-Adema J, Scheele F, et al: Supervisor leadership in relation to resident job satisfaction. BMC Med Educ 16:194, 2016 27480528

Wallbank S, Robertson N: Midwife and nurse responses to miscarriage, stillbirth and neonatal death. Evid Based Midwifery 6(3):100–106, 2008

Watling CJ, Kenyon CF, Zibrowski EM, et al: Rules of engagement: residents' perceptions of the in-training evaluation process. Acad Med 83(10)(Suppl):S97–S100, 2008 18820513

Watling C, Driessen E, van der Vleuten CPM, et al: Learning from clinical work: the roles of learning cues and credibility judgements. Med Educ 46(2):192–200, 2012 22239333

Wimmers P, Schmidt H, Splinter T: Influence of clerkship experiences on clinical competence. Med Educ 40(5):450–458, 2006 16635125

Chapter 2

Psychotherapy Supervision Research

A Status Report and Proposed Model

C. Edward Watkins Jr., Ph.D.

Jennifer L. Callahan, Ph.D., ABPP

"Assuming that clinical supervision is useful is not enough..."

Simpson-Southward, Waller, and Hardy (2017, p. 1242)

Research matters, and research matters greatly in psychotherapy supervision: To ever advance beyond merely "assuming usefulness," supervision science is needed. The first supervision study appeared over 60 years ago (Bernard and Goodyear 2019). Through the decades, a host of supervision subjects has been examined, the whole of supervision science has increasingly burgeoned, and the supervision knowledge base has ever expanded (Inman et al. 2014). But what has been learned so far about psychotherapy supervision? What do the empirical data say? Does supervision really make a difference? Those questions are considered in what follows. In this chapter, we 1) provide a concise summary, a status report, of what appear to be some of the most salient research observations, findings, and conclusions about psychotherapy supervision, and, building on that status report, 2) propose a unifying model that might be useful in trans-theoretically advancing future supervision research. Although drawn exclusively from the research literature of psychotherapy supervision, the material presented here may have relevance across other forms of supervision as well (e.g., nonpsychotherapy clinical supervision, administrative or scholarly supervision).

Key Points

- Research strongly suggests that supervision works—and works well—at least for supervisees.

- Supervision/patient outcome studies present mixed and inconsistent findings; any firm, definitive conclusions about supervision's impact on patients cannot be drawn at this time.

- Becoming a therapist can be profitably conceived as an unfolding developmental process, and supervision seems most process facilitative when guided by an ethos of developmental accommodation.

- The supervisor-supervisee relationship appears to be a (if not the) crucial mediating variable that holds the power to make or break the supervision process.

- Multicultural variables have an impact on the supervision experience, and supervisors appear best served when they are aware of that reality and use that awareness to accordingly inform their supervisory practice.

- Criticisms of supervision research have focused on small sample sizes, limited availability of longitudinal data, dearth of valid supervision measures, overreliance on self-report measures, limited availability of process studies, and limited focus on client outcome.

- Supervision research benefits most from the empirical embrace of methodological pluralism.

- The generic model of psychotherapy supervision might serve as a heuristic trans-theoretical framework, facilitating research inquiry across disparate models of supervision.

Supervision Research Then and Now

Supervision research has long been recognized as highly challenging to conduct—for example, because of the supervision relationship's triadic nature—and programmatic research has been quite limited. The current state of supervision research has even been likened to psychotherapy research in the 1950s and 1960s, with measurement and effectiveness issues being paramount (Milne et al. 2012). Although supervision research studies have generally increased decade after decade, the actual number of supervision studies produced each year is estimated to still be only about 10 or so (Ladany and Inman 2008). With that being the case, unfortunately, much is still not understood or understood well about supervision (Inman et al. 2014; Watkins 2014a). Perhaps, as Milne and colleagues (2012) have opined, "[W]e are currently about 'half-way there,' working on the 'search for scientific rigour...'" (p. 144).

But even being only "half-way there," supervision research still has much of value to offer: It does not lack for gains in incrementally building an informed and informative evidence base, particularly with regard to studies conducted across the last generation of supervision scholarship (Callahan and Watkins 2018). If that evidence base is examined closely, what emerge as supervision's most robust findings? What are some safe and strong statements that could now be made about the current status of supervision understanding and practice? Furthermore, what defining observations can be made about supervision research now and into the future? Several such robust findings, safe statements, and defining observations have been identified:

1. *Supervision works, at least for supervisees.* Research evidence has increasingly suggested that supervision has positive and direct effects on supervisees. Some of those positive effects include enhanced supervisee self-awareness, enhanced treatment knowledge, and enhanced skill acquisition. Bernard and Goodyear (2019) make clear that a host of studies demonstrate supervision's effectiveness in stimulating supervisees' development of case conceptualization skills, intervention skills, and effectively using self in the treatment situation. Supervision's favorable impact on supervisees is well established.

2. *Supervision studies about patient outcome present mixed and inconsistent findings and do not allow for any firm, definitive conclusions to be drawn about supervision's impact on patients at this time.* Over two decades ago, Ellis and Ladany (1997) proposed that the real acid test for supervision comes down to this: Does supervision result in favorable patient changes? That question, yet to be decisively answered, looms ever large in this age of accountability, and calls have been increasingly made for the supervision/patient outcome issue to be substantively addressed (Simpson-Southward et al. 2017; Watkins 2011a): "[T]he effectiveness question *must* be compellingly addressed if supervision is to ever advance beyond 'the reasonable but unproven practice stage' and convincingly justify itself..." (Watkins 2011b, p. 63, emphasis added). Outcome studies have often been faulted on myriad methodological grounds, and even data from those very few sound studies have been mixed (Ellis and Ladany 1997; Freitas 2002; Watkins 2011a). But within the past decade, a set of three rigorous and robust supervision outcome studies—all reporting a modest supervisor effect on patient outcome—has emerged and at least provides some promise for future study in this area (Callahan et al. 2009; Rieck et al. 2015; Wrape et al. 2015). These studies, in which patient recovery status was coded as an outcome variable, perhaps provide a model of inquiry that could prove useful in ultimately unraveling the supervisor/patient outcome conundrum. Until then, the current reality remains: supervision has yet to conclusively, definitively, and decisively pass its real acid test.

3. *Becoming a therapist is an unfolding developmental process, and supervision may be most acutely valuable early on as beginning therapists struggle with that very process of becoming.* Therapists do not come ready-made. Instead, research suggests that 1) therapists develop over time, sometimes agonizingly so, increasingly building their base of treatment skills/competencies and consolidating a sense of therapist identity; and

2) supervision appears highly facilitative of that therapist development process and may have its greatest value early on—when beginning therapists/supervisees are at their most vulnerable and lacking in critical treatment fundamentals (Orlinsky and Ronnestad 2005; Ronnestad and Skovholt 2013). The notion of therapist development is now considered endemic to supervision and an important concept globally: supervisors ideally strive to understand the unfolding developmental process of each supervisee and accordingly tailor or customize supervision to then best match the supervisee's evolving learning needs (Bernard and Goodyear 2019; Inman et al. 2014; Watkins et al. 2018).

4. *The supervision relationship seemingly holds a place of supreme significance in making supervision work, and supervisors appear best served when they are highly attentive to and strive to consistently cultivate and maintain a constructive working relationship with their supervisees.* Although the supervisory relationship involves various components (e.g., real relationship, transference-countertransference configuration) (Watkins 2015b), the alliance component has received the most empirical attention. Defined as the shared bond, shared goals, and shared tasks, the supervisor-supervisee alliance appears to be supervision's most robust, empirically supported common factor. Features that are often used to describe a favorable alliance include the following: empathic, respectful and warm, facilitative and collaborative, flexible, affirming and encouraging, interested and engaged, effective for providing useful feedback, and constructively challenging (Watkins 2011b, 2016, 2018a). Features that are often used to describe an unfavorable alliance include the following: disengaged, intrusive, preoccupied, lack of interest and commitment, insensitive, disaffirming and discouraging, authoritarian or laissez-faire in style, demeaning, critical and judgmental, characterized by critical and nonsupportive behaviors, and unethical (Watkins 2011b, 2016, 2018a). When a favorably perceived supervisor-supervisee alliance is in place, favorable outcomes tend to co-occur; conversely, unfavorably perceived alliances and unfavorable outcomes tend to co-occur. For example, favorably perceived alliances have correlated with such desirable supervision variables as greater judged effectiveness of and higher satisfaction with supervision, more job satisfaction and less burnout, higher sense of supervisee self-efficacy and well-being, increased supervisee willingness to self-disclose during supervision, more availability of supervisee coping resources, and more supportively perceived gender events and discussions of culture during supervision (Watkins 2014b, 2015a). Unfavorably perceived alliances have correlated with such undesirable supervision variables as more frequent occurrences of negative supervision events; higher degree of supervisee stress, exhaustion, and burnout; and greater amount of reported supervision role conflict and role ambiguity (Watkins 2014b, 2015a). Across more than 60 studies, spanning over three decades, the supervisory alliance has generally functioned as hypothesized. The supervisor-supervisee alliance may well be the evidence-based anchor that grounds supervision practice, and, according to Ladany et al. (2016), "arguably the foundation for effective supervision" (p. 24). Furthermore, wherever inadequate or harmful supervision occurs, the alliance is most likely compromised or perhaps has never even been put in place (cf. Ellis et al. 2014).

5. *Multicultural variables can indeed affect supervision process and outcome, and supervisors appear best served when they are aware of that reality and forever strive to make multiculturalism an integral part of their supervision practice.* Multicultural variables include

race/ethnicity, gender, sexual orientation, disability, age, socioeconomic status, religion and spirituality, international status, and their intersections. Every encounter is in some way a multicultural encounter (Bernard and Goodyear 2019). Willingness to consider multicultural differences and their potential impact has been increasingly recognized as critical to good supervision practice: Supervisors ideally strive to 1) incorporate multicultural sensitivity and understandings into the supervisor-supervisee dyad and 2) infuse multicultural sensitivity and understandings into discussions about the therapist-patient dyad (Watkins 2014a). Research suggests that insensitivities, misunderstandings, micro-aggressions, and rupturing events surrounding multicultural variables can indeed occur in supervision, that a solid supervisory alliance is critical for constructive and productive multicultural supervision encounters, and that the supervisor is preeminently pivotal in throwing the door wide open on multiculturalism and making it a critical part of the supervisory experience (see, e.g., Inman et al. 2014; Soheilian et al. 2014). Supervisees appear to very much desire engaging in multicultural discussions in supervision, and supervisors are perfectly positioned to make it so (cf. Soheilian et al. 2014; Tohidian and Quek 2017).

Limitations of the Research

Despite research advances, a repeating chorus of limitations and pressing needs has generally defined much supervision research and continues to do so. Past and current criticisms of supervision research have focused on small sample sizes, lack of longitudinal data, limited availability of valid supervision measures, overreliance on self-report measures, limited availability of supervision process studies, and limited attention to client outcome (e.g., Hill and Knox 2013; Inman et al. 2014; Lambert and Ogles 1997; Watkins 1998, 2014a, 2014b). It has long been understood, and commonly acknowledged, that supervision research needs to 1) engage in proper scale validation procedures (e.g., adapting a psychotherapy measure for supervision study), 2) conduct multisite studies that make for larger sample sizes and more robust findings, 3) study the supervision process over time, 4) consider the possibility of discipline-specific supervision effects, and 5) use a multimethod, multitrait approach to the data collection/analysis process (e.g., self-report and observational; Callahan and Watkins 2018; Hill and Knox 2013; Inman et al. 2014; Watkins 2018c). Although efforts continue to be made to address these limitations and needs, they "remain as ever pressing and eminently salient for psychotherapy supervision now" (Watkins 2012, p. 201).

Supervision research benefits most from a pluralistic approach to the investigative endeavor, drawing on quantitative, qualitative, and case study methodologies to inform empirical efforts. Any supervision study ideally proceeds by asking, What particular research method best answers the particular supervision question under study? Supervision in many respects remains a relatively new area of study. A pluralistic approach to research opens up the possibilities of broadening and widening the supervision knowledge base (Hill and Knox 2013; Watkins 2014b). Rigorous examples across the spectrum of methodological possibilities show that to be so (e.g., Arczynski and Morrow 2017). Pluralism is highly recommended as *the* preferred path to pursue in best advancing supervision research (Hill and Knox 2013; Watkins 2014b).

Future Directions: A Proposed Model for Supervision Research Study

As supervision research continues to accumulate and advance, might a unifying model of supervision study be of benefit in guiding future empirical efforts? Could a supervision research framework—a way of organizing the supervision experience so as to more specifically capture some of its most common, most meaningful trans-theoretical essentials—be proposed for heuristic purposes? Such a framework, the authors contend, is much needed. Analogizing from Orlinsky and Howard's (1987) generic model of psychotherapy (GMP), we propose the generic model of psychotherapy supervision (GMPS; Watkins 2018a, 2018b) as one such framework for potentially meeting that need. The GMPS is presented in Figure 2–1. Just as the GMP has provided a useful framework for organizing and critically evaluating hundreds of psychotherapy process-outcome research studies and thousands of process-outcome findings (see the last four editions of the *Handbook of Psychotherapy and Behavior Change* [e.g., Lambert 2013]), the authors hope that the GMPS can come to serve the very same purpose for supervision.

The Input part of the model reflects much of the *supervision as system* aspect of supervision, with particular emphasis given to what the supervisor and supervisee bring to the supervision situation and other setting and social influences on that situation. Input variables largely smooth the way for supervision, or can do just the opposite.

The Process part of the model reflects much of the *supervision as relationship* aspect of supervision. The crucial variables of Process, trans-theoretical in nature, are a) the supervisor-supervisee contract or agreement; b) supervision operations (or the cycle of intervention that gets enacted between supervisee and supervisor); c) the supervision bond; d) supervisee and supervisor self-relatedness, referring to the openness and non-defensiveness of the involved parties; e) in-session impact, referring to supervisory session effects; and f) temporal patterns (an embedded though not visibly reflected variable), recognizing the effect of time itself on the supervision experience. Process captures the synergistic work of the supervisory relationship and intervention in action.

The Output part of the model reflects much of the *supervision as developmental process* aspect of supervision, with particular emphasis given to changes or growth that can happen for both supervisee and supervisor. Output captures those outcome variables that ideally reflect supervisory impact.

Much as Orlinsky and Howard's (1987) generic psychotherapy model has helped us to think more completely and more complexly about psychotherapy, perhaps this analogized supervision model might similarly help us think more completely and more complexly about psychotherapy supervision. We present the GMPS in that spirit. Supervisors appear far more alike than different in the supervisory essentials in which they engage, and the GMPS is an effort to show how that is so.

Questions for the Supervision Researcher

■ How does supervision work? What are the mechanisms of action involved?

■ To what degree do the different factors (e.g., interventions, relational conditions) of the supervision situation actually contribute to its unfolding process?

- What is the effect of supervision model upon supervision practice?

- Does supervision affect patient outcomes? If so, how and why?

- How does supervisor training impact the supervision process and its outcomes?

Additional Resources

Hill CE, Knox S: Training and supervision in psychotherapy, in Bergin and Garfield's Handbook of Psychotherapy and Behavior Change, 6th Edition. Edited by Lambert MJ. Hoboken, NJ, Wiley, 2013, pp 775–811

Inman AG, Hutman H, Pendse A, et al: Current trends concerning supervisors, supervisees, and clients in clinical supervision, in Wiley International Handbook of Clinical Supervision. Edited by Watkins CE Jr, Milne D. Oxford, UK, Wiley, 2014, pp 61–102

References

Arczynski AV, Morrow SL: The complexities of power in feminist multicultural psychotherapy supervision. J Couns Psychol 64(2):192–205, 2017 27918171

Bernard JM, Goodyear RK: Fundamentals of Clinical Supervision, 6th Edition. Upper Saddle River, NJ, Merrill, 2019

Callahan JL, Watkins CE Jr: The science of training III: internship, supervision, and competency. Train Educ Prof Psychol 12(4):245–261, 2018

Callahan JL, Almstrom CM, Swift JK, et al: Exploring the contribution of supervisors to intervention outcomes. Train Educ Prof Psychol 3:72–77, 2009

Ellis MV, Ladany N: Inferences concerning supervisees and clients in clinical supervision: an integrative review, in Handbook of Psychotherapy Supervision. Edited by Watkins CE Jr. New York, Wiley, 1997, pp 447–507

Ellis MV, Berger L, Hanus AE, et al: Inadequate and harmful clinical supervision: testing a revised framework and assessing occurrence. Couns Psychol 42:434–472, 2014

Freitas G: The impact of psychotherapy supervision on client outcome: a critical examination of 2 decades of research. Psychother 39:354–367, 2002

Hill CE, Knox S: Training and supervision in psychotherapy, in Bergin and Garfield's Handbook of Psychotherapy and Behavior Change, 6th Edition. Edited by Lambert MJ. Hoboken, NJ, Wiley, 2013, pp 775–811

Inman AG, Hutman H, Pendse A, et al: Current trends concerning supervisors, supervisees, and clients in clinical supervision, in Wiley International Handbook of Clinical Supervision. Edited by Watkins CE Jr, Milne D. Oxford, UK, Wiley, 2014, pp 61–102

Ladany N, Inman AG: Developments in counseling skills training and supervision in Handbook of Counseling Psychology, 4th Edition. Edited by Brown SD, Lent RW. Hoboken, NJ, Wiley, 2008, pp 338–354

Ladany N, Friedlander ML, Nelson ML: Supervision Essentials for the Critical Events in Psychotherapy Supervision Model. Washington, DC, American Psychological Association, 2016

Lambert MJ (ed): Bergin and Garfield's Handbook of Psychotherapy and Behavior Change, 6th Edition. Hoboken, NJ, Wiley, 2013

Lambert MJ, Ogles BM: The effectiveness of psychotherapy supervision, in Handbook of Psychotherapy Supervision. Edited by Watkins CE Jr. New York, Wiley, 1997, pp 421–446

Milne D, Leck C, James I, et al: High fidelity in clinical supervision research, in Supervision and Clinical Psychology: Theory, Practice and Perspectives, 2nd Edition. Edited by Fleming I, Steen L. London, Routledge, 2012, pp 142–158

Orlinsky DE, Howard KI: A generic model of psychotherapy. Int J Eclect Psychother 6:6–27, 1987

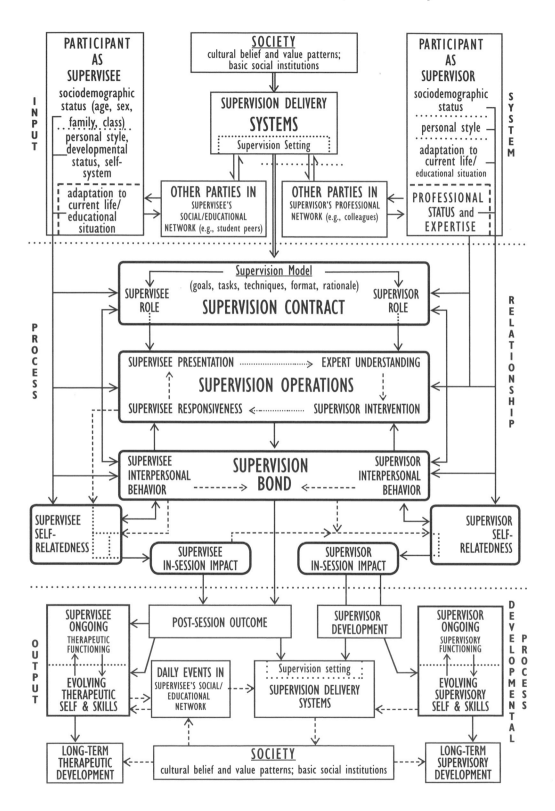

Figure 2–1. Generic model of psychotherapy supervision: interrelation of input, process, and output variables. *(opposite)*

Source. Adapted from Watkins CE Jr: "The Generic Model of Psychotherapy Supervision: An Analogized Research-Informing Meta-Theory." *Journal of Psychotherapy Integration* May 24, 2018. Copyright 2018, American Psychological Association. Used with permission.
Generic supervision model adapted from the generic psychotherapy model; see Figure 1 in Orlinsky DE, Ronnestad MH, Willutzki U: "Fifty Years of Psychotherapy Process-Outcome Research: Continuity and Change," in *Bergin and Garfield's Handbook of Psychotherapy and Behavior Change*, 5th Edition. Edited by Lambert MJ. Hoboken, NJ, Wiley, 2013, pp. 307–389. Copyright 2013, John Wiley Publishers. Adapted with permission.

Orlinsky DE, Ronnestad MH: How Psychotherapists Develop: A Study of Therapeutic Work and Professional Growth. Washington, DC, American Psychological Association, 2005

Rieck T, Callahan JL, Watkins CE Jr: Clinical supervision: an exploration of possible mechanisms of action. Train Educ Prof Psychol 9:187–194, 2015

Ronnestad MH, Skovholt TM: The Developing Practitioner: Growth and Stagnation of Therapists and Counselors. New York, Routledge, 2013

Simpson-Southward C, Waller G, Hardy GE: How do we know what makes for "best practice" in clinical supervision for psychological therapists? A content analysis of supervisory models and approaches. Clin Psychol Psychother 24(6):1228–1245, 2017 28421642

Soheilian SS, Inman AG, Klinger RS, et al: Multicultural supervision: supervisees' reflections on culturally competent supervision. Couns Psychol Q 27:379–392, 2014

Tohidian NB, Quek KMT: Processes that inform multicultural supervision: a qualitative meta-analysis. J Marital Fam Ther 43(4):573–590, 2017 28299797

Watkins CE Jr: Psychotherapy supervision in the 21st century. Some pressing needs and impressing possibilities. J Psychother Pract Res 7(2):93–101, 1998 9527954

Watkins CE Jr: Does psychotherapy supervision contribute to patient outcomes? considering 30 years of research. Clin Supervisor 30:235–256, 2011a

Watkins CE Jr: Psychotherapy supervision since 1909: some friendly observations about its first century. J Contemp Psychother 41:57–67, 2011b

Watkins CE Jr: Psychotherapy supervision in the new millennium: competency-based, evidence-based, particularized, and energized. J Contemp Psychother 42:193–203, 2012

Watkins CE Jr: Clinical supervision in the 21st century: revisiting pressing needs and impressing possibilities. Am J Psychother 68(2):251–272, 2014a 25122988

Watkins CE Jr: The supervisory alliance: a half century of theory, practice, and research in critical perspective. Am J Psychother 68(1):19 55, 2014b 24818456

Watkins CE Jr: The alliance in reflective supervision: a commentary on Tomlin, Weatherston, and Pavkov's critical components of reflective supervision. Infant Ment Health J 36(2):141–145, 2015a 25640088

Watkins CE Jr: Extrapolating Gelso's tripartite model of the psychotherapy relationship to the psychotherapy supervision relationship: a potential common factors perspective. J Psychother Integration 25:143–157, 2015b

Watkins CE Jr: A unifying vision of psychotherapy supervision: part I—productive and unproductive supervision relationships. J Unified Psychother Clin Sci 4:21–35, 2016

Watkins CE Jr: The Generic Model of Psychotherapy Supervision: an analogized research-informing meta-theory. Journal of Psychotherapy Integration May 24, 2018a [Epub ahead of print]

Watkins CE Jr: Psychotherapy supervision: the educational practice of hope, promise, and possibility. Keynote address delivered at the International Conference: Supervision in Psychotherapy, Timisoara, Romania, June 2018b

Watkins CE Jr: A unifying vision of psychotherapy supervision: part III. meta-values, meta-principles, and meta-roles of the contextual supervision relationship model. J Unified Psychother Clin Sci 5:23–40, 2018c

Watkins CE Jr, Davis EC, Callahan JL: On disruption, disorientation, and development in clinical supervision: a transformative learning perspective. The Clinical Supervisor January 15, 2018 [Epub ahead of print]

Wrape ER, Callahan JL, Ruggero CJ, et al: An exploration of faculty supervisor variables and their impact on client outcome. Train Educ Prof Psychol 9:35–43, 2015

Part 2 Supervision Formats

Chapter 3   Supervision Formats

Elise Gibbs, Psy.D.

Kathleen M. Corcoran, Ph.D.

Supervision comes in many shapes and sizes. Clinical supervision, as defined by Milne (2007), is "the formal provision, by approved supervisors, of a relationship-based education and training that is work focused and which manages, supports, develops and evaluates the work of colleagues" (p. 15). In this chapter, we outline the various permutations of supervision in terms of structure and style, along with important considerations for each.

Key Points

- Supervision can be delivered in a variety of formats, in terms of both structure and style.

- When deciding on the format of supervision, a training program should consider a variety of factors, including the needs of the supervisee, the setting, the supervision requirements for program accreditation, the length of the training experience, and the preferences/abilities of the supervisors.

- Rather than being a single distinct activity, supervision is a dynamic process that may shift in structure or intensity over the course of a training experience.

Supervision Formats

Individual Supervision

Individual supervision is the most common format of supervision in training programs and involves a supervisee meeting with his or her assigned supervisor on a regular, individual basis to discuss cases. Individual supervision is often 1 hour in length each week, and the agenda for each meeting is mutually decided on by the supervisee and supervisor. If the supervisee has video-recorded content such as a recording of a psychotherapy session, this may be reviewed in supervision.

Potential benefits of the one-on-one format include the opportunity for more focus on specific training objectives, a greater sense for quality control of patient care, and a dyadic relationship between supervisor and supervisee that is often preferred by both (Milne and Oliver 2000). Another benefit of individual supervision is the general familiarity that most have with this modality compared with other formats. Individual supervision is asynchronous; thus, a potential drawback is the delay between the supervisory feedback and the time of the supervisee's behavior. Another potential drawback is the potential for a problematic interpersonal fit between supervisee and supervisor, which may be less paramount in larger group settings for the overall functioning of supervision (see Chapter 36, "Ruptures in the Supervisory Alliance").

Group Supervision

Group supervision typically involves a small group of supervisees and at least one supervisor meeting on a regular basis to discuss cases. The structure of the group meeting may vary depending on the needs of the supervisees and/or the preference of the supervisor(s). Supervisees may be assigned a specific meeting date during which they are expected to present a case to the group for general feedback on their conceptualization and treatment plan. They may also bring specific questions that they have about the case to be answered in a group discussion during the meeting. Group supervision can also involve discussion of a theme or issue relevant to all supervisees.

Group supervision may be a more efficient mode of training for a program in which there is a high ratio of supervisees to supervisors. Another benefit of group supervision is the opportunity for supervisees to experience both individual and vicarious learning (Milne and Oliver 2000). A potential drawback of group supervision is the possibility for peer competition, which may have a negative impact on learning and require more effort from the supervisor to manage if detected (Milne and Oliver 2000). Special attention must be given to ensure that video review and specific management of cases occur in a group format (Sudak et al. 2015) and that the time is balanced appropriately across the supervisees. Some supervisors have noted challenges in providing constructive or critical feedback in a group setting, where it is more difficult to determine how the supervisee received the feedback.

Live Supervision

Live supervision occurs when the supervisor watches the supervisee perform clinical care directly. This can be accomplished in vivo or through use of a one-way mirror,

Health Insurance Portability and Accountability Act (HIPAA)–compliant video conferencing technology, or the "Bug in the Ear" or "Bug in the Eye" (BITE) method (Gallant et al. 1991; Rizvi et al. 2016). When a one-way mirror is used, supervisors may be able to call into a telephone in a psychotherapy session and provide feedback. With BITE, technology is incorporated for the supervisor to provide feedback either visually through text or audibly through an earpiece for the supervisee.

Live supervision allows for clear, immediate feedback on the supervisee's behavior with patients, which can, in turn, allow for more immediate learning for the trainee and the potential for patients to benefit from the supervisor's expertise (Rousmaniere 2016). A potential drawback to live supervision is the increased anxiety that may arise in response to live feedback, which could interfere with a supervisee's learning (Costa 1994). Live supervision also requires the specific technology and/or space mentioned above, the absence of which could preclude it as an option within a training program. This form of supervision, especially when immediate feedback is provided to the supervisee, creates a different experience of treatment for the patient. Patients may experience this positively (e.g., feeling more cared for or in more expert hands) or negatively (e.g., feeling interrupted or questioning their provider's expertise), and thus patient reaction may be an important piece of information for the patient's case formulation and should be considered when this form of supervision is being considered.

Peer Supervision

When a supervisee supervises another supervisee, this would be classified as *peer supervision*. Peer supervision tends to be used as a supplementary supervision experience to complement the required supervision with a licensed, nonpeer supervisor. This may also be referred to as *peer-assisted learning* (PAL) (Silbert and Lake 2012). Peer supervisors may or may not have a formal evaluative role of the supervisee within the training program. Martin et al. (2018) posit that peer supervision should be instead labeled *peer consultation* to "avoid conveying a medical-legal duty of care."

There are many benefits to peer supervision. First, there is an opportunity for multiple levels of teaching within one interaction if the senior supervisee providing supervision to a junior colleague is observed by a supervisor and subsequently given feedback on their performance (Blanchard 2015). Second, peer supervision has been described as enjoyable and beneficial by supervisees, especially because of the peer supervisor's understanding of the supervisee's perspective and knowledge level (Silbert and Lake 2012). Another benefit of peer supervision is the relative ease with which it may be organized, assuming the peer supervisor has more flexibility than the supervisor. Peer supervision is closest in style to peer consultation (Martin et al. 2018), which could benefit supervisees by familiarizing them to this style of career-long learning. However, for peer supervision to be an effective and quality use of time, peer supervisors must also receive supervision of their supervision.

Drawbacks include the potential for subpar supervision quality if the peer supervisor lacks sufficient expertise or experience without appropriate oversight. It is also possible that peer supervision is more vulnerable to the potential for multiple relationships, if the peer supervisor and supervisee overlap within other training settings or have a preexisting relationship that could interfere with the supervisory framework.

Team Supervision

Team supervision occurs when a group of providers on a specific team meet for group supervision. This may be a multidisciplinary group; for example, all the providers (psychologists, psychiatrists, clinical social workers, nurses, and others) who treat patients in a mood disorders clinic may meet for team supervision on a regular basis. These supervision meetings may look very similar in structure to group supervision, and often case assignment within that team is part of the supervision agenda.

A benefit of team supervision is the opportunity for scaffolding of new supervisors through modeling from senior supervisors within the meeting (Milne and Oliver 2000). There is also an opportunity for a greater sense of professional collaboration and support for those involved, and the wider variety of perspectives within the team may benefit the entire team's learning. Drawbacks include the potential for interpersonal difficulties within a larger team and the potential for the difference in ability levels of team members to be so large that it interferes with the process. For example, if one team member is a novice, it may be frustrating to others and inefficient if most of the supervision meetings focus on helping this particular team member. Additionally, because a team may have clinical, supervision, and administrative items to cover, these meetings could feel rushed or incomplete if timing and structure are not managed well. These meetings may benefit from increased length if all clinical, supervision, and administrative items are focused on in the team meeting.

Supplemental Supervision

A supervisee may benefit from additional supervision outside of the required supervision designed by their training program. This may arise as a result of a training gap that would be best filled by a supervisor who is not the supervisee's primary supervisor. Many institutions have adjunct faculty members who may offer this type of supervision. A benefit of supplemental supervision is the opportunity for the supervisee to experience a wider variety of supervisory styles and perspectives. Drawbacks include the added time burden of additional supervision and the potential for the training program to have less oversight over this relationship if problems arise.

Supervision of Supervision

Supervision is its own competency and should be a focus of training (Falender et al. 2004). Supervising supervision can look identical to supervision of direct patient care in terms of format or style. Supervisors may meet in a group setting to discuss their supervisees with a more senior supervisor. Video review of supervision sessions may also be incorporated. Supervision training is a very important yet largely neglected part of clinicians' professional training (Falender et al. 2004). Thus, supervision of supervision may be an especially challenging undertaking if most supervisors did not receive this type of formal training themselves. It may be viewed by some as unnecessary given the historical lack of training in this domain. However, the importance of supervision training and competency has been the focus of increased attention (Falender and Shafranske 2014; Falender et al. 2004).

Levels of Supervision

In addition to differences in format, supervision can be classified in terms of supervisor activity or level of involvement. There are multiple models of classification in the literature to describe the various levels of supervision. One, described by Galanter et al. (2016), is described below.

Direct Supervision

Direct supervision occurs when the supervisor is physically present with both the supervisee and the patient. Live supervision, a format mentioned in the preceding section, is direct in nature by definition. This is most typical for trainees early in their development, although direct supervision is not widely used in psychiatry training programs. Galanter et al. (2016) posited several factors for its limited use, including "following the status quo, which in psychiatry was oversight supervision and had been perceived as being effective in most situations, the desire to foster supervisee's autonomy, to preserve the perception of confidentiality, and limited guidelines and regulations regarding direct supervision" (p. 161). Direct supervision can also result in direct patient care on the part of the supervisor if care is taken over by the supervisor and the supervisee is asked to observe (Kennedy et al. 2007). This approach could also be referred to as *responsive oversight* and may occur in the context of severely ill patients or concern about the supervisee's level of competence.

Indirect Supervision

Indirect supervision occurs when the supervisor is available at the hospital or clinic to provide direct supervision on an as-needed basis. Per the Accreditation Council for Graduate Medical Education (ACGME) program requirements, this is referred to as "indirect supervision with direct supervision immediately available" (Accreditation Council for Graduate Medical Education 2017, p. 32). It can also extend to "indirect supervision with direct supervision available" (Accreditation Council for Graduate Medical Education 2017, p. 32), in which the supervisor is not physically present within the hospital or other site of patient care but is available for supervision through technological means such as phone or email. This level of supervision is often used for supervisees once they have demonstrated a certain level of skill, making this increased independence developmentally appropriate for their training.

Oversight Supervision

Oversight supervision occurs when the supervisor reviews information about the care of the patient after the patient encounter is completed (Accreditation Council for Graduate Medical Education 2017, p. 32). Such oversight can be routine or responsive in nature and may entail reviewing psychotherapy notes, lab results, assessment reports, or video recordings. This form of supervision may also be referred to as "backstage oversight" (Kennedy et al. 2007) and could include supervision activities of which the supervisee is unaware (such as reading the patient's chart). Oversight supervision is used frequently with advanced trainees and in certain settings such as "night float," where direct supervision is not possible (see Chapter 15, "Night Float: Working With Supervisees Remotely").

Alternative Modes of Delivery

Finally, there are different modes of supervision delivery. Any of the previously mentioned formats of supervision can be delivered in a variety of ways. The most common mode of supervision delivery is in person at the training site. However, modern technology has created new opportunities for novel delivery of supervision.

Videoconferencing

Videoconferencing, also known as *telesupervision*, has been used as a way to delivery supervision to clinicians in rural areas (Wood et al. 2005). In a small pilot study of group telesupervision, Reese et al. (2009) found that supervisees rated telesupervision similarly to in-person supervision in terms of their satisfaction generally and in terms of the supervisory relationship. Supervisees in this study shared their belief that some emotional elements of supervision were lost via videoconferencing that would have been apparent in person. They also expressed a preference that telesupervision be used as adjunctive to in-person supervision, rather than as a stand-alone format.

Telesupervision is beneficial in terms of addressing geographical limitations for rural populations and for unexpected situations in which the supervisor may not be able to present at the physical training site. Additionally, telesupervision may facilitate the incorporation of other forms of media into supervision given that both parties are already engaged on some type of computer or device, such as training videos or websites (Wood et al. 2005). A drawback of telesupervision is the potential for technological glitches, such as loss of internet connectivity that could delay or interrupt the supervision session. Additionally, any videoconferencing technology used in the context of patient care needs to be HIPAA-compliant, a requirement that limits the number of programs available for this mode of delivery and may increase potential cost (see Chapter 4, "Virtual or Hybrid Supervision").

Specific Challenges and Strategies

- **My program has too few supervisors for the number of supervisees who need training.** Consider arranging for group supervision or telesupervision. If the ratio of supervisor to supervisee is so high that adequate supervision may not be feasible, consider advocating for increased hiring of supervisors. It is also possible to use multiple modes of supervision to help enhance the training experience, for example, by holding weekly group supervision meetings with multiple trainees, supplemented by less frequent individual supervision meetings to address the unique training needs of each trainee.

- **Supervising in a group format has been difficult because one trainee is really struggling.** It can be challenging to address gaps in competence or issues of professionalism when conducting group supervision. Consider utilizing different strategies within group supervision that are known to be effective, such as role-plays and videotape review, allowing the trainee to observe other members of the group in action. While the group is watching videotapes, stop the videotape during important learning moments and ask each member of the group how they would respond, and use this to facilitate a conversation about key areas of growth you think are important for the trainee. If this is not sufficient, consider building in individual supervision meetings with all trainees on a monthly basis to provide time for individual feedback. Alternatively, speak to the supervisee directly about your observations and arrange for additional oversight, either with you or with a separate individual supervisor.

- **I worry that my supervisees aren't exposed to enough therapy cases during their training.** While individual supervision allows the supervisor to provide close oversight of each supervisee's cases, and to "dive deep" with each supervisee, it does limit the number of patient presentations to which a supervisee will be exposed. Group supervision allows for increased exposure to a variety of cases throughout the training experience and might be a good option to include once supervisees have acquired foundational skills.

Questions for the Supervisor

■ Which format of supervision would best meet the needs of my supervisees?

■ What resources are available within my setting (e.g., how much time is protected for supervision, both for supervisors and for supervisees), and how might this affect my decision about choosing a supervision format?

■ Are there benefits of combining supervision formats, such as providing a mix of individual and group supervision?

Additional Resources

Falender CA, Shafranske EP: Clinical supervision: the state of the art. J Clin Psychol 70:1030–1041, 2014

Milne D: An empirical definition of clinical supervision. Br J Clin Psychol 46:437–447, 2007

Oliver DM: Flexible formats of clinical supervision: description, evaluation and implementation. J Ment Health 9:291–304, 2000

Rousmaniere T: Using technology to enhance clinical supervision and training, in The Wiley International Handbook of Clinical Supervision. Edited by Watkins CE, Milne DL. New York, Wiley, 2014, pp 204–237

References

Accreditation Council for Graduate Medical Education: Program requirements. Section 11.B.1.a. July 1, 2017. Available at: http://acgme.org/Specialties/Program-Requirements-and-FAQs-and-Applications/pfcatid/21/Psychiatry. Accessed August 6, 2018.

Blanchard DS: Peer-teaching: an important skill for all medical students and doctors? Perspect Med Educ 4(1):6–7, 2015 25605494

Costa L: Reducing anxiety in live supervision. Couns Educ Superv 34:30–40, 1994

Falender CA, Shafranske EP: Clinical supervision: the state of the art. J Clin Psychol 70(11):1030–1041, 2014 25220545

Falender CA, Cornish JA, Goodyear R, et al: Defining competencies in psychology supervision: a consensus statement. J Clin Psychol 60(7):771–785, 2004 15195339

Galanter CA, Nikolov R, Green N, et al: Direct supervision in outpatient psychiatric graduate medical education. Acad Psychiatry 40(1):157–163, 2016 25424638

Gallant JP, Thyer BA, Bailey JS: Using bug-in-the-ear feedback in clinical supervision: Preliminary evaluations. Res Soc Work Pract 1:175–187, 1991

Kennedy TJ, Lingard L, Baker GR, et al: Clinical oversight: conceptualizing the relationship between supervision and safety. J Gen Intern Med 22(8):1080–1085, 2007 17557190

Martin P, Milne DL, Reiser RP: Peer supervision: International problems and prospects. J Adv Nurs 74(5):998–999, 2018 28792603

Milne D: An empirical definition of clinical supervision. Br J Clin Psychol 46(Pt 4):437–447, 2007 17535535

Milne D, Oliver V: Flexible formats of clinical supervision: description, evaluation and implementation. J Ment Health 9:291–304, 2000

Reese RJ, Aldarondo F, Anderson CR, et al: Telehealth in clinical supervision: a comparison of supervision formats. J Telemed Telecare 15(7):356–361, 2009 19815905

Rizvi SL, Yu J, Geisser S, et al: The use of "bug-in-the-eye" live supervision for training in dialectical behavior therapy: a case study. Clin Case Stud 15:243–258, 2016

Rousmaniere T: Technology for evidence-based cognitive behavioural supervision: new applications and research to improve organizational support. The Cognitive Behaviour Therapist 9:e28, 2016

Silbert BI, Lake FR: Peer-assisted learning in teaching clinical examination to junior medical students. Med Teach 34(5):392–397, 2012 22471912

Sudak DM, Codd RT 3rd, Ludgate JW, et al: Teaching and Supervising Cognitive Behavioral Therapy. New York, Wiley, 2015

Wood JA, Miller TW, Hargrove DS: Clinical supervision in rural settings: a telehealth model. Professional Psychology: Research and Practice 36(2):173–179, 2005

Chapter 4   Virtual or Hybrid Supervision

Peter Yellowlees, M.B.B.S., M.D.

Technological changes are currently transforming the U.S. health and education markets (Yellowlees and Shore 2018). One of the areas that they have been transforming for a number of years is the area of professional supervision, and this change is now well past the tipping point: Hybrid (or virtual) supervision involves use of a combination of in-person and one or more online approaches within supervision. This is already standard practice for many supervisors and supervisees. The formal literature on clinical supervision is relatively small, and little research has been undertaken given how commonly technologies are used for supporting the supervisory process. In this chapter I discuss the process and technologies used in hybrid supervision and conclude with guidelines for both supervisors and supervisees.

Key Points

- Communication technologies are ubiquitous and are already widely used for all types of supervision.

- Hybrid supervision (online and in-person) is likely to become the standard of practice for many supervisory relationships in the future.

- Virtual supervision enables and supports more flexible, accessible and egalitarian supervisor-supervisee relationships.

- There is a need for more research in this area, especially on the significance and use of the "virtual space" that exists between supervisors and supervisees.

- Hybrid approaches to supervision can potentially be undertaken across languages and cultures given that geographic access barriers will likely soon be reduced through the use of automated translation systems.

What Technologies Are Being Used in Hybrid Supervision?

Many technologies are currently being used in psychiatry (American Psychiatric Association 2018; see also the American Telemedicine Association website [www.american-telemed.org]). These technologies can be divided into those that have become a standard part of daily practice and those that are currently not in widespread use or deployment, but which will likely become common in the future. Most can be used either synchronously (in real time) or asynchronously (in delayed time).

The base technologies currently in use for clinical, educational, and research supervision include the following:

1. *Email or secure messaging.* These asynchronous technologies are especially useful for administrative issues such as creating agendas prior to supervision and meeting notes after sessions, as well as for easy communication between or after sessions.
2. *Videoconferencing.* Live interactive videoconferencing usually occurs in real time (synchronous) and is already widely adopted for clinical purposes, with over a million individual psychiatric patients treated using telepsychiatry in the United States in 2016 (Yellowlees and Shore 2018). Videoconferencing is also commonly used for supervision and other educational experiences, including individual supervision, small groups, and large international conferences (Smith et al. 2012). If clinical cases or patient material is being discussed, this technology must meet Health Insurance Portability and Accountability Act (HIPAA) standards. Sometimes video recordings of patients can be played and reviewed during real-time videoconferencing supervision sessions, and such sessions can also be recorded so that they can be viewed by others at a later time (asynchronously).
3. *Web-based applications.* Web-based applications are currently being widely deployed for education, and many incorporate synchronous and asynchronous communication capacities, allowing them to be used as an adjunct to supervision, or communication technologies, such as video or texting, as the tools through which supervision may occur.
4. *Mobile devices.* Mobile phones are the ubiquitous mental health technology of the twenty-first century and encompass all the traditional functions of phone systems along with texting, apps, and many monitoring, recording, and note-taking capacities. Such devices have the ability to free supervisors and supervisees from their offices or desktops, enabling supervision communication to occur literally anytime, anywhere.
5. *Electronic medical records (EMRs).* These can be shared for hybrid or online clinical supervision, and many already incorporate access to a range of educational and de-

cision support materials. Videoconferencing and instant messaging capacities are currently being introduced that will likely make these EMRs "one-stop shops" for clinical supervision in the near future.

Emergent technologies are those that are not yet in widespread and consistent use in supervision, or more widely in psychiatric clinical practice, but are currently being piloted in limited settings. These include virtual reality and massive multiplayer systems (Yellowlees et al. 2012), social networking environments, artificial intelligence, the creation of avatars, and the use of geospatial tracking and systems (Yellowlees and Shore 2018). All these technologies, and others, will doubtless find roles in supervision in the future.

Advantages of Hybrid Supervision

The integration of communications technologies into supervisory practice allows supervisor and supervisee relationships to be both in person and online, and it is likely that the future standard of supervisory practice will be a "hybrid" relationship, which has major advantages over a purely in-person educational experience. Not surprisingly, this follows the trend that has occurred in clinical practice, in which increasing numbers of patients and practitioners have established "hybrid" relationships, meeting and communicating both in person, and by video, email, messaging, and telephone, where and when it is most convenient for both (Yellowlees et al. 2015).

Enhanced Empathy

Yellowlees and Shore (2018) have noted how the addition of an online component may increase the ability of both supervisor and supervisee, as well as doctor and patient, to empathize with each other and form a meaningful, trusting therapeutic dyad and interaction. The addition of interactions via videoconferencing, e-mail, text messaging, and telephony leads to improved access and interactions at times and in places where it was previously not possible to do so, and is exciting and rewarding for both. The incorporation of a "virtual environment" between the teacher and the student enables them to interact more intimately, while at the same time supports more objective observation by both, using the extra electronic distance and "virtual space" within the sessions (Yellowlees and Shore 2018).

Expanded Reach

Using these hybrid approaches, supervision can potentially be undertaken across languages and cultures as geographic access barriers are dramatically reduced through the use of technology, especially when there is access to automated translation systems that are increasingly being incorporated into videoconferencing environments. The use of such translation systems may in the future make comprehension across different languages better via videoconferencing than it is in person through interpreters, because these systems are constantly being improved and becoming more accurate through the incorporation of machine learning. Martin et al. (2018) reviewed most of the formal studies of technology supported supervision, systematically examining the factors that influence the quality and effectiveness of telesupervision for health professionals. They noted that clinical supervision via technology has been particularly helpful in providing professional support for isolated professionals, such as occurs in Australia, and that it also promotes networking and professional interaction of health practitioners who work outside metropolitan areas. They commented that while the use of technology in clinical supervision is increasing, there is a lack of clear guidelines on what factors make it effective and of high quality.

Reduced Power Differential

In videoconferencing environments, clinicians and patients have a more equal power relationship, in which either may reserve the right to decide whether to have the next component of the relationship play out in person or online, immediately or in the future (Chan et al. 2015). Similar dynamics may occur in clinical supervision, where the power hierarchy between supervisee and supervisor is frequently flattened. This is particularly obvious from the perspective of the supervisee who may well feel less inhibited by an experienced supervisor on video compared with in person. If the supervisee also has the well-described disinhibition that occurs frequently among video technology users (Yellowlees and Shore 2018), this combination of power flattening and disinhibition may lead to the unintended consequence of disrespect or misunderstandings if these elements are not acknowledged and understood by all involved.

Enhanced Communication

The converse of this concern is the interesting finding by Martin et al. (2018), who, in a review article on the factors that influence quality in supervision, concluded that telesupervision enhanced communication between the supervisor and the supervisee. They described how the process forced supervisees to verbalize and communicate better, leading to supervisors giving better and more detailed instruction and explanations, while supervisees asked more questions.

Enhanced Safety

It is known that interactions over videoconferencing involve more eye contact compared with in-person interactions, but that simultaneously the actual physical distance and separation between patient and therapist also creates a type of psychological distance and greater sense of separation (Yellowlees and Shore 2018). Yellowlees et al. (2015) have discussed the concept of this "virtual space," which is a combination of the increased physical distance and psychological distance that arise by virtue of the videoconferencing medium, but that between them provide more mutual safety for the participants and counter-intuitively support an increased sharing of intimacy. Kocsis and Yellowlees (2018) extended this concept, noting how in telepsychotherapy, the patient may be able to be more honest, and to describe important material more candidly, because of the "protection" afforded by the virtual space, while still maintaining intimacy-fostering eye contact. It seems that what has been learned in the telepsychotherapy experience and from the associated literature may well apply very directly to the supervisor-supervisee relationship, although more research on this topic is certainly needed.

Important Considerations in Hybrid Supervision

Tendency for Disinhibition

Other caveats about moving to this hybrid relationship style of supervisory practice concern the need for both supervisors and supervisees to ensure that appropriate professional boundaries—ethical, physical, technical, and time-related—as well as confidentiality of the process itself, are maintained. There is a well-described tendency toward disinhibition that can not only accompany videoconferences but also be seen in email interactions. It is only too easy to press "reply," or worse "reply all," after writing an emotion-charged response on some issue, and then later to regret it. Supervisors need to think about the sort of educational practice they wish to have and discuss this with their supervisees, perhaps going as far as creating some simple "rules" of communication and engagement for all the various technologies that they use to interact directly with students (Yellowlees and Shore 2018).

Confidentiality

The importance of maintaining confidentiality is key. In the health industry, if patients are to be discussed in supervision, then whatever technology is used must meet HIPAA standards. Technology standards, though, are only part of the issue, and it is vital that both parties to any communication be aware of everyone who is in the room at both ends of the interaction, because it is all too easy to have people, possibly family members at home, sitting to the side "off screen." Windows and doors must also be shut at both ends so that the conversation cannot be heard outside of the rooms where the electronic communication is taking place. The lifelong development of professional competencies and skills for telepsychiatry, as well as the importance of training in media communication skills across a range of technologies, is detailed by Yellowlees and Shore (2018), and such training issues are identical to those needed for supervisors and supervisees.

Themes That Contribute to High-Quality Telesupervision

Martin et al. (2018) identified eight themes that contribute to effective and high-quality telesupervision: supervisee characteristics, supervisor characteristics, supervision characteristics, the supervisory relationship, communication strategies, prior in-person contact, environmental factors, and technological considerations (see Table 4–1 for descriptions). They concluded that telesupervision can be a feasible and acceptable form of supervision if it is set up well, but noted that this is an area where much more research is required to strengthen the level of existing evidence, and in particular to examine the cost-effectiveness of this approach.

TABLE 4–1.   **Eight themes that contribute to effective and high-quality telesupervision**

Theme	Description
Supervisee characteristics	Clinical practice experience; insight into one's own needs, open to learning via distance supervision; personality that is flexible, pragmatic, and relaxed
Supervisor characteristics	Experience of context of supervisee's practice; good skills as facilitator and organizer in group settings
Supervision characteristics	Structured sessions; use of minutes and agenda, with topic designation prior to sessions; mutual contractual expectations, preparation and length and time of meetings
Supervisory relationship	Strength of working alliance; immediacy, continuity, and accessibility of relationship
Communication strategies	More formal speaking; longer speech blocks if timing of interaction is significant, allowing both supervisee and supervisor to get comfortable using video
Prior in-person contact	Enhanced mutual trust and respect
Environmental factors	Quiet space; access to phone and soundproof private environments
Technological considerations	Ability to operate technologies and minimize, and at the very least tolerate, background noise, audio lags, and distractions (usually reduce over time)

Source.   Adapted from Martin et al. 2018.

Guidelines for Being an Effective Hybrid Supervisor

There is certainly a unique feeling about some aspects of virtual supervision, whether it is hybrid or completely conducted online, and as in any good supervisory relationship, the structure of the experience, the use of specific supervisory approaches and techniques, and the mutual engagement of the involved dyad are of great importance. A number of strategies are suggested for any supervisor, as described below.

Increase Planning and Organization

Before and after sessions, it is helpful to use email to discuss agendas, provide specific written feedback, and confirm discussion topics and agreed-on actions. Email discussion in-between sessions can also be helpful in allowing both supervisee and supervisor to be fully accountable to themselves and each other.

Be Careful in Use of Oral Communication Skills

Direct conversations are often easier via video than in person, especially regarding difficult or potentially stigmatizing topics, because the distance allows both parties to be more open and honest with each other, with less potential embarrassment. This distance, if not appreciated, can unfortunately lead to difficulties, because it is relatively easy on video to come across as either overbearing or insensitive, perhaps partly because of the relative lack of perceived feedback that can occur during a video conversation.

Effectively Use Body Language and Media Skills

It is well known that on video, an increased use of body language and verbal intonation, perhaps 110% of usual, is generally helpful and can make both individuals appear more lively, rather like TV news anchors (Yellowlees and Shore 2018). It is important not to be excessively disinhibited, on the other hand, and a way of monitoring this is to keep the small "picture in picture" video window open at all times, allowing a continuous self-view to the supervisor. Without this extra body language some people may appear excessively reserved or flat on video. It is strongly suggested that supervisors who are going to use videoconferencing regularly take a media skills course of the type offered by many journalists and media commentators.

Be Prepared to Be Flexible and Use Multiple Technologies and Approaches

This is especially important when hybrid supervision is occurring, with the use of multiple technologies over months or years. The combination of synchronous (telephony, videoconferencing, or in-person meetings) and asynchronous (texting or e-mail) communications approaches can make the supervisory process more enlightening and effective. It also allows an almost continuous "conversation" to occur over time via different technologies as part of the supervision process, rather than needing to have all interactions occur at once during a single physical in-person session.

Develop the Capacity for Prudent Mediation and Facilitation of Groups

Prudent mediation and group facilitation are skills that are typically learned in the in-person world but that are highly transferable online for group supervision, where they can be put to use to make groups run much more smoothly. Managing several video inputs at once requires the facilitator to take a fairly structured process that may well involve setting a running agenda during the meeting, by giving warning that person A will speak next, then person B, then a representative from site C, so that all group members are able to have input. This is especially the case if the video feeds are voice activated, or if there is some time delay with poor network connections, because it ensures that unplanned interruptions, which can be very disruptive and lead to rapid changes in video pictures through the voice activation systems, are minimized.

Guidelines for Being an Effective Hybrid Supervisee

Supervisees may well find hybrid supervision to be a much more natural approach than do supervisors, especially if the supervisees are what has been described as "digital natives" (Yellowlees and Shore 2018), who are typically younger than 30 years and have never experienced life without the internet. They still need to take note of all the strategies described above for supervisors and the following extra issues.

Be Tolerant

Your supervisor may possibly lack technological sophistication, so it is important to be tolerant. However technologically savvy the supervisor, just because of generational differences he or she may have some difficulty managing multiple technologies or will not immediately understand how the much younger and more technologically sound supervisee may want to share documents or file work in apparently unusual places online. Remember that the supervisor may be much more comfortable receiving documents as email attachments rather than via cloud-based services, and that he or she may still want to print them out to read and review. Check in with the supervisor to learn his or her preferences for communication and document sharing, rather than assume he or she has a similar level of technological knowledge.

Be Proactive and Respectful in the Relationship

Be proactive and respectful but not excessively demanding or intrusive. Remember that while a supervisee may be comfortable communicating with friends and colleagues at midnight on Sunday, the supervisor may be less so and will not necessarily respond within half an hour. So be accountable, keep to agreed timelines, and be respectful of the fact that the supervisor may well be dealing with multiple other students at the same time, so cannot be expected to respond instantly.

Specific Challenges and Strategies

- **My videoconferencing froze or was of poor quality during a session.** Reboot at both ends. Check that the camera and audio at both ends are working and that the hardware has not failed. Remember that audio is more important than video, and takes less bandwidth, and so tends to be preserved ahead of video if there is a bandwidth problem. You can usually continue supervision with audio only, but not with video only. Spend some time piloting the software prior to using it for supervision to iron out any difficulties.
- **My supervisee keeps sending me too many emails.** Set up some written rules with the supervisee that determine how long it will take you to respond, when you will respond, and what the maximum number of emails or attachments you will review is. Discuss any challenges that arise during supervision, and if the supervisee continues to have difficulty following your written guidelines, this becomes a professionalism issue that needs to be addressed.
- **I would rather see my supervisor in person, but she seems to be using technologies to avoid meeting with me.** Set up regular appointments in advance and check your supervisor's office hours and availability. Discuss your preferences for supervision with your supervisor and try to work out a mutually agreed-on solution. If the issue continues, consider discussing this with your program directors.

Questions for the Supervisee

- What are your expectations for supervision using technology?

- How many sessions on average will be online compared with in-person and how often will they occur?

- Do you have access to a relatively new PC, laptop, tablet, or smartphone, and which are you most likely to use for virtual supervision sessions?

- Have you used videoconferencing to communicate with your family and friends and are you comfortable with using it?

- Do you have a private setting you can use for videoconferencing sessions?

Additional Resources

American Psychiatric Association. Telepsychiatry Toolkit. Available at: https://www.psychiatry.org/psychiatrists/practice/telepsychiatry/telepsychiatry-toolkit-home
American Telemedicine Association. www.americantelemed.org

References

American Psychiatric Association: Telepsychiatry toolkit. 2018. Available at: https://www.psychiatry.org/psychiatrists/practice/telepsychiatry/telepsychiatry-toolkit-home. Accessed August 6, 2018.

Chan S, Parish M, Yellowlees P: Telepsychiatry Today. Curr Psychiatry Rep 17(11):89, 2015 26384338

Kocsis BJ, Yellowlees P: Telepsychotherapy and the therapeutic relationship: principles, advantages and case examples. Telemed J E Health 24(5):329–334, 2018 28836902

Martin P, Lizarondo L, Kumar S: A systematic review of the factors that influence the quality and effectiveness of telesupervision for health professionals. J Telemed Telecare 24(4):271–281, 2018 28387603

Smith AC, White MM, McBride CA, et al: Multi-site videoconference tutorials for medical students in Australia. ANZ J Surg 82(10):714–719, 2012 22957836

Yellowlees PM, Shore J: Telepsychiatry and Health Technologies: A Guide for Mental Health Professionals. Arlington, VA, American Psychiatric Association Publishing, 2018

Yellowlees PM, Holloway KM, Parish MB: Therapy in virtual environments—clinical and ethical issues. Telemed J E Health 18(7):558–564, 2012 22823138

Yellowlees P, Richard Chan S, Burke Parish M: The hybrid doctor-patient relationship in the age of technology—telepsychiatry consultations and the use of virtual space. Int Rev Psychiatry 27(6):476–489, 2015 26493089

Part 3   Supervision Techniques

Chapter 5   Working With Transcripts

An Underutilized Supervisory Approach

Sallie G. De Golia, M.D., M.P.H.

Katherine E. Williams, M.D.

Debra L. Safer, M.D.

Working with transcripts is an underutilized strategy for providing oversight and education within the context of psychotherapy supervision. In a survey of Canadian psychotherapy coordinators, De Roma and colleagues (2007) reported that case discussion/presentation was the most commonly utilized psychotherapy supervisory method (42%), followed by video recording (12%), live supervision (10%), and audio recording (9%). It is not surprising that transcripts were not listed, as very little literature exists on the specific use of verbatim transcripts (Arthur and Gfroerer 2002). Given that objective methods of discussing case material within supervision have been demonstrated to enhance therapist competence (Miller et al. 2004), it is important to include verbatim transcripts in the supervision toolbox. In this chapter, we explore the benefits and drawbacks of using verbatim transcripts and offer strategies to effectively use transcripts within supervision.

Key Points

- Benefits of working with transcripts outweigh the downsides.

- Transcripts allow for an effective and expedited, albeit limited, review of the clinical session.

- Transcripts may be used to reinforce knowledge through assigning specific tasks.

- Transcripts offer a content catalogue of sessions.

Benefits of Using Transcripts

Supervisee Benefit

One of the most significant benefits of transcripts is that the supervisee uses three learning modalities. The supervisee views the session video (visual and auditory) and transforms it into written form (kinesthetic), thus greatly increasing his or her potential for learning (Dwyer 1978). Through the transcribing process, supervisees undergo a reflective process as they recognize what the patient *actually* said, which was perhaps not perceived (either consciously or unconsciously) during the session itself, as well as how they *actually* responded to a patient response. Supervisees become re-immersed in the experience, but now—by rewatching the video and typing the actual words—through a heightened visual and literary engagement.

Even when supervisees are asked to transcribe only a small section (10 minutes) of a session, they must spend more time reflecting on what was actually said than they would by presenting the video alone. In addition to reflecting more deeply on the transcribed section, they also may consider alternative responses, identify questions for the supervisor, and process their feelings about the experience in advance of supervision. Furthermore, supervisees may be less willing to rewatch a video unless asked to choose a section to transcribe.

Another valuable benefit of a transcript is that it is easier for the supervisee to reflect on a written document than to keep track of dialogue and nonverbal material on a video or audio recording. Transcripts are far easier to annotate and index. Furthermore, given how much faster one can read a transcript than watch a video, if one wants to develop a library of sessions, the transcript allows easy access for review. Importantly, the supervisee can also more easily keep track of supervisor comments related to specific points within the transcript (e.g., by inserting them onto the transcript) to which he or she can more easily refer back, compared with a video or audio recording.

Supervisor Benefit

From the supervisor's perspective, the use of transcripts can be ideal. First, given time constraints, it is far faster to read through a verbatim transcript than to watch a video section prior to supervision. This allows the supervisor to obtain a more accurate view of the session, even without an accompanying video portion, compared with recall or process notes, in which the supervisee can intentionally or unintentionally omit information. A transcript, like a video, allows for mutual exploration of a session, which may lead to an enhanced alliance between the supervisor and supervisee. A transcript also allows for the supervisor to identify teaching points in advance of a supervisory session, formulate responses to supervisee questions, and identify trouble spots worth viewing, enabling greater efficiency for in-depth discussions without leaving teaching to chance.

By reviewing the transcript, the supervisor can identify where the supervisee failed to follow a patient and might explore the nature of this in-depth with the supervisee. For example, perhaps something about the patient's affect or nonverbal cues caused a disconnect or countertransference. Similarly, the supervisor may be able to highlight the supervisee's distortion or countertransference more clearly with the transcript than by watching a video. To identify the missing nonverbal material, the supervisor and supervisee might review the tape. This may lead to a rich discussion about the importance of nonverbal material in the work with patients. Furthermore, if an entire session is transcribed and reviewed in advance, the supervisor may be able to identify sections of particular worth that the supervisee may not be aware of when selecting a section to review.

Finally, transcripts could serve as an archive of the patient's improvement over time. But very importantly, transcripts allow the supervisor to prepare feedback for the supervisee that is more specific, directed, and sensitive—an essential part of learning and improvement.

Intrinsic Value of Transcript

The fact that a transcript can be reviewed separately from a video allows for review of the literal material spoken by the patient, without the distraction of nonverbals material, intonations, or other potentially diverting elements. This language or "data" used by the patient can be more closely analyzed, allowing for closer observance of inconsistencies, fluency, slips of the tongue, use of associations, concreteness versus abstractions, and shifts in topics. Although misinterpretation of the material is still possible, even when paired with the video, inconsistencies between verbal content and affect provide potent information to the supervisee regarding how a patient might be misunderstood in his or her outside life.

Supervision Session Benefit

When the supervisee is asked to transcribe and present a question based on the transcript, the focus of the supervisory session becomes more directed. The supervisee must take time to reflect on his or her own learning objectives. Given the time constraints of supervision sessions, simple video reviews may be less efficient because of a greater likelihood for distractions and tangents. Often, when video recordings are used, the supervisee and/or supervisor may not review the tape prior to supervision and either start with the beginning of the session or skip through to various clips—which may waste supervisory time.

The "gold standard" is to pair transcripts with video for a closer reenactment of the actual "live" clinical session. This combination allows for more efficient use and deeper analysis of the video by enabling swifter identification, in advance, of trouble areas or potential teaching points. The video can be readily fast-forwarded to specific key points annotated in the transcript. Finally, even if time runs out in supervision for completing review of the video, the previewed transcript has allowed the supervisor to identify important take-home points, ensuring that key teaching points are not missed.

Drawbacks of Using Transcripts

There are a few, yet substantive, drawbacks to using transcripts. The first drawback is important to readily acknowledge: Transcripts take time to prepare. Since most beginning supervisees are likely trainees, the time pressures are particularly significant, given the multiple demands of residency, including managing call and/or night float. However, with ever-advancing technological options, digital recordings with speed-play options enable transcripts to be done more quickly than previous methods involving tape recorders.

In addition, especially for a beginning trainee, writing out a verbatim dialogue between oneself and the patient may feel painful without the ability to transform the information into a more palatable utterance or insight. Furthermore, when transcripts are *not* paired with a video, they provide only part of the therapist-patient experience. Even when this nonverbal material (e.g., a patient sigh or nervous laugh) is noted, the fuller meaning of the actual words is not realized without the accompanying nonverbal signals or verbal nuances.

Finally, transcripts must be safeguarded from breach of confidentiality through avoiding the use of identifying information such as names; ensuring encrypted computer or server storage; and distributing transcripts via encrypted flash drives, secured emails, HIPAA-approved websites, or other secure mechanisms.

How to Work With Transcripts

Firstly, explain to supervisees the powerful benefits of transcripts because they will no doubt balk at the time perceived to create a transcript. After supervisees have completed one or two transcripts, they often recognize the transcript's utility and value. They also become faster at creating them.

Select Segment to Transcribe

Start with asking the supervisee to select 10 minutes of a video to transcribe. This usually takes 30–60 minutes to transcribe depending on the supervisee. Request that the supervisee identify a question and/or point of curiosity or confusion within the session. Examples might include "Why did the patient respond this way?" "What did the patient mean by this?" or "How do I go deeper into the affect in this section?"

Ask the supervisee to send the transcript along with his or her question/learning goals in advance of the session to allow the supervisor time to review and develop teaching points. Remind the supervisee about the importance of removing identifying information and sending the transcript through secure e-mail or HIPAA-approved platforms. Given the richness of even a 10-minute segment, it is critical that the supervisor address the supervisee's question and hold back on other teaching points until time allows. If the supervision takes place in a small-group setting, ask the supervisee to send the transcript to all members in advance.

Review the Transcript

Start each review session by responding to the supervisee's stated question(s). As time allows, watch the video with the transcript for a richer analysis of the question(s) at hand. You might then ask: "What was your intent?" "What was the impact of your intervention?" "Did it appear to work (or not) and why?" or "Are their alternative ways to get at what you were hoping for?" Once the supervisee's questions have been adequately addressed, the supervisor might want to point out other teaching points identified in the transcript.

Additional Uses of Transcripts

Consider assigning tasks to the supervisee depending on the educational goals or particular needs of the supervisee. A supervisor could ask the supervisee to annotate the transcript in advance to identify affect or affect-laden words (particularly when the patient's affect does not match the verbal response); examples of transference, resistance, use of defenses, parallel process, enactment, ethical dilemmas, cultural impact, intent and/or types of interventions used (clarification vs. confrontation), or evidence of core beliefs, conflicts, or introjects; how the responses support the goals of the patient; or how the section relates to the proposed formulation.

The transcript, like the video, could be used as a prompt to discuss alternative responses. With more advanced supervisees, the supervisor might ask how one might respond to different patient responses given different theoretical frameworks, comparing and contrasting different ways to approach the same therapeutic content. For example, how would the supervisee integrate goals within the section of cognitive behavioral therapy, how might this material apply to the cyclical maladaptive pattern for time-limited dynamic psychotherapy, and/or, if dynamic psychotherapy is being used, what unconscious conflict might the patient be experiencing?

Specific Challenges and Strategies

- **My supervisee refuses to transcribe.** Make sure you have explained fully the benefits of transcribing. Supervisors might transcribe their own sessions, if they have not done this before, to experience the benefits firsthand. Your explanation will be much more persuasive if you fully buy in to the process! If the supervisee still refuses, assess the barriers. If it is a question of time, start with a small task—request that he or she transcribe only 1 or 2 minutes of a session and proceed from there.
- **My supervisee is too embarrassed to share a transcription.** Have the supervisee transcribe the part of a session with which the supervisee feels comfortable and summarize the parts that he or she feels too embarrassed to transcribe. If the supervisee is too embarrassed to even summarize, then have him or her describe what made the interaction so embarrassing. Building the supervisee's confidence about the parts that went well and empathy for the difficulty experienced will help him or her feel understood. Also, assess the learning climate and supervisory alliance for safety and confidentiality. Adjustments may be needed to establish a safer climate for the learner. Even very experienced therapists find themselves falling into reenactments without realizing it. These are teaching moments.
- **How can a 10-minute segment do justice to the overall theme or flow of the session?** The overall session should certainly be addressed during supervision; however, a segment often reflects the overall themes and provides concrete examples of ways skills can be more readily assessed and addressed and feedback given.

Questions for the Supervisee

- Where did I feel most stuck in the session?

- What bothered me the most about the session?

- Did I feel disconnected in any place?

- Where did I notice my countertransference?

Questions for the Supervisor

- What does my supervisee have most difficulty with, and how can I use the transcripts repetitively to help with that competency?

- What would my supervisee be most interested in exploring in a transcript?

- Have I set an agenda for the session to address the supervisee's questions adequately, identify teaching, and feedback points?

References

Arthur GL, Gfroerer KP: Training and supervision through the written word: a description and intern feedback. Fam J (Alex Va) 10(2):213–219, 2002

De Roma VM, Hickey DA, Stanek KM: Methods of supervision in marriage and family therapist training: a brief report. N Am J Psychol 9:415–422, 2007

Dwyer FM: Strategies for Improving Visual Learning: A Handbook for the Effective Selection, Design, and Use of Visualized Materials. State College, PA, Learning Services, 1978, pp 1–20

Miller WR, Yahne CE, Moyers TB, et al: A randomized trial of methods to help clinicians learn motivational interviewing. J Consult Clin Psychol 72(6):1050–1062, 2004 15612851

Chapter 6   Working With Process Notes

Dana Wideman, Ph.D.

In most psychoanalytic and many psychodynamic psychotherapy training programs, writing process notes is a *conditio sine qua non* of supervision. They serve as a communication about the patient from the supervisee to the supervisor while also being a learning tool about the process of psychotherapy. A deeper appreciation of the unconscious dynamics is gained through the experience of writing and reading the notes. In a written form, the whole session can also be condensed into a manageable unit (Sarnat 2016). In this chapter, after defining and presenting the benefits of process notes, I focus on how to create and use them in individual and group supervision. The difficulties related to writing and presenting the notes, as well as the specific strategies for dealing with these challenges, will be discussed.

Key Points

- Process notes provide not only a narrative account of the session but also rich clinical material on the therapist's conscious experience and its interpretation.

- Process notes are a source of information on the unconscious processes between the therapist and the patient.

- Process notes help the supervisor discover the unconscious dynamics of the patient's psyche.

- Process notes are useful in unearthing the therapist's unconscious material.

- Process notes can be used in both individual and group supervision.

Definition of Process Notes

On the surface, process notes claim to be a recording of what happened in the session from the point of view—and memory—of the therapist. They are not verbatim text based on an audio or video recording. They tend to be of the "he said, she said" variety. On that level, they are meant to present the patient's narrative of his or her concerns and the therapist's interventions, which can then be explored and possibly alternative responses offered within a particular theoretical frame of reference. On another level, they represent the clinical material as metabolized through the therapist's own psyche (e.g., "The patient seemed angry or in need of reassurance and was putting pressure on me to answer his question").

Attending to a presumably less conscious level, therapists are also asked to record their own internal reactions occurring at any particular moment in the session: associations, thoughts, fantasies, feelings, and bodily sensations. These countertransference reactions can then be used to think about unconscious processes: projections, projective identifications, and unconscious communications. The focus is on unearthing the unconscious processes in the belief that they are responsible for most of our human trials and tribulations while, by definition, they are outside of our awareness. Process notes are an attempt to capture these unconscious processes in the here and now of a session.

Benefits of Process Notes

Supervisors and supervisees infer unconscious processes when they attend to the written process notes and can register previously unknown, not-remembered, not-noticed material that can shed a new light on what may be occurring at the unconscious level. In the process of writing, the supervisee goes through the material once again and is better able to attend to its different strata. It is significant what is remembered, what is forgotten, what is attended to, what is understood and misunderstood, what associations arise, and what slips of the tongue are made when writing and when presenting. Process notes represent a mode of learning about the patient's and the supervisee's unconscious as they both interact and influence each other. It is a world of microanalytic events that represent a pattern. One can hear them in a recording, but there is also something to be said about material that can be looked at back and forth when analyzing mutual responses. Aware that the patient is the best supervisor, the supervisee examines the text for how his or her interventions were understood, and responded to, and how the supervisee reacted, both consciously and unconsciously, to these responses.

Creation of Process Notes

Some authors (Epstein and Wallerstein 1958) suggest that process notes be written in a way that seems most useful to the supervisee, which is certainly flexible and open minded. It may also be useful to ask for a write up of at least a few sessions with certain recommendations in mind. The issue is not accuracy per se, but the therapist's rendition of the session, which is meant for exploration, not evaluation. The following suggestions to the supervisee may help with this process:

1. Write the notes as soon as possible after the session; it is best to do it the same day, because a lot is forgotten by the next day.
2. Write the account in a "he said, she said" form and include any associations, images, fantasies, feelings, and bodily sensations that arose during the session and are being experienced at the time of writing (and/or dictating).
3. Try *not* to write notes during the session, because it interferes with being present and attentive to what is occurring here and now. Sometimes writing provides a distance that may be useful to some supervisees, particularly beginners, in containing their high level of anxiety.

Use of Process Notes

Process notes are used slightly differently in individual and in group supervision sessions.

Individual Supervision

The supervisee is requested to provide a copy of the process notes (so the supervisor can follow the text) and asked to read them out loud. If the supervisee is aware of any currently arising reactions/afterthoughts to the presented material, he or she is encouraged to share them. In response, the supervisor shares his or her associations, thoughts, and feelings and sometimes suggests an alternative hypothesis and/or a possibility of a different intervention. The discussion of the supervisee's reactions to the supervisor's ideas follows. The process should be one of exploration fueled by curiosity and not one characterized by prescriptive statements ("You should do this..."). Both the supervisor and supervisee hypothesize what may be happening on different levels. The following serves as an example:

> The supervisee reports that the patient had unexpectedly brought him a gift, a box of chocolates. The supervisee felt confused, yet he awkwardly and quite hesitantly accepted the gift. He mumbled a thank you but did not explore the patient's thoughts or feelings about this gift. Later, as the supervisee was writing the description of the patient handing the chocolates, he recalled thinking that the chocolates might make him ill. He was surprised and could not understand what made him so uncomfortable. When he read the notes in the supervision session, the supervisor was very interested in the supervisee's feelings of confusion and the thoughts that the chocolates would make him sick. Perhaps he was picking up emotionally something the patient was afraid to feel. The supervisee was not typically so awkward. The supervisor and the supervisee wondered if the gift could have been a complicated undoing of the patient's anger with the therapist. The supervisee remembered that it did feel a bit like "a bribe." They both arrived at a hypothesis that the gift might have been meant to ward off disowned angry feelings towards the therapist which were not safe to express. "I only bear gratitude toward you, want to give you something good, not bad" could summarize this attitude. In the next session, the therapist brought up his curiosity about the gift of chocolates and wondered when the patient decided to give them to him. Surprisingly, the patient revealed that he had purchased the chocolates during the therapist's recent vacation. The patient was surprised by this himself, as he remembered feeling annoyed that the therapist was away on vacation "again." This resulted in the patient being able to begin to discuss his angry and mixed feelings toward the therapist. In future sessions, the therapist will be more attuned to the patient's underlying angry feelings so he can eventually address them. The incident with the chocolates became something that the therapist and patient could refer back to explore the patient's anxiety about angry feelings.

Group Supervision

The presenter is asked to provide the group members with a copy of the process notes, read them aloud, and then share any reactions arising in the moment of reading. The presenter reads the notes until the supervisor finds a good stopping point: a change of direction of the content of the material, a moment when the supervisor wishes to stress a response signifying an underlying unconscious process or draw attention to transference, or other relevant teaching opportunities. Group members are encouraged to share their unfiltered reactions to the presented material. The supervisor then asks them to propose hypotheses about what may be going on with the patient and the therapeutic relationship. The presenter is encouraged to share his or her responses to the group's reactions and ideas, and the participants discuss emerging hypotheses. It is also interesting to explore how different members could be representing different parts of the patient and/ or various aspects of the therapist/patient relationship on the unconscious level—the concept of parallel process (Epstein and Wallerstein 1958; Rosbrow 1997).

During discussions of the process notes, it is important to analyze the here-and-now of the patient-therapist dynamics. The group considers the dominant feeling, movement of anxiety and defenses, transference, countertransference, unconscious fantasies, and beliefs, as well as who reacted to what and possibly why.

It cannot be denied that writing process notes is a very time-consuming task and often felt as a burden. However, it often turns out to be a meaningful, rewarding experience, because it provides an opportunity to revisit a session but with more inner space to explore, contemplate, and discover something new. It is also a good training in therapeutic receptivity as this process presupposes that the therapist is not only empathic but also receptive to the patient's conscious/unconscious communications. To fully appreciate the richness and depth of the therapeutic process as experienced via process notes, it may be worthwhile at least once during the training, to video record the session, write process notes, and then watch the video recording.

Storage of Process Notes

The Health Insurance Portability and Accountability Act of 1996 (HIPAA) stresses keeping process notes separate from progress notes and the patient's official chart because they are only meant for the therapist and the supervisor. They allow supervisees to be as open as possible about their countertransference reactions without worrying that the record may be seen by the patient, another clinician or used in formal proceedings. Process notes are exempted from formal proceedings but can, though only in very rare circumstances, be subpoenaed in legal cases (Health Information Privacy 2017).

Specific Challenges and Strategies

- **My supervisee has a hard time with process notes.** Presenting process notes can feel very exposing and be fraught with anxiety for the supervisee. As a result, a supervisee may resist engaging in this task. Although the purpose of the notes is to explore and learn, they may be viewed as an opportunity to criticize the supervisee's clinical work. In such cases, the process notes are sometimes used to justify the therapist's interventions and even to misrepresent what happened in the session. Creating a safe, accepting environment cannot be emphasized enough. Not only might issues within therapy contribute to the resistance, but unresolved issues in the supervisor-supervisee relationship can also be part of this resistance.

- **My supervisee isn't bringing in completed process notes.** Sometimes the supervisee may bring only partial notes, claiming to have not had time to write them or to have not been able to sufficiently remember the session. In these moments, it can be useful to review all the recommendations regarding writing process notes and discuss how these could be fulfilled. Transference and countertransference could be visited if bringing insufficient notes is deemed to be a manifestation of reluctance (fueled by anxiety) to bring fuller material to the supervision session similar to the patient's reluctance to reveal more of himself of herself. Insufficient process notes could also be an expression of unresolved issues between the supervisor and supervisee that the supervisor would inquire about and address.

- **The process notes are lacking in sufficient detail to make them useful for processing.** Insufficient detail can manifest as not having the notes prepared; bringing partial, incomplete, or unclear notes; or bringing notes that consist primarily of a patient's long narrative without acknowledging the therapist's interventions. As a result, the supervisor is left in the dark as to the process of the session. The supervisor might address these difficulties by wondering if the supervisee is fearful of being judged and/or found wanting. The supervisor might analyze his or her own behavior as to whether it may have contributed to this anxiety and the defense against it. On another level, these all may also be taken up as the therapist's unconscious reactions to what is going on in the patient-therapist relationship.

Questions for the Supervisee

■ Do you know the difference between process notes and progress notes?

■ What are your challenges or difficulties in writing these notes?

■ Are there any difficulties in presenting your notes in our session?

■ Does it feel safe to record and present your interventions, reactions, feelings, and associations?

■ Are you learning more, and in more depth, about the patient, yourself, and the therapeutic process by writing the process notes?

■ Would you like to change the structure of process notes to one that would feel more useful to you?

Additional Resources

American Psychological Association: DVD Relational Psychodynamic Psychotherapy Supervision. Washington, DC, American Psychological Association, 2015. Available at: http://www.apa.org/pubs/videos/4310942.aspx.

Casement P: Towards autonomy: some thoughts on psychoanalytic supervision, in Psychodynamic Supervision: Perspectives of the Supervisor and the Supervisee. Edited by Rock M. Northvale, NJ, Jason Aronson, 1997, pp 263–284

References

Epstein R, Wallerstein R: The Teaching and Learning of Psychotherapy. New York, Basic Books, 1958

Health Information Privacy: Does HIPAA provide extra protections for mental health information compared with other health information? September 21, 2017. Available at: https://www.hhs.gov/hipaa/for-professionals/faq/2088/does-hipaa-provide-extra-protections-mental-health-information-compared-other-health.html. Accessed August 7, 2018.

Rosbrow T: From parallel process to developmental process: a developmental plan/formulation approach to supervision, in Psychodynamic Supervision: Perspectives of the Supervisor and the Supervisee. Edited by Rock M. Northvale, NJ, Jason Aronson, 1997, pp 213–238

Sarnat J: Supervision Essentials for Psychodynamic Psychotherapies. Washington, DC, American Psychological Association, 2016

Chapter 7   Role-Play

Kim D. Bullock, M.D.

Use of role-play as an active learning and pedagogical technique has been reported across a wide range of disciplines and applications. Simply defined in learning environments, role-play is any practice that involves having students and teachers take on specific roles and act them out for the purpose of learning. While role-play is commonly used as a therapeutic device in psychiatry, there is little mention in the literature of its use as a tool for teaching psychiatry (King et al. 2015).

Role-play has recently been reported as being better suited for adult learners than traditional teaching methods, especially in today's fast-paced learning environments. Three learning outcome domains have evidence of efficacy when role-play pedagogy is applied: affective, cognitive, and behavioral (Rao and Stupans 2012). Although no controlled trials exist, review of the literature supports role-play as superior to other teaching methods in terms of long-term retention and ability to elicit self-reflection. In the largest extensive literature review of how medical students learn communication skills, it was concluded that passive instructional methods should not be used in communication trainings because experiential methods that involve role-play are superior and recommended for this type of learning (Aspegren 1999). Much of psychiatric supervision involves the instruction of implicit and explicit communication skills; thus, role-play techniques ought to be considered a staple teaching skill for supervisors (Baile and Blatner 2014). In this chapter, instructions on how to conduct role-plays will be provided as well as descriptions of the strengths and caveats of using this method in psychiatric learning environments.

Key Points

- Role-play in psychiatric supervision involves three steps: 1) modeling, 2) reversing roles, and 3) reflecting and correcting.

- At each step, the autonomy of the supervisee should be preserved by providing choices, orienting to the process, and asking permission to engage in role-play techniques.

- The supervisor should make sure to give specific, corrective feedback along with generous praise without relying on the supervisee or other observing group members to do this.

- Role-play enhances learning by locating and targeting specific skills deficits, enhancing trust and safety, and facilitating skills generalization.

- Role-play can have efficiencies in resource utilization, risk reduction, and compassion building.

- The supervisor should dialog with his or her teaching institution about ways to implement, support, and normalize role-play.

What Is Role-Play?

Role-play is a unique skill that can augment the more passive and necessary declarative knowledge learning a trainee receives thru lectures, didactics, and observation. Active learning is a complementary type of skills acquisition that is especially important in procedural, behavioral, cognitive, emotional, and implicit skills training (Bennett-Levy et al. 2009). Although much of medical training, from internship through residency rotations, could be argued as being experiential, this is very different than role-play. Most trainees report feeling as if they are "imposters" or pretending at some points during their training. This "trial by fire" is not considered part of role-play. Role-play takes active learning to a whole other level beyond "fake it till you make it."

When to Use Role-Play

Role-play is most useful for teaching the application of concepts, principles, and procedures into real-world interactions with patients. Examples include teaching supervisees how to validate patients and improve the therapeutic alliance, how to uncover core beliefs, and how to deliver motivational interviewing or set the structure of a session. Teaching the nuts and bolts of how to repair therapeutic alliance ruptures is another example where role-play can be incorporated. This technique also expedites teaching of operationalized procedures such as setting the agenda, refocusing on the process, or externalizing voices to name just a few. Skills can be developed for setting limits, addressing transference or therapy-interfering behaviors. Role-play also can be used to help a supervisee explore and develop different styles of interacting with patients outside his or her normal repertoire.

How to Do a Role-Play

The role-play method presented here can be broken down into three parts that can be modified for use in almost any setting (Figure 7–1). As with any procedural learning, it is recommended that supervisors watch a skilled supervisor model this method. Ironically, it may be most useful for supervisors to practice the role-play using the role-play method. Role-plays can be performed in one-on-one learning environments or in groups with multiple observers. Below is a three-step model developed for performing role-plays in a psychiatric supervision.

Step 1: Modeling

Modeling can be considered its own stand-alone technique. Modeling is best performed using the specific problem that a supervisee is asking help with. This avoids teaching unneeded areas that may not be relevant to the trainee or that have already been learned. The adult learner knows where skills deficits exist and usually is most motivated to focus on these deficits and knows exactly where these areas manifest during specific moments of therapy. The supervisor targets specific moments when a supervisee wants help and feels the need for help can be an important motivational method. Questions such as "Was there a specific moment in time during one of your recent therapy sessions where you had a question or were unsure?" may be useful. The supervisee is asked to describe the problem and provide a discrete example as it showed up in the room with the patient. Next, the supervisor provides validation and empathy about the problem itself to create an environment of emotional safety. To preserve autonomy and maximize engagement, the supervisor orients the supervisee to the modeling step and asks explicit permission to do the modeling step of the role-play method. If the supervisee is hesitant or refuses, then the supervisor explores the obstacles. If the supervisee agrees, then the supervisor proceeds to orienting and explaining the modeling process. Then, the supervisee is asked to simulate the problematic communication with the patient by playing the role of patient. The supervisor should play the role of psychiatrist with the patient. During this simulation, it may be helpful for the supervisor to take notes on exactly what is said by the supervisee playing the patient to facilitate the next step of role reversal. The simulation is concluded when the supervisor completes demonstration of the desired skill or teaching goal. After the demonstration, the supervisor checks in with the supervisee and any other observing learners about what was observed, asking questions like "What was that like?" "What did you notice?" and "What did you like and dislike in my responses to the patient?" The supervisor and supervisee then reflect on the process and skill being taught. In this conversation, the supervisor can highlight the procedures and learning points he or she wants to make. It is often a nice time to link more declarative knowledge concepts to the procedures and applications modeled. The demonstration can be repeated, or problematic spots be addressed, if more modeling is needed or requested by the supervisee.

Step 2: Role Reversal

Reversing roles so that the supervisee now plays himself or herself can be the most emotionally challenging yet effective part of role-play learning. One can talk about riding a

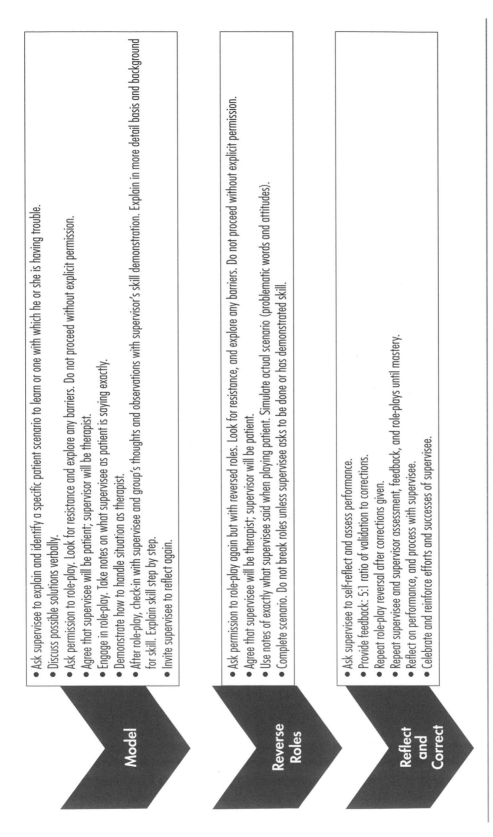

Model

- Ask supervisee to explain and identify a specific patient scenario to learn or one with which he or she is having trouble.
- Discuss possible solutions verbally.
- Ask permission to role-play. Look for resistance and explore any barriers. Do not proceed without explicit permission.
- Agree that supervisee will be patient; supervisor will be therapist.
- Engage in role-play. Take notes on what supervisee as patient is saying exactly.
- Demonstrate how to handle situation as therapist.
- After role-play, check-in with supervisee and group's thoughts and observations with supervisor's skill demonstration. Explain in more detail basis and background for skill. Explain skill step by step.
- Invite supervisee to reflect again.

Reverse Roles

- Ask permission to role-play again but with reversed roles. Look for resistance, and explore any barriers. Do not proceed without explicit permission.
- Agree that supervisee will be therapist; supervisor will be patient.
- Use notes of exactly what supervisee said when playing patient. Simulate actual scenario (problematic words and attitudes).
- Complete scenario. Do not break roles unless supervisee asks to be done or has demonstrated skill.

Reflect and Correct

- Ask supervisee to self-reflect and assess performance.
- Provide feedback: 5:1 ratio of validation to corrections.
- Repeat role-play reversal after corrections given.
- Repeat supervisee and supervisor assessment, feedback, and role-plays until mastery.
- Reflect on performance, and process with supervisee.
- Celebrate and reinforce efforts and successes of supervisee.

FIGURE 7–1.   Three easy steps to role-play.

bike—model riding a bike—but not until one rides a bike can riding a bike be learned. The role-play should again be introduced and described ahead of time and explicit permission gathered before it is performed. Often supervisees feel too unskilled to engage in this part of the role-play, and cognitive distortions need to be addressed. Motivational interviewing may be helpful by exploring the challenges of role reversal. Similarly, safety and trust must be established, especially in a group setting. Most of medical training involves avoiding or even hiding errors or deficits. Role reversal may be a radically different way of learning for a supervisee. Performance anxiety issues are expected and should be addressed. Once permission is granted for role reversal, remind the supervisee who is who and proceed using the exact scenario, words, and attitudes of the patient that were modeled by the supervisee in the previous step. At times, supervisees may be tempted to break role with laughter or feelings of doing poorly. The supervisor should try not to allow a supervisee to break role until some amount of the scenario or skill has been demonstrated. Most often supervisees are performing much better than they perceive. Being firm about not allowing a supervisee to escape the discomfort if he or she is performing well is important. If a supervisee is really stuck or overwhelmed, the supervisor can ask, "Do you want to switch roles again and I will model this?" Then supervisors can immediately return to Step 1 and perform the modeling for those areas where the supervisee is having trouble. This is an important learning efficiency in that time is spent on repetitions only where the trainee is having problems. Precise skills deficits are diagnosed and treated quickly. If return to Step 1 is necessary, the roles should be reversed as quickly as possible so that the modeling of the desired behavior is accessible and in short-term memory.

Step 3: Reflection and Correction

Once the supervisor ends the role reversal, it is important to reflect first with the supervisee and then with other observers in the room, if present. The most common mistake supervisors make when using role reversal is to rely on the group or the supervisee to provide feedback. The group and the supervisee may notice important aspects of a concept being taught but often overestimate their own insight and are not usually familiar with the specific application of the skills being introduced. The supervisor should make sure to have the last word on the feedback and correct any inaccuracies in the feedback. Highlighting the strengths that the supervisee demonstrated is in many cases useful to reinforce continuing in this often emotionally uncomfortable technique and to increase participation in further repetitions. The supervisor should emphasize the effort, willingness, and courage supervisees display in performing the role play or the skill. Often, a supervisor sharing his or her own failures while learning the skill can be extremely validating and motivating for supervisees who might perform multiple iterations of the role reversals without success before achieving a target objective. Normalizing that most supervisees do not learn skills in one practice session is important. Different supervisees will need a different number of repetitions to learn and master concepts and skills. The supervisor should acknowledge learning differences and the need to personalize learning by being persistent and "failing frequently." Modeling and role reversal can be repeated as many times as desired. These are powerful tools for creating confidence and continuing the learning process. Often role-play is the most painful but powerful of the learning techniques a trainee ever experiences. The supervisor-supervisee alliance is crucial for success given the emotional vulnerability and disclosure of weaknesses that must be tolerated.

Strengths of Role-Play

Role-play methods are active in nature and can increase the arousal and engagement of both supervisors and supervisees and improve the under-engaged learning environment. Conversely it can also help the over-aroused, over-engaged anxious supervisee or supervisor by facilitating play-based learning, fostering trust, strengthening bonding, and promoting relaxation that can help working memory and learning. A variety of reasons exists for why role-play enhances learning, as discussed below.

Precision Targeting and Treatment of Skills Deficits

What is most remarkable about role-play is the speed and efficiency at which it uncovers a supervisees' deficits. It allows a supervisor to see exactly what needs to be corrected. The supervisor can also modulate the interaction to reveal the boundaries of the skills deficits or the boundaries of the skills acquisition that need to be generalized. During modeling, the supervisee can customize and control what aspect of the problematic scenario to play up as well as target new areas of learning. For instance, if a supervisee wants to learn how to deal with erotic transference but realizes it is unlikely that this will occur in any of his or her current cases, a role-play can extend the current circumstances to target this scenario. The supervisee can be in control of what is being learned as much as the supervisor. This form of engagement is more balanced and interactive than traditional learning.

Increased Trust and Safety

Our brains are hardwired from childhood to learn through "play," and role-play is often a surprisingly natural and familiar process once implemented. Learning proceeds more effectively in a climate of trust and safety. Alliance between supervisee and supervisor is critical to learning outcomes. This sense of safety and self-disclosure of vulnerabilities in a supportive nonjudgmental and unconditionally caring way allow a process of trust building that is vital to supercharged learning experiences. The attachment process can, in itself, become a reinforcement of learning and create supervisees who are hungry and eager for supervision.

Decreased Resource Utilization

Role-play allows direct observation of a trainee's skills without the usual resource demands. The use of audio recordings or video equipment can be eliminated if needed, and role-plays are easier to set up than some other methods of supervision, such as one-way mirror observation or cotherapy with a patient. Doing role-play in groups can also be very efficient in terms of time. Modeling by a supervisor can occur just once for an entire group of supervisees. Supervisees can witness the iterative process of fellow trainees, and this can speed up the time it takes for their own learning when it is their time for reversing roles.

Risk Reduction

Role-play minimizes risk for patients, trainees, and supervisors alike. Much of learning involves making mistakes, taking risks, receiving feedback, and going through multiple trial-and-error iterations. A trial-and-error approach in the imaginary world has no consequences and avoids the devastating effects possible in the real world such as ruptures in the therapeutic relationship. Role-plays can also be used prophylactically to prevent or treat many crises in the clinical setting. Supervisors can more accurately assess skills and teach more effectively with role-play methods, thereby decreasing liability and malpractice issues attached to these type of teaching activities. Additionally, role-play allows supervisees to face their most embarrassing moments or mistakes within the confines of the role-play environment rather than at the bedside or within the therapeutic relationship.

Empathy and Compassion

Embodiment of another person in a role-play, especially as patient, allows one to reprogram implicit biases and see things from another's point of view. This forced empathy that elicits mirror neuron networks may create opportunities for supervisees to enhance critical thinking skills and problem solving by looking at the problem from a different angle as well as understand the feelings and motives of another. Empathy building can enhance the therapeutic alliance, an effect that is known to impact outcomes in a multitude of psychiatric settings. Empathy leads to compassion, which can be helpful for modulating emotions elicited in countertransference and throughout treatment. Thus, role-play methods may also have the unintended but positive side effect of increasing the therapeutic alliance and addressing transference issues via increasing empathy and compassion.

Specific Challenges and Strategies

- **My supervisee appears to be very weak in the skill I'm teaching and seems overwhelmed by the role-play.** Role-play can be counterproductive for supervisees who have weak skills or are unprepared or for those suffering with anxiety or mood problems, as well as burnout. Be sure to orient and provide necessary knowledge and modeling prior to asking a supervisee to engage in role-play. If a supervisee feels overly embarrassed and emotionally overwhelmed, this can lead to poor performance, loss of confidence, giving up, and avoidance on an entire skill set. Assess the readiness for a supervisee to embark on role-play and continue to assess the emotional well-being of a supervisee throughout the technique and adjust accordingly.

- **My supervisee is self-disclosing personal problems and asking for help during role-play.** Sometimes supervisees' own psychological issues may get blurred into the supervision that centers on personal communication and beliefs. The perception of a dual role as supervisor and therapist can easily be misinterpreted by a supervisee. It is important for the supervisee and the supervisor to acknowledge and agree that the supervision is not a therapeutic relationship. When "pretend" activities become emotionally flooding, the line can start to disappear, putting participants at risk because of emotional stress and putting the trainer and the organization at risk due to liability issues. Be aware of the limits of your role-play in terms of helping a supervisee with psychological issues.

- **Is my usual hour per week for supervision enough time to include role-play techniques?** The amount of time necessary for a supervisor to deliver and prepare for role-play can be enormous for complex skills training delivery. Mastery of both the skill and the pedagogical technique is necessary. Be confident in the skills and method being taught and have adequate time to deliver. It is recommended that this type of teaching not be scheduled for any less than 60 minutes for a single role-play. The more time available the better. The brief "role-plays" (2–5 minutes) often done during supervision are considered a form of modeling.

- **What if my colleagues aren't supporting role-play techniques?** Introducing the technique of role-play as a common practice in the field of active psychiatric training requires institutional prerequisites; the educational institution must be supportive of this pedagogical approach like other forms of supervision. Otherwise, role-play may be perceived as a pedagogical method that is only entertaining and engaging and represents an odd and uncommon style of teaching. This may be challenging if the culture of supervision is such that role-play has not been implemented in the program or training in this methodology has not been made available. Therefore, continuous collective dialogue at the organizational and institutional level is highly recommended.

Questions for the Supervisee

- Do you have any experience in doing role-plays in supervision? If so, what was your experience like? If not, do you have any concerns about using this technique?

- Was there a specific moment in time during one of your recent therapy sessions where you had a question or were unsure, and would benefit from doing a role-play?

- What did you like least and best about the role-play process in supervision?

- What grade would you give yourself on the role-play? What did you do well, and where do you need to improve?

Additional Resources

Allen D: Role play in training for clinical psychology practice: investing to increase educational outcomes. Clinical Psychology Supervision Observation Report, 2006. Available at: https://www.scribd.com/document/64316786/Role-Play-in-Training-for-Clinical-Psychology-Practice-Investing-to-Increase-Educative-Outcomes. Accessed August 7, 2018.

References

Aspegren K: BEME Guide No. 2: Teaching and learning communication skills in medicine-a review with quality grading of articles. Med Teach 21(6):563–570, 1999 21281175

Baile WF, Blatner A: Teaching communication skills: using action methods to enhance role-play in problem-based learning. Simul Healthc 9(4):220–227, 2014 24614796

Bennett-Levy J, McManus F, Westling BE, et al: Acquiring and refining CBT skills and competencies: which training methods are perceived to be most effective? Behav Cogn Psychother 37(5):571–583, 2009 19703329

King J, Hill K, Gleason A: All the world's a stage: evaluating psychiatry role-play based learning for medical students. Australas Psychiatry 23(1):76–79, 2015 25512966

Rao D, Stupans I: Exploring the potential of role play in higher education: development of a typology and teacher guidelines. Innov Educ Teach Int 49(4):427–436, 2012

Chapter 8

Modeling, Rehearsal, and Feedback

A Simple Approach to Teaching Complex Skills

Joanna Jarecki, M.D.

Susan McNair, M.D.

Jennifer Ruzhynsky, M.D., M.A.

Priyanthy Weerasekera, M.D., M.Ed.

Psychiatry residents need to develop competence in interviewing skills, negotiating goals, assessing risk, forming therapeutic alliances, conducting several psychotherapies, and managing agitation or aggression with de-escalation techniques. These are all sophisticated skills that cannot be learned simply through reading or accumulating theoretical knowledge. *Modeling–rehearsal (practice)–feedback* (Figure 8–1) has been demonstrated to be the key method for learning skills (Peters et al. 1978). It is important that this method be situated for the learner within a context. In this chapter, we present a discussion of modeling-rehearsal and feedback from a practical perspective so that the clinical supervisor can incorporate these techniques in supervision.

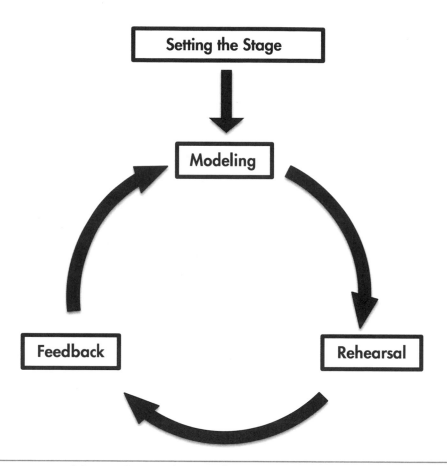

FIGURE 8–1. Modeling–rehearsal (practice)–feedback.

Key Points

- Set the stage for learning by providing a meaningful context and setting specific learning goals.

- Remember that modeling is an essential first step in teaching a complex skill. It provides the learner with a visual demonstration of the key ingredients of the skill.

- Model skills a) directly with patients b) indirectly through role-playing, or c) through the use of technology (audio, video, or online resources).

- Give the learner the opportunity to rehearse each skill repeatedly.

- Observe rehearsal (directly or with the use of audio/video technology) for valid assessment of learner's competence.

- Provide feedback in a safe and respectful environment. This supports the intended goal of learning rather than evaluation.

- Make feedback specific, goal directed, constructive, and timely. Provide it regularly to support ongoing optimal learning.

Providing Context

Providing the context for what will be observed or practiced, as well as discussing goals, is important for skill development. The supervisor should provide a rationale to the supervisee as to why learning the skill is important. It is important to specify the situations in which the skill is to be used, describe how it can be modified, and emphasize that learning the skill will take time. Supervisors can ensure adequate instruction by making time for a brief discussion with the trainee before any modeling or rehearsal experience occurs.

Modeling

Modeling is essential in the initial conceptualization of any skill. A supervisor can model (or demonstrate) specific skills with a patient or through a role-play. If live modeling is limited, supervisors can consider the use of technology such as audio or video recordings and online websites. Various videos exist on video-sharing sites such as YouTube and Vimeo. Supervisors should watch these videos first to ensure that students are receiving good-quality modeling (see "Additional Resources" later in this chapter).

Modeling provides the learner with a visual demonstration of the key ingredients essential in a specific skill. Systematic modeling breaks down the necessary components of a complicated set of skills so that they can be learned separately and, later, integrated into complex behavioral chains (Rosenbaum et al. 2001). Although rarely presented to learners, modeling is one of the simplest aspects of the cycle to implement. Trainees should be encouraged to observe their supervisors perform the specific skills that they need to learn. Such observation should be made on several occasions, as repetition is a central part of learning (Ericsson et al. 1993). When possible, the supervisor should allow the trainee to watch more than one expert person performing the skill.

After modeling, the supervisor should make time to debrief with the trainee to address the supervisee's observations and questions.

Rehearsal

In rehearsal the learner practices the specific skill. Without practice (and feedback), learning does not occur (Mazor et al. 2011). Repeated practice with feedback leads to the development of competence, mastery, and expertise. It is therefore essential that in training, opportunities exist for both deliberate practice with feedback, and graduated independent practice. The latter is essential for the development of confidence and a sense of autonomy.

The Accreditation Council for Graduate Medical Education emphasizes direct observation of residents performing skills and considers this essential for the reliable and valid assessment of resident competence (Jardine et al. 2017). Trainee performance of skills in psychiatry (e.g., interviewing, forming an alliance) cannot be inferred from a case presentation. Whenever possible, rehearsal should be directly observed either live in the room or through a one-way mirror; if this is not possible, trainees can record their rehearsal using video- or audio-recording equipment, with patient consent. Patients are generally happy to give consent for this, knowing that the purpose of the recording is to improve the trainee's skills.

Feedback

Feedback is essential to learning (Mazor et al. 2011). When providing feedback, the supervisor discusses his or her observations regarding the learner's performance in rehearsal and provides suggestions for further development of the skill. Research demonstrates several essential methods for giving effective feedback.

1. Establish a respectful environment before feedback begins (Ramani and Krackov 2012). The supervisor should communicate clearly that the purpose of feedback in this context is primarily to improve performance, rather than to evaluate or judge.
2. Make feedback specific and goal directed (Peters et al. 1978). It should be based on *direct observation* and reinforce or correct observed behaviors (Ramani and Krackov 2012). A global statement about performance, such as "That was great!," is less useful than noting a specific point of competence or excellence and providing a rationale for why it was successful. For example: "When the patient spoke about feeling fearful in her home, you nicely explored whether there are specific individuals she is fearful of, and whether she is planning or has gone to any means to protect herself. You collected all of the information necessary for the risk assessment, but in a gentle and empathic manner that maintained rapport and connected the questions to the patient's concerns. This was skillfully done." Similarly, it is important to provide constructive feedback with specific suggestions for how the learner can improve their skills instead of stating, "That was a poor interview." For example:

   > When you asked the patient how he felt about his wife's death, he replied by saying "Fine," yet his affect immediately shifted and became depressed and tearful. Instead of taking the content of his response at face value, it may have been helpful to gently note and explore this change in affect, as well as the discrepancy between the two aspects of his response. For example, you could have said, "I hear you say 'Fine,' but I hear the sadness in your voice, and I can see the tears in your eyes."

3. Maintain a balance between positive and corrective feedback, because too much of one or the other can undermine the effectiveness of the feedback itself (Jardine et al. 2017).
4. Provide feedback in a timely and regular manner. Supervisors should attempt to devote adequate time to feedback as close to the rehearsal as possible (Ramani and Krackov 2012). Research also demonstrates an inverted U-curve relationship between feedback frequency and performance, with very low and very high feedback frequency leading to poor performance (Lam et al. 2011). Therefore, it is essential that feedback be given at a moderate frequency to ensure an optimal level of performance. Once feedback has been given, it is important to allow time for the learner's reaction and reflection to the feedback (Jardine et al. 2017).
5. Develop an action plan regarding how the learner will use this feedback (Jardine et al. 2017). Feedback is most effective if it is actively incorporated to inform ongoing learning and development.

In addition to direct feedback between supervisor and learner, trainees can also learn from one another's skills development and benefit from observing peers rehearsing and receiving corrective feedback. This increases learning and suggests an advantage for group supervision (Rohbanfard and Proteau 2011).

Training proceeds through further iterations of parts or all of this sequence as needed. Gradually learners will demonstrate increasing levels of skill and competence in more complex situations, with a decreased need for involvement and feedback from their supervisor.

Specific Challenges and Strategies

- **I don't have time to use the model-rehearsalfeedback approach.** Although this model may seem simple, time constraints and the need for service often interfere with the implementation (Hauer et al. 2011). Supervisors often do not feel that they have sufficient time to allow residents to observe their skills, to complete an entire observed interview, or to provide specific feedback on everything that they observed in a skills rehearsal session. As a result, learners have few opportunities for observed practice; in most cases they function independently, even at junior levels of training (Hauer et al. 2011). Instead of focusing on an entire assessment interview as one "skill," consider breaking down the skill into component parts, each of which may be a focus for a briefer and more concentrated cycle of modeling, rehearsal, and feedback. Rather than an entire interview or patient encounter, focus on specific components of an interview for observation and feedback, such as opening the interview, risk assessment, trauma history taking, and depression screen.
- **I don't know if I feel confident about using the model-rehearsal-feedback approach; I was never taught how to do this during *my* training.** Supervisors may feel uncomfortable with having learners observe their skills. Many supervisors would not have had the opportunity to observe experts when they were training, or to have had their own skills observed by supervisors with feedback, and so this can be an unfamiliar process. Modeling-rehearsal-feedback is a skill set that ideally needs to be modeled and rehearsed for supervisors, and feedback needs to be received. Supervisors themselves can model learning from experience and demonstrate a willingness to reflect on their own practice. Supervisors can receive feedback on their teaching skills by pursuing continuing education or having other supervisors/educators observe their teaching. Feedback from *learners* regarding the supervision process is also important and should be solicited to inform continuing development of supervision skills.

Questions for the Supervisor

- ■ Have I worked out skills-focused goals for learning with the trainee?

- ■ Have I broken down the skills into component parts?

- ■ Have I set adequate time for learner skills development?

■   Have I modeled these skills for the trainee?

■   Have I observed the trainee rehearsing the skill?

■   Have I provided specific constructive feedback regarding the skill?

Additional Resources

Use of Videos

Dong C, Goh PS: Twelve tips for the effective use of videos in medical education. Medical Teacher 37:140–145, 2015

Online Resources in Medical Education

American Psychological Association: APA PsycNET Streaming Videos. Available at: http://www.apa.org/pubs/databases/streaming-video/index.aspx.

Beck Institute: Online training. Available at: https://beckinstitute.org/get-training/online-training.

Psychotherapy Training e-Resources (PTeR): https://pter.mcmaster.ca.

Weerasekera P: Psychotherapy Training e-Resources (PTeR): on-line psychotherapy education. Acad Psychiatry 37(1):51–54, 2013 23338876

References

Ericsson K, Krampe RT, Tesch-Romer C: The role of deliberate practice in the acquisition of expert performance. Psychol Rev 100:363–406, 1993

Hauer KE, Holmboe ES, Kogan JR: Twelve tips for implementing tools for direct observation of medical trainees' clinical skills during patient encounters. Med Teach 33(1):27–33, 2011 20874011

Jardine D, Deslauriers J, Kamran SC, et al: Milestones guidebook for residents and fellows. ACGME, 2017. Available at: https://www.acgme.org/Portals/0/PDFs/Milestones/MilestonesGuidebookforResidentsFellows.pdf. Accessed August 16, 2018.

Lam CF, DeRue DS, Karam EP, et al: The impact of feedback frequency on learning and task performance: challenging the "more is better" assumption. Organ Behav Hum Decis Process 116:217–228, 2011

Mazor KM, Holtman MC, Shchukin Y, et al: The relationship between direct observation, knowledge, and feedback: results of a national survey. Acad Med 86(10)(Suppl):S63–S67, quiz S68, 2011 21955772

Peters GA, Cormier LS, Cormier WH: Effects of modeling, rehearsal, feedback, and remediation on acquisition of a counseling strategy. J Couns Psychol 25:231–237, 1978

Ramani S, Krackov SK: Twelve tips for giving feedback effectively in the clinical environment. Med Teach 34(10):787–791, 2012 22730899

Rohbanfard H, Proteau L: Learning through observation: a combination of expert and novice models favors learning. Exp Brain Res 215(3–4):183–197, 2011 21986667

Rosenbaum DA, Carlson RA, Gilmore RO: Acquisition of intellectual and perceptual-motor skills. Annu Rev Psychol 52:453–470, 2001 11148313

Chapter 9   Video Recordings

Learning Through Facilitated Observation and Feedback

Sallie G. De Golia, M.D., M.P.H.

Video-based observation offers an ideal method for teaching, evaluating, and providing feedback to supervisees whether in a clinical or a nonclinical (e.g., teaching) setting. Its advantages and limitations have been well described throughout the literature (Abbass 2004; Betcher and Zinberg 1988; Benschoter et al. 1965; Chodoff 1972; Goldberg 1983). However, few supervisors have been formally educated on how to use video recordings in supervision, a particularly important format given the era of competency-based supervision in which observing performance is critical for assessing competence as well as providing effective and accurate feedback to supervisees (Accreditation Council for Graduate Medical Education 2018; Falender and Shafranske 2007).

In this chapter, I focus predominately on video use within individual and group clinical supervision; however, video can also be effectively utilized in supervising teaching or leadership skills or in any venue where a supervisor and/or supervisee would like to observe performance directly or a supervisor wants to provide specific feedback when live observation is not possible.

Key Points

- Ensure institutional commitment through resources, administrative and supervisor support, and clear guidelines.

- Prepare supervisee and/or supervision group on process.

- Support reactions to being taped.

- Debrief through using the play-pause-discuss method in a sensitive and supportive manner.

- Encourage self/group reflection about the process and learning experience.

- Facilitate identifying and implementation of new/modified behaviors.

- Address system barriers.

Purpose for Using Video

Teaching

Video use in supervision can be an effective teaching and oversight tool. Given that learning is more effective when it occurs in the context of the actual activity (Godden and Baddeley 1975), reviewing one's direct performance by video recording presents an excellent educational modality for teaching and providing feedback. The process helps supervisees develop observational, assessment, and analytic capacities. It allows the supervisor to focus on complex concepts, skills, and/or attitudes and break them down into smaller steps for the supervisee.

When used in the context of peer or group supervision, the process can lead to a culture of supportive and collaborative learning. By sharing work, supervisees not only learn from their own mistakes but are able to observe and analyze peer's styles and techniques in practice. The process also models continuous learning, especially if the supervisor shares his or her own videos. In the context of peer supervision, supervisees develop skills in facilitation of video-recording review, are able to practice providing feedback to peers, and learn to receive meaningful feedback.

Furthermore, video recording allows for more accurate oversight. Often the supervisor is not required to meet with a supervisee and his or her psychotherapy patient within the context of residency training. Video recording enables the supervisor to actually see what is happening within a treatment session without reliance on imperfect recall.

Support Tool

In the context of group supervision, supervisees learn from one another and can receive support from peers and supervisors after a particularly challenging encounter. This allows learners to feel less alone and more competent and/or secure. Also, the experience may lead to increased empathy on the part of supervisees toward their patients as the supervisees address their own vulnerability of being "seen" by supervisors, not unlike a patient's experience within therapy (Funkenstein et al. 2014).

Evaluation

Video observation is a way in which to directly observe a supervisee's performance. This may reduce any supervisor bias and/or allow for more accurate performance assessment by reducing supervisee distortion from recall and/or interpretation, as well as allow for visualizing nonverbal signals. In the context of group supervision, everyone is able to observe the same behaviors, which reduces subjectivity.

Feedback

By directly observing performance in action, the supervisor can provide meaningful and specific feedback to a supervisee within the context of a comfortable and supportive space, free from patient pressures or work demands. The feedback is more accurate because it is based on observed performance, not just recall from the supervisee.

Video feedback has been demonstrated to have an impact on learner behavior (Beckman and Frankel 1994; Chou and Lee 2002; Edwards et al. 1996; Huhra et al. 2008; Maguire et al. 1986), as well as patient outcomes (Diener et al. 2007), to enhance supervisee insight (Alpert 1996; Falzone et al. 2005), and to be superior to verbal feedback in teaching clinical skills (Ozcakar et al. 2009). Furthermore, in one implementation report, supervisees were also less likely to disagree with assessments when the assessments were conducted through video observation, reported significant change in their behaviors, and perceived their supervisors as more supportive and fairer when the assessment was based on observations (Kane et al. 2015).

Institutional Support

For video recording to be meaningful, the program and institution need to actively commit and support the video-recording process. Without it, the program will be at risk of failure. Investment in technology, encrypted safeguards, ongoing technical support, supervisor and supervisee training, and ongoing administrative monitoring must all be established and maintained. Various articles have explored the development and maintenance of the logistical aspects of video recording (Harvard University, Center for Education Policy Research 2015; Muench et al. 2013; Rousmaniere and Renfro-Michel 2016).

Before engaging in video supervision, programs must develop procedures for consenting patients, Health Insurance Portability and Accountability Act (HIPAA)–approved transfer of and access to the recordings, video storage, data destruction, and guidelines for loss or breach of video-recorded material. Despite U.S. Department of Health and Human Services guidance for securing protected health information (such information needs to be encrypted using valid encryption processes), professional organizations have not yet established formal policies, recommendations, or standardized practice guidelines for storing video-recorded material. Only individual program guidelines exist (Funkenstein et al. 2014).

Preparation for Video Use

Supervisees

Supervisees, particularly novices, tend to feel anxious and vulnerable about being video recorded. Supervisors—or in the case of trainees, the training program—should help supervisees understand the benefits of video recording, not only for the supervisee but, if appropriate, for the patient. The program might schedule training times when supervisees can practice setting up video equipment before seeing a patient. The supervisee should be informed about how to trouble-shoot technical problems and whom to call if problems arise. Once the supervisee is comfortable with the equipment, the supervisor or program staff should carefully review guidelines on who has access to video recordings and how the recordings will be used, stored, and/or destroyed. In the case of clinical supervision, protecting patient safety and confidentiality should be a fundamental concern.

Next, within the clinical setting, the patient consent procedure should be reviewed. Basic principles include seeking permission to record and disclose information to a supervisor, informing about the purpose including the pros and cons for taping without pressuring the patient, informing the patient that he or she may request that the recording (or consent) be stopped at any time without consequences to treatment, and disclosing the secure storage and elimination procedure. If the supervisee intends to use the tape beyond the originally consented scope (e.g., for teaching purposes), additional consent will be necessary. In the case of a nonclinical setting, it should be determined who, if anyone, needs to be consented. It may be possible to video record the supervisee without involvement of others; however, if images or voices of others are captured on tape, it is best to consent the participants.

The supervisor should consider role-playing the consent process to develop this competency and hopefully reduce reluctance to consent before having the supervisee perform it "live." Supervisees should understand that by video recording routinely, they (and their patients) will become accustomed to the process and feel less self-conscious.

Supervisor

The supervisor needs to be informed of the benefits of using video and how to securely access the videos (a significant benefit to off-site supervisors). Expectations for videotaping, including whether it will be required or recommended within supervision and how it will be monitored, should be reviewed. Supervisors should also be trained on how to use videos in teaching and supervision as well as any associated evaluation form.

Strategies for Using Video

Several strategies can be used to enhance the use of videotaping in supervision. Typically, a supervisee selects a portion of a tape to be reviewed. Supervisors may choose to review a tape on their own time and provide feedback during the supervision session and/or written feedback, or they may review the tape during the session with the supervisee. If reviewing an entire tape, they may also review the tape prior to the session and select parts of the tape to review more carefully with the supervisee. Thoughtful attention to the approach and process in which video recordings are incorporated into supervision is important to the successful use and impact of this teaching method.

The steps discussed below (and shown in Figure 9–1) describe an approach to group supervision, but the same concepts apply to individual supervision as well.

Step 1: Establish a Supportive Learning Climate

As in any supervisory experience, a safe and comfortable working alliance will allow for more self-discovery and deeper learning and will help create a place where learners can take more risks. Particularly situations in which one's work will be viewed and shared directly, supervisees tend to feel anxious, exposed, and apprehensive about the situation, particularly if peers are involved. The environment must feel safe for sharing.

Step 2: Prepare the Group

The entire process of viewing a supervisee's video clip and debriefing session should be intentional and structured. Discuss the purpose of viewing videos in the context of supervision: to support supervisee learning and development. Reassure the supervisee that the goal is not to judge the supervisee's work but rather to foster self-reflection and improvement.

Before determining who will present a tape, set ground rules for the process. Review who will be seeing the tape, who will be facilitating the session, and how the tape will be utilized within the supervisory session. Assuming that the tape is used for teaching purposes, ensure that the tape will be used not for summative but rather for formative evaluation. The goal is to promote growth and learning. Remind the supervisee that all tapes should be destroyed following supervision use, unless the program has other purposes consistent with consents for storage. Also review how to give appropriate feedback with the goal of improving performance (see Chapter 1, "Elements of Supervision"). Be prepared to manage the "culture of nice" that can develop in a peer setting where supervisees avoid giving corrective feedback for fear of hurting their colleague's feelings. The usefulness of this kind of feedback is often limited.

The supervisor's role is that of a facilitator. The supervisor serves to guide supervisees in viewing their work, helping them reflect on what they hoped would happen, what they observe, potential reasons for any discrepancy, and brainstorming alternative strategies. In a collaborative manner, the supervisor helps identify areas of growth. By effectively performing this role, the supervisor models how to review one's own work, provide feedback and facilitate a process among peers.

Ask the supervisee to select a video clip of his or her choosing. This can be any 10-minute clip a supervisee felt he or she performed well in, demonstrated a new skill, felt challenged or stuck, experienced an alliance rupture, or identified as a good teaching segment, perhaps reflecting a concept described in a recent didactic. This approach helps the supervisee think critically and what he or she hopes to learn from the supervision session. Allowing supervisees to select their own clip also increases perceptions of fairness in an observation (Kane et al. 2015) and enhances agency for their own learning process. Even if supervisees tend to select their perceived "best work," there will be enough content to provide both positive and corrective feedback (Kane et al. 2015). Have supervisees identify a question they may have regarding the selected clip. For example, "What did I miss?" "How could I have deepened the rapport?" "Why did the patient respond in a

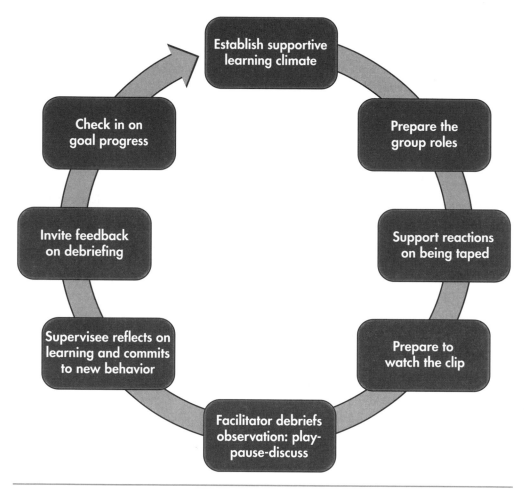

FIGURE 9–1.   Key steps in supervision of video recording.

given way?" "Why do I feel so frustrated here?" "How do I respond to the patient's emotion?" "How does this segment relate to the formulation of the case?"

Instruct peer observers to observe the video but to allow the supervisee to take the lead.

Step 3: Support Reactions on Being Taped

Before reviewing the clip, ask about how the supervisee felt about being recorded and watching the clip (if this occurred). This will help diffuse some of the anxiety associated with the video recording process and access to their work. Once this has been done a few times with the same supervisee, you may not need to spend much time on this process.

Step 4: Prepare to Watch the Clip

Ask the supervisee to give some background before showing the 10-minute clip, including a brief review of the case formulation, the nature of the particular session, the supervisee's intended goals in the clip, and how you (and the peer group) could be helpful to the supervisee.

Now have the group watch the clip. Make sure to preset the video to the selected clip so delays are avoided. Inform the supervisee and the other observers that they can pause the video at any point. Consider letting the supervisee control the remote; this allows the supervisee to exercise some control over a process in which he or she may feel very vulnerable, at least initially.

Step 5: Debriefing: Play-Pause-Discuss

The key to this process is to let the supervisee discover what he or she did well in the segment and what may have been suboptimal or a missed opportunity. It is less effective to tell supervisees what they should or should not have done.

Always allow the supervisee to describe what he or she observed on the video in a descriptive manner without interpretation before others participate. This allows the supervisee to feel more comfortable and in control. Stay close to the data on the video clip as well as connected to the supervisee's goals. Invite peer observers to also describe the data without interpretation. This approach helps develop the supervisee's observation skills. In addition, it provides you with important information about the observation skills of the other supervisees.

The segment may involve multiple goals. Ask the supervisee what the intended goal(s) was in the segment and whether he or she felt it was attained. You might ask questions like "Did the intervention have the intended impact? If not, what went awry?" "Tell me about your decision to…" "What were you thinking at a given moment?" "How did that match up to what you had anticipated?" "When you said 'x,' what did you mean?" "How do you think that went?" Furthermore, allow the supervisee to brainstorm alternative approaches to achieve the intended goal. In a group setting, open the discussion to the other observers trying to keep the discussion close to the supervisee's question or goal at hand. Repeat this process by using the play-pause-discuss method throughout the selected segment. Monitor the number of critical comments made so as not to overwhelm the supervisee, and restrict the feedback to the supervisee's goals identified for the segment.

At the end of the clip, consider asking the supervisee to reflect on what he or she learned from reviewing the video clip. If time permits, consider asking each observer to reflect on the presented clip. What came to mind for each person? Following the observers' comments, allow the supervisee, whose clip has been shown to respond to the thoughts and questions of colleagues.

If a supervisee shows a segment as an example of a teaching point, ask the supervisee to explain his or her understanding of a given concept. Show the segment that the supervisee believes demonstrates the concept. Then consider asking the supervisee if there are aspects that diverge from the concept and, if so, how and why: "Are there aspects about the concept that are not adequately portrayed or remain confusing?" Invite the group to join the discussion. Allow the supervisee to field questions and articulate his or her understanding.

Step 6: Reflect on Learning and Commit to New Behavior

Complete the debrief by asking the supervisee to reflect on what he or she learned from the discussion. If time permits, open this process to all observers, because each one may have learned something different. On the basis of what was learned, ask the supervisee to commit to trying a new or modified behavior during the next session based on what was learned during the observation and debriefing session. The supervisee will report back on this commitment at the start of the next session.

Step 7: Ask for Session Feedback

Finally, ask the supervisee for feedback regarding the review session. This will provide you and the observers important information on how to proceed in future reviews. After the session, it is advised to keep notes on what was discussed and the new supervisee goal(s) in order to remind yourself at the start of the next session.

Step 8: Review Progress on Goals

At the subsequent session, if the supervisee has already undergone video review, ask if he or she made any progress on goals identified at an earlier review session.

Barriers to Video Recording

Barriers to incorporating videotaping into supervision include a lack of institutional support through funding, administrative support, or other resources; unclear administrative and supervision procedures; lack of supervisor encouragement (or requirement) to using video recording; and lack of supervisor/supervisee training on how to consent, use equipment, and facilitate video use and debrief (Edwards et al. 1996). Poor technical service response to difficulties, including uploading problems, sound quality, or other obstacles, may be enough to discourage trainees or supervisors from utilizing this teaching method. Supervisors may not value video use because of their clinical or supervision orientation, perceived time requirements, security issues, or because they do not want to learn a new teaching method. Finally, supervisee anxiety and vulnerability in the face of supervisors and/or peers may lead to reluctance in obtaining consent from a patient and failure to record or bring videos to supervision. This resistance may also be due to feeling inadequate about the consent process and uncomfortable with the specific patient (e.g., paranoid, overly anxious). It is important to proactively address barriers. Maintaining a supportive, nonjudgmental, and learner-centered environment can help supervisees feel more comfortable with the process. Supporting faculty through addressing their concerns and needs regarding the process is also important. Finally, a supervisor's reluctance or inability to allow the supervisee to guide the process and keep it learner-centered will impede an otherwise meaningful and potentially transformative learning experience.

Specific Challenges and Strategies

- **My supervisee never has a video ready for review.** Explore with the supervisee what he or she thinks might be the reason for not having a video. Perhaps the supervisee has an overly anxious or paranoid patient who reluctantly consented to be recorded but puts up resistance each time the supervisee tries to record their interaction. Recording may not be appropriate for this patient. On the other hand, it may be that the supervisee feels very uncomfortable about recording for fear of exposure of perceived incompetence. Most supervisees feel somewhat uncomfortable about recording—even the most senior supervisors who record their sessions. Try to process their discomfort with them and remind them of the value of recording. Whether it is a reluctant patient or supervisee, you might suggest starting by using only audio recording, or video recording without having the patient or supervisee captured in the image. As patient and supervisee feel more comfortable, slowly work toward including their image within the recording. Also, assess the supervisory learning climate and alliance (see Chapter 1). Is it a safe environment in which supervisees can safely express limitations and be vulnerable?

- **My supervisee broke into tears during the play-pause-discussion section.** Take a deep breath. Allow the supervisee some space, then check-in gently. Ask the supervisee what may have just happened. Was he or she responding to a comment? Anxious about what was seen on the tape? Feeling vulnerable? Did the clip bring up some unresolved feelings within the supervisee? The supervisor should reflect on the quality of the discussion. Was there too much corrective feedback? Too much feedback? Were the comments intrusive? Was there not enough validation and support? Encourage the supervisee to express his or her feelings and what may have triggered them and validate, validate, validate. A recorded supervisee is in a very vulnerable position—particularly if the supervision session is within a group of peers. Carefully support the supervisee through the process, but do not avoid giving corrective feedback as necessary, within reason. Limit the amount of feedback offered. Remind the supervisee that the goal of video recording is for supervisee improvement and growth.

- **The supervisor doesn't believe in videotaping.** Some supervisors will not want to engage in video recording with their supervisee. Make sure the program has provided appropriate orientation to the video recording program to ensure the supervisor understands the purpose and benefits of taping. If the supervisor still resists, and the program requires or strongly encourages video recording as a mode of teaching, resistant supervisors may need to be replaced with those who are willing to video record. Perhaps the resistant supervisors could be moved into supervision environments where video recording is not used or required.

Questions for the Supervisee

- What would you like help on in this segment?

- What did you find most challenging in this video segment?

- Was there anything that confused you in this segment?

- What did you feel you came away with from this discussion?

Additional Resources

Best Foot Forward: A tool-kit for fast forwarding classroom observations using video. Best Foot Forward Project. Center for Education Policy Research, Harvard University. Available at: https://cepr.harvard.edu/video-observation-toolkitAccessed. Accessed August 7, 2018.

Rousmaniere T, Renfro-Michel E: Using Technology to Enhance Clinical Supervision. Alexandria, VA, American Counseling Association, 2016

Consent Process

Funkenstein A, Kessler K, Schen C: Learning through the lens: ethical considerations in videotaping psychotherapy. Harv Rev Psychiatry 22(5):316–322, 2014

Review Process

Kane TJ, Gehlbach H, Greenberg M, et al: The Best Foot Forward Project: substituting teacher-collected video for in-person classroom observations: first-year implementation report. Center for Education Policy Research, Harvard University. Available at: http://cepr.harvard.edu/files/cepr/files/l4a_best_foot_forward_research_brief1.pdf. Accessed on August 7, 2018.

Steinert Y: Twelve tips for using videotape reviews for feedback on clinical performance. Medical Teacher 15(2/3):131–139, 1993

References

Abbass A: Small-group videotape training for psychotherapy skills development. Acad Psychiatry 28(2):151–155, 2004 15298869

Accreditation Council for Graduate Medical Education: The Psychiatry Milestone Project. 2018. Available at: www.acgme.org/Portals/0/PDFs/Milestones/PsychiatryMilestones.pdf?ver=2015-11-06-120520-753. Accessed on March 17, 2018.

Alpert MC: Videotaping psychotherapy. J Psychother Pract Res 5(2):93–105, 1996 22700270

Beckman HB, Frankel RM: The use of videotape in internal medicine training. J Gen Intern Med 9(9):517–521, 1994 7996296

Benschoter RA, Eaton MT, Smith P: Use of videotape to provide individual instruction in techniques of psychotherapy. J Med Educ 40(12):1159–1161, 1965 5839291

Betcher RW, Zinberg NE: Supervision and privacy in psychotherapy training. Am J Psychiatry 145(7):796–803, 1988 2454590

Chodoff P: Supervision of psychotherapy with videotape: pros and cons. Am J Psychiatry 128(7):810–823, 1972 5009256

Chou C, Lee K: Improving residents' interviewing skills by group videotape review. Acad Med 77(7):744, 2002 12114164

Diener MJ, Hilsenroth MJ, Weinberger J: Therapist affect focus and patient outcomes in psychodynamic psychotherapy: a meta-analysis. Am J Psychiatry 164(6):936–941, 2007 17541054

Edwards A, Tzelepis A, Klingbeil C, et al: Fifteen years of a videotape review program for internal medicine and medicine-pediatrics residents. Acad Med 71(7):744–748, 1996 9158342

Falender CA, Shafranske EP: Competence in competency-based supervision practice: construct and application. Prof Psychol Res Pr 38:232–240, 2007

Falzone RL, Hall S, Beresin EV: How and why for the camera-shy: using digital video in psychiatry. Child Adolesc Psychiatr Clin N Am 14(3):603–612, xi, 2005 15936676

Funkenstein AB, Kessler KA, Schen CR: Learning through the lens: ethical considerations in videotaping psychotherapy. Harv Rev Psychiatry 22(5):316–322, 2014 25188735

Godden DR, Baddeley AD: Context dependent memory in two natural environments: on land and under water. Br J Psychol 66:325–331, 1975

Goldberg DA: Resistance to the use of video in individual psychotherapy training. Am J Psychiatry 140(9):1172–1176, 1983 6614223

Harvard University, Center for Education Policy Research: Best Foot Forward: a tool-kit for fast forwarding classroom observations using video. Best Foot Forward Project, 2015. Available at: https://cepr.harvard.edu/video-observation-toolkit. Accessed on August 7, 2018.

Huhra RL, Yamokoski-Maynhart CA, Prieto LR: Reviewing videotape in supervision: a developmental approach. J Couns Dev 86(4):412–418, 2008

Kane TJ, Gehlbach H, Greenberg M, et al: The Best Foot Forward Project: Substituting teacher-collected video for in-person classroom observations: first year implementation report. Center for Education Policy Research, Harvard University, 2015. Available at: http://cepr.harvard.edu/files/cepr/files/l4a_best_foot_forward_research_brief1.pdf. Accessed August 7, 2018.

Maguire P, Fairbairn S, Fletcher C: Consultation skills of young doctors: I—Benefits of feedback training in interviewing as students persist. Br Med J (Clin Res Ed) 292(6535):1573–1576, 1986 3719282

Muench J, Sanchez D, Garvin R: A review of video review: new processes for the 21st century. Int J Psychiatry Med 45(4):413–422, 2013 24261274

Ozcakar N, Mevsim V, Guldal D, et al: Is the use of videotape recording superior to verbal feedback alone in the teaching of clinical skills? BMC Public Health 9:474–478, 2009 20021688

Rousmaniere T, Renfro-Michel E: Appendix C: recommendations for video recording counseling sessions, in Using Technology to Enhance Clinical Supervision. Alexandria, VA, American Counseling Association, 2016, pp 281–283

Chapter 10

Deliberate Practice for Clinical Supervision and Training

Tony Rousmaniere, Psy.D.

Deliberate practice is a term introduced by K. Anders Ericsson and colleagues in the science of expertise (Ericsson et al. 1993). Defined as "the individualized training activities specially designed by a supervisor or teacher to improve specific aspects of an individual's performance through repetition and successive refinement" (Ericsson and Lehmann 1996, pp. 278–279), deliberate practice involves an intensive training process with repetitive skill-building exercises informed by expert feedback and performed throughout a professional career. Professionals from a wide range of fields, from music to athletics to chess to medicine, rely on deliberate practice to achieve expert performance (Ericsson and Pool 2016). Professionals use deliberate practice to acquire and maintain their skills throughout their entire career, from beginning training to seasoned professionals. In this chapter, I review the theory of deliberate practice and explore how it can be applied to clinical supervision and training.

Key Points

- Research suggests that traditional methods of clinical training have limited impact on clinical skill acquisition and client outcome.

- Deliberate practice is a trans-theoretical model of training that focuses on acquisition of specific clinical skills.

- Active learning methods, such as behavioral rehearsal in psychiatric simulations (role-plays), are emphasized.

- Skill acquisition is enhanced through repetition and higher levels of effort.

- Homework (behavioral rehearsal in simulations) is used as an integral part of learning.

- Performance is assessed by evaluating client outcome, rather than fidelity or adherence to treatment models.

- Deliberate practice is used throughout an entire professional career.

Deliberate Practice in Medical Education

Traditional medical education has not focused on deliberate practice (McGaghie and Kristopaitis 2015). Rather, students' primary learning activity has been supervised clinical experience organized around a series of clinical training sites (internships, residencies, and fellowships). However, studies have raised questions about the limitations of supervised clinical experience for aiding the acquisition of specific clinical skills. For example, three studies in the 1990s that examined specific clinical skills found that licensed physicians were no more skilled than medical students at performing a range of medical interventions such as cardiac auscultation and evaluating heart sounds (McGaghie and Kristopaitis 2015).

In recognition of these limits, researchers have explored how to use deliberate practice to enhance the effectiveness of medical education. This change involves increasing the focus on repetitive behavioral rehearsal of specific clinical skills.

Deliberate practice in medical education settings means that learners are engaged in difficult, goal-oriented work, supervised by teachers, who provide feedback and correction, under conditions of high achievement expectations, with revision and improvement (McGaghie and Kristopaitis 2015, p. 223).

In contrast to the classic medical training adage of "see one, do one, teach one," deliberate practice can be summarized as "see one, do many more, and keep doing it until you get it right." (Rousmaniere 2016, 2019). A 2011 meta-analysis of 14 studies comparing traditional medical education with skill-focused exercises using deliberate practice and clinical simulations found that deliberate practice and simulation-based training (role-plays) greatly outperformed traditional medical education (McGaghie et al. 2011).

Deliberate practice can help supervisees who understand their treatment model (e.g., cognitive-behavioral therapy, psychodynamic psychotherapy) but still cannot apply it with their patients. Deliberate practice maximizes time spent on simulation-based behavioral rehearsal, rather than teaching theory or talking about skills. Unless a supervisee is practicing a skill, the learning is theoretical, not behavioral. For example, if in a

1-hour class 20 minutes is spent explaining a technique, 10 minutes watching a demonstration of the skill, 10 minutes in discussion, and another 20 minutes in role-play of the skill (with each supervisee doing 5 minutes), then each supervisee has 5 minutes of substantive skill development. A better ratio is 2:1 or 1:1 discussion to practice versus 11:1 as in the above example. This stands in contrast to traditional psychotherapy training, where passive learning (lecture) or theoretical learning (discussion) is paramount (Rousmaniere 2016, 2019).

Deliberate practice facilitates skill development and maintenance throughout an entire career. Just as musicians, athletes, chess masters, and pilots practice the same basic skills throughout their careers, clinicians should never stop practicing. Furthermore, deliberate practice is not mindless repetition, but a constant attempt to push oneself to upset one's homeostasis. Aim for continual improvement rather than automaticity. If it doesn't feel hard, then the supervisee is not advancing his or her skills.

Deliberate Practice in Psychiatric Training

Deliberate practice is currently not commonly utilized in psychiatric training or most other disciplines of mental health training. Scott Miller was the first researcher to propose that deliberate practice could benefit mental health training (Miller et al. 2007). More recently, other researchers have examined how deliberate practice can improve the effectiveness of psychotherapy supervision and training (Chow et al. 2015; Rousmaniere 2016; Rousmaniere et al. 2017; Tracey et al. 2014).

How to Supervise Using Deliberate Practice

Deliberate practice for psychotherapy follows the procedure presented below (and outlined in Figure 10–1).

1. *Supervisee presents a case to the supervisor.* The supervisee should pick a patient who is stalled or at risk of deterioration or dropout. A video of a therapy session or role-play of a challenging moment in therapy is used.
2. *Supervisor identifies one to three microskills.* Examples of skills are not interrupting or talking over the patient; reflecting the patient's experience; and inviting the patient to explore their thoughts or feelings.
3. *Supervisee practices.* The supervisee practices in role-play with supervisor or by talking at the video. The supervisor might say: "Notice whenever you feel the urge to interrupt or talk over the client. Instead, press your lips together. Simultaneously, notice any complex feelings or anxiety you may have."
4. *Repeat this process sufficient times.* The goal is for the skill to become more comfortable and expand the supervisee's capacity for self-awareness and mindfulness while working with his or her patients.
5. *Consolidate skills via homework.* Deliberate practice alone or with a partner is where most development happens in other fields. The supervisee should aim for 1 hour of practice per month in 15- to 20-minute chunks, in which the supervisee practices in role-play with a colleague or does deliberate practice homework exercises with their videos (see "Specific Challenges and Strategies" below).

Deliberate Practice for Psychotherapists
www.drtonyr.com

1 **Present case to consultant**
- Pick a client who is stalled or at risk of deterioration or dropout
- Use video of therapy session (use encrypted drive) or role-play of challenging moment in therapy

2 **Identify 1–3 microskills**
- Include both skill and psychological capacity
- Example: "Notice whenever you feel the urge to interrupt or talk over the client. Instead, press your lips together. Simultaneously, notice any complex feelings or anxiety you may have."

3 **Practice with consultant**
- In role-play or talking at your video
- Be mindful of complex feelings, anxiety, countertransference, etc. within yourself and with consultant

4 **Repeat sufficient times**
- Skill should become more comfortable
- Expand your capacity for self-awareness and mindfulness while working with your clients

5 **Homework**
- Solitary Deliberate Practice is where most development happens in other fields
- Aim for 30 minutes of practice in 10- to 15-minute chunks between each consultation

FIGURE 10–1. Creating your own deliberate practice routine.

Specific Challenges and Strategies

- **My supervisee doesn't know what skills to focus on in deliberate practice.** Focus on small, incremental skill components. Try to isolate the smallest components of skills—microskills—that are just beyond their ability. For example, in traditional training a supervisor may suggest that a supervisee "listen more carefully" to a client. In deliberate practice, the supervisor will isolate a microskill within "listening carefully," such as "Watch the video of this patient and count how many times you talk over the patient" or "Watch the video and count how many seconds you allow to pass after the patient stops talking before you respond" or "Watch this video and carefully note your internal experience when the patient is expressing anger. Write down how often that makes you feel uncomfortable."

- **My supervisee complains that she does not have enough supervision time.** As in many other fields, clinical expertise comes from many hours of solitary deliberate practice, or practicing with a colleague. Meeting with supervisors or consultants is essential for feedback and performance appraisal, but logistical variables (notably, money) limit how much expert feedback clinicians can access. The good news is that practicing alone or with a colleague is free! The bad news is that it requires considerably more effort and willpower than practice with an expert.

Questions for the Supervisee

■ What clinical skills are you having a hard time acquiring?

■ Are there any clinical populations or specific presentations (e.g., anxiety, psychosis) with which you perform less effectively?

■ Have you told your supervisor about your clinical challenges and asked her or him to help you more in those areas?

■ Do you feel comfortable revealing your clinical weaknesses?

■ Do you know anyone who could help you, in the role of an auxiliary supervisor, mentor, or supervisor, acquire more clinical skills?

■ What would motivate you to invest time, energy, and money into a careerlong process of clinical skill development?

Questions for the Supervisor

■ What clinical skills do my trainees have a hard time acquiring?

■ How much do I engage in simulated behavioral rehearsal in supervision?

■ Do I assign homework for supervisees? (Not reading homework, which focuses on learning theory, but instead behavioral rehearsal homework, which focuses on skill acquisition.)

■ Can I help my supervisees find auxiliary supervisors, mentors, or supervisors to further develop their clinical skills?

■ Am I helping my supervisees prepare for a career-long process of clinical skill development?

Additional Resources

Deliberate Practice Benefit to Mental Health Training

Rousmaniere TG: Deliberate Practice for Psychotherapists: A Guide to Improving Clinical Effectiveness. New York, Routledge, 2016

Rousmaniere TG: Mastering the Inner Skills of Psychotherapy: A Deliberate Practice Manual. Seattle, WA, Gold Lantern Books, 2019

Rousmaniere TG, Goodyear R, Miller SD (eds): The Cycle of Excellence: Using Deliberate Practice to Improve Supervision and Training. London, Wiley, 2017

Theory and Science of Deliberate Practice

Ericsson KA, Pool R: Peak: Secrets From the New Science of Expertise. New York, Houghton Mifflin Harcourt, 2016

Deliberate Practice in Medical Education

McGaghie W: Advances in medical education from mastery learning and deliberate practice, in The Cycle of Excellence: Using Deliberate Practice to Improve Supervision and Training. Edited by Rousmaniere TG, Goodyear R, Miller SD, et al. London, Wiley, 2017, pp 249–264

Use Across a Range of Other Fields

Ericsson KA, Charness N, Feltovich PJ, et al: The Cambridge Handbook of Expertise and Expert Performance. Cambridge, UK, Cambridge University Press, 2006

Deliberate Practice Video Exercises and Other Resources

www.dpfortherapists.com

References

Chow DL, Miller SD, Seidel JA, et al: The role of deliberate practice in the development of highly effective psychotherapists. Psychotherapy (Chic) 52(3):337–345, 2015 26301425

Ericsson KA, Pool R: Peak: Secrets from the New Science of Expertise. New York, Houghton Mifflin Harcourt, 2016

Ericsson KA, Krampe RT, Tesch-Romer C: The role of deliberate practice in the acquisition of expert performance. Psychol Rev 100(3):363–406, 1993

Ericsson KA, Lehmann AC: Expert and exceptional performance: evidence of maximal adaptation to task constraints. Annu Rev Psychol 47:273–305, 1996 15012483

McGaghie WC, Kristopaitis T: Deliberate practice and mastery learning: origins of expert medical performance, in Researching Medical Education. Edited by Cleland JA, Durning SJ. Hoboken, NJ, Wiley Blackwell, 2015, pp 219–230

McGaghie WC, Issenberg SB, Cohen ER, et al: Does simulation-based medical education with deliberate practice yield better results than traditional clinical education? A meta-analytic comparative review of the evidence. Acad Med 86(6):706–711, 2011 21512370

Miller SD, Hubble MA, Duncan BL: Supershrinks: learning from the field's most effective practitioners. The Psychotherapy Networker 31(6):26–35, 56, 2007

Rousmaniere TG: Deliberate Practice for Psychotherapists: A Guide to Improving Clinical Effectiveness. New York, Routledge, 2016

Rousmaniere TG: Mastering the Inner Skills of Psychotherapy: A Deliberate Practice Manual. Seattle, WA, Gold Lantern Books, 2019

Rousmaniere TG, Goodyear R, Miller SD, et al (eds): The Cycle of Excellence: Using Deliberate Practice to Improve Supervision and Training. London, Wiley, 2017

Tracey TJG, Wampold BE, Lichtenberg JW, et al: Expertise in psychotherapy: an elusive goal? Am Psychol 69(3):218–229, 2014 24393136

Chapter 11 Live Supervision

Behind the One-Way Mirror

Douglas S. Rait, Ph.D.

Live supervision is most closely associated with state-of-the-art training centers in couples and family therapy because it represents the most immediate, compelling way to help supervisees rapidly learn both observational and technical skills. Imagine a couples therapy session conducted by a beginning therapist. Behind a one-way mirror are the supervisor and members of the supervision group, observing the session and quietly discussing their reactions, hypotheses, and ideas about what next steps might help the couple. At a crucial moment in the contentious session, the husband begins to withdraw, and the supervisor quickly calls the supervisee on the phone and points out, "You just joined so nicely with the wife, but the husband might feel a little left out. Find a way to make contact with him before you pursue their conflict further." The therapist then moves her chair closer to the husband, who reengages, and the couple completes a successful conversation.

In this way, live supervision can feel suspenseful, electrifying, and visceral for the patients, supervisee, supervisor, and supervision team. Change happens in an instant, and the feedback is immediate. One obvious way that live supervision differs from other modalities is that the supervisor directly observes the session from behind the mirror, watching the drama of therapy unfolding in real time. Yet, the added benefit of live supervision is that the supervisor can also communicate directly with the supervisee who is conducting the therapy through a phone (or, in some settings, an ear piece, or "bug in the ear"). Feedback can therefore be delivered at precise moments where the supervisee's learning, as well as the patient's, couple's, or family's experience, may be expanded.

In addition, live supervision flexibly allows for the supervisor to occasionally join the therapist in the treatment room, for the supervisee to take breaks during the session to consult with the supervisor, and for a small team of supervisees to join the supervisor behind the mirror. Live supervision can therefore provide a needed nudge, even a push, to help the therapist in the room to first see and then redirect entrenched relational patterns. As illustrated above, live supervision also permits the introduction of probes, experiments, challenges, and support in the therapeutic process that can produce instantaneous outcomes. It can be exciting and galvanizing for the therapist, the supervision group, and the supervisor to work closely together in drawing inferences from the clinical data, generating hypotheses, devising interventions, and testing them, all within the span of a single therapeutic hour.

Key Points

- Live supervision allows for real-time observation, case formulation, and hypothesis development and testing.

- Live supervision allows for the collaborative development of clinical interventions and the opportunity to rapidly integrate immediate feedback from these interventions into the supervisee's working hypotheses and formulation.

- Live supervision offers real-time feedback for the supervisee's clinical skills, including joining and alliance maintenance, tracking and identifying systemic patterns, and implementing specific interventions.

- Live supervision creates the opportunity for the supervisor to responsibly attend to the patients' needs as well as the supervisee's training needs.

- Live supervision encourages the formation of a supportive, collaborative clinical team that can reduce anxiety and isolation for supervisees working with challenging cases and, at the same time, permit learning for all team members.

Contexts for Live Supervision

Couples and Family Therapy

Live supervision has many benefits for treatment involving couples or families. Couples and family therapy can feel demanding to even the most experienced therapists. Because there are multiple participants in couples or family treatment, simply meeting with a couple or family can be trying, especially for the beginning supervisee. Couples and family sessions tend to be noisier and more openly conflictual than the modal individual psychotherapy meeting. In addition to contending with the difficulties in managing the multi-sourced therapeutic conversation, the supervisee immediately recognizes that not every family member comes to treatment with equal motivation, similar goals, or agreed-on beliefs about how to change. The intent of live supervision is to add clarity to this complexity, direct the supervisee's attention and therapeutic focus, and encourage the supervisee's ability to move freely and intervene creatively.

Individual Therapy

While live supervision has been most closely associated with clinical training in couples and family therapy, some of its concepts and practices have been shown to be applicable to the individual therapy context as well with some modification (Kivlighan et al. 1991; Reardon et al. 2014). One of the main advantages of live supervision is that supervisees can more rapidly practice and apply specific intervention skills. According to Berger and Dammann (1982), supervisory feedback is immediately available, the supervisor can provide in vivo modeling for the supervisee, the supervisor can help to shape the supervisee's behavior by offering incremental suggestions, and there can be a synergistic effect with each supervisory intervention building on previous supervisory interventions.

Role of Supervisor

The supervisor often experiences many competing goals and responsibilities in conducting live supervision. First, the supervisor is present behind the one-way mirror to ensure that the patient, couple, or family is receiving the highest quality care while meeting with a relatively inexperienced clinician. Second, the supervisor holds an important role as a primary educator and mentor to the supervisee. Third, if there is a team behind the mirror with the supervisor, the supervisor is often providing commentary and sharing decision-making dilemmas and choice points with team members.

Supervision Structure

The structure of live supervision is often unfamiliar to trainees. Each supervision session begins with a presession discussion in which the supervisee's formulation, hypotheses, and plan for the session are considered. The treatment room is equipped with a one-way mirror and an observation room with phone hook-up so that the supervisor (and observing team, if one is working with a small group) can communicate directly with the trainee therapist in the room. Individual patients, couples, and families are notified about the observation arrangement in advance and sign informed-consent forms before their initial session.

Opportunities to use the time and space flexibly are one of the strengths of live supervision. The supervisor can call in to the supervisee by phone, the supervisee can choose to take a break to consult with the supervisor and team behind the mirror, or the supervisor may decide to enter the room to gather more information, support the supervisee's intervention, model a technique, help to generate intensity, or shift the focus of the session. Following the session, the team often meets briefly to discuss the session, what worked well, and what to focus on in the next meeting. Because of the immediacy of the learning, trainees often describe the experience of live supervision as riveting and invaluable. The context and format of live supervision are also new to most patients, couples, and families, and patients commonly report that they appreciate having a clinical team made up of their therapist in the room and a team behind the one-way mirror devoted to their care.

Approach to Live Supervision

Establish a Trusting, Supportive Supervision Relationship

Because live supervision involves the direct observation of the supervisee's work, it invariably asks the clinician to take significant personal risks. Supervisees may worry about showing their work in front of the supervisor and team, especially when working in a modality that feels new. As a result, understanding the level of comfort and learning the goals of each trainee are essential first steps in establishing trust within the clinical team. Inquiring about each trainee's willingness to stretch and develop greater comfort in the areas of tolerating intensity and conflict, creating opportunities for honest emotional exchange, and directly identifying and confronting dysfunctional patterns of behavior is also important at the outset. The relationship between the supervisor and supervisee is strengthened when the supervisee develops the trust and confidence that such risks can be taken and that the supervisor will help the supervisee manage the situation by calling in or entering the room should conflict escalate to an unsafe level.

Discuss and Establish Clear Guidelines for When and How the Supervisor Will Intervene

It is helpful to clarify when and how the supervisor might intervene. For supervisees to feel empowered, engaged, and responsive in the room requires bicameral thinking: on the one hand, they must operate freely and confidently as the couple or family's therapists; on the other hand, they know that the supervisor is there to enhance the learning and growth of the entire therapeutic system (family and therapist). Ideally, the supervisee feels the trust and support of the supervisor to take risks, experiment, and ask for help. A secure bond with the supervisor ideally encourages the supervisee's autonomy rather than constrains it. Assuming that there has been good communication about the plan for the session and how to deal with anticipated challenges, the supervisor can also rely on the supervisee's judgment and clinical choices, thereby reducing the need to call in too often.

The supervisor should strive to identify clear objectives for phoning in to the supervisee, asking for a break, or entering the room. A well-timed phone call can encourage the supervisee to return to an important unanswered question, pay closer attention to a pattern of interaction noted behind the mirror, to initiate an enactment, or to deliver a specific intervention. A phone call can also be used to interrupt an escalation between family members or to celebrate a successful interaction. In general, when feedback is being given, it is best for the supervisor to connect, provide genuine support, and be both clear and concise. At times, the supervisor may recommend taking a midsession break in order to allow the supervisee to rethink the direction of a session based on new information or to think through how to address a tricky, stubborn impasse. Finally, the supervisor may choose to enter the room to regulate the level of intensity in the session, model a technique, or help restore the supervisee's authority.

Emphasize the Importance of Bilateral Feedback

As noted, communication with the supervisee should be direct, supportive, and clinically beneficial. However, a collaborative learning system values learning that goes both ways; wise supervisees learn from the supervisor, and the wise supervisor learns from the supervisees. Expanding one's own self-awareness as a supervisor about what types of feedback may be too vague, insufficiently instructive, or potentially unsupportive is critical. Asking for input from the supervisee and the clinical team can therefore be instrumental in reducing the tendency to adopt a "supervisor always knows best" position that will invariably preclude the greatest possible learning.

Impact of Live Supervision

Because of the immediate opportunity for learning, live supervision is especially helpful in expanding the supervisee's broad technical skills, such as developing the therapeutic alliance, honing observational skills, experimenting with technical and interventional skills, and expanding the supervisee's emotional and behavioral range.

Alliance-Building Skills

Unlike in individual psychotherapy, managing the therapeutic alliance represents one of the unique differences that new supervisees face in working with couples and families, and live supervision can be invaluable in supporting this educational goal (Rait 2000). In couples and family therapy, the supervisor can help the supervisee to appreciate and develop different types, or levels, of alliance, including a relationship with each individual family member, the various subsystems within the family (e.g., the couple or siblings), and the couple or family as a whole. While video-based supervision can identify specific relationships that the supervisee is having difficulty developing and maintaining, live supervision often can be helpful in encouraging the supervisee to do something specific "in the moment" to create more connection and trust, reduce anxiety or inhibition, and foster more playfulness with a particular family member. For example, a supervisor might ask the supervisee to move closer to a member of a couple while also asking the person to do something he or she might find challenging, "Talk to him about why you are so afraid of his anger."

Observational Skills

Noticing and identifying patterns and tracking, as well as elaborating, content themes are some of the observational skills a supervisee can develop through the use of live supervision. Because there is so much to attend to in couples and family treatment, live supervision can help the supervisee to immediately see durable patterns that are reflective of the couple's or family's organization or structure in the form of boundaries, alliances and coalitions, and hierarchy. Supervisees also learn to look for patterns of complementary—that is, interdependent roles, such as caretaker and sick person, novice and expert, pursuer and distancer. With a brief phone call or by entering the treatment room as a consultant, the supervisor can point out these complementary patterns as they occur, giving the supervisee a useful way to reframe and then interrupt these patterns of behavior (Rait and Glick 2008).

Technical and Interventional Skills

Learning therapeutic technique can also be enhanced with live supervision. Supervisees can be coached on the spot to expand their capacity to listen and to join, especially with family members who may be hard to reach. Supervisees may also be encouraged to stage enactments, or interactions between family members, in the room. For example, when calling in, the supervisor might ask the therapist to address a mother, "You have something important to say to your son. Can you tell him now?" These in-session enactments allow the clinician to observe, support, and interrupt patterns that may be inhibiting problem resolution or individual expression. Because many clinicians who are beginning to work with couples and families find direct therapeutic confrontation to be especially difficult, live supervision can also help them to provide support for individual family members while challenging dysfunctional patterns of interaction. Instead of reflecting back to the wife in a couple, "You seem very sad," the supervisor might ask the supervisee to address the husband differently: "Your wife seems so very sad. Can you speak to her in a way that does not depress her?"

Emotional and Behavioral Range

Just as supervisees can be encouraged to be more direct, they can also be helped to create an atmosphere of warmth, softness, and authenticity in the moment. For example, through the phone (or "bug in the ear"), the supervisor might urge a supervisee to emphasize a moment of tenderness in an interaction, gently saying something like, "Did you hear what your very caring wife said? Say it to him again. Say that lovely thing to him again." Although this type of intervention could be recommended after reviewing video of a session, the learning in live supervision is instantaneous and immediately expands the therapist's therapeutic range and repertoire.

Specific Challenges and Strategies

- **I'm worried about sharing my work in front of my supervisor and team.** Understanding the level of comfort and learning the goals of each trainee are essential first steps in establishing trust within the clinical team. Inquiring about each trainee's willingness to stretch and develop greater comfort in the areas of tolerating intensity and conflict, creating opportunities for honest emotional exchange, and directly identifying and confronting dysfunctional patterns of behavior is also important at the outset. The relationship between the supervisor and trainee is strengthened when the trainee develops the trust and confidence that such risks can be taken and that the supervisor will help the supervisee manage the situation by calling in or entering the room should conflict escalate to an unsafe level.
- **At the beginning, I wasn't sure when the supervisor would call.** In live supervision, the supervisor must constantly balance the needs of the case, the supervisee's education, and the collaborative team learning environment. Throughout the presession, session, and postsession discussion, finding the right stance and rhythm in the supervisory relationship is essential, as the supervisor's primary responsibility should always be to protect and support the supervisee's authoritative position in

the treatment room and to help the patient, couple, or family move toward their therapeutic goals. As a result, the supervisor must manage his or her own anxiety and resist the temptation to call in too frequently, potentially disempowering the supervisee in front of the family and the clinical team (Schwartz et al. 1988).

- **My supervisor's comments were so helpful, I kept waiting for him to call in rather than think for myself.** Good live supervision hopefully augments what the supervisee is doing rather than replaces it. Occasional calls or brief midsession breaks should enhance the supervisee's understanding of what is happening in the treatment room, help to refine clinical hypotheses, as well as highlight potential interventions. Sometimes the supervisor will be very directive, while at other times the supervisor might offer a simple set of options from which the therapist in the room can choose. Remembering to generally leave the initiative in the supervisee's hands is a good rule of thumb for beginning supervisors.

Questions for the Supervisee

■ What specific concerns do you have about live supervision?

■ How do you feel about having your work observed by me or the team?

■ What type of specific attention and help would you like in the upcoming session?

■ Would you be comfortable with my entering the room if I thought it would be helpful to model an intervention?

Additional Resources

Liddle H, Breunlin D, Schwartz R (eds): Handbook of Family Therapy Training and Supervision. New York, Guilford, 1988

References

Berger M, Dammann C: Live supervision as context, treatment, and training. Fam Process 21(3):337–344, 1982 7128770

Kivlighan D, Angelone E, Swafford K: Live supervision in individual psychotherapy: effects on therapist's intention use and client's evaluation of session effect and working alliance. Prof Psychol Res Pr 22:489–495, 1991

Rait DS: The therapeutic alliance in couples and family therapy. J Clin Psychol 56(2):211–224, 2000 10718604

Rait D, Glick I: A model for reintegrating couples and family therapy training in psychiatric residency programs. Acad Psychiatry 32(2):81–86, 2008 18349325

Reardon C, May M, Williams K: Psychiatry resident outpatient clinic supervision: how training directors are balancing patient care, education, and reimbursement. Acad Psychiatry 38(4):476–480, 2014 24664608

Schwartz R, Liddle H, Breunlin D: Muddles in live supervision, in Handbook of Family Therapy Training and Supervision. Edited by Liddle H, Breunlin D, Schwartz R. New York, Guilford, 1988, pp 183–193

Chapter 12 Cotherapy

Observing and Modeling in Real Time

Angela Lee, A.B.

Shani Isaac, M.D.

Dorothy Stubbe, M.D.

Anita R. Kishore, M.D.

Cotherapy is defined as psychotherapy conducted by two therapists concurrently (Tanner et al. 2012). Most commonly employed in the setting of group, family, or couples therapy, the cotherapy model allows real-time supervision for practitioners training in the science and art of psychotherapy. Most other training modalities require the trainee to present the therapeutic interaction to his or her supervisor through process notes or video clips. The supervisor is reliant on what the trainee reports, and this makes detecting a trainee's skill deficits extremely challenging. Integrating cotherapy into psychotherapy training allows for direct and unedited observation of a trainee's therapeutic interactions, and an opportunity for the trainee to directly observe and experience the supervisor's therapeutic style. Cotherapy thereby enhances training by facilitating efficient detection and discussion of a trainee's blind spots, while concurrently offering therapeutic modeling by the supervisor. In a 1995 survey, program directors rated cotherapy as the best method of supervision (Romans et al. 1995).

Another distinguishing feature of cotherapy is the presence of three therapeutic relationships in the room: those between the faculty member and the patient, between

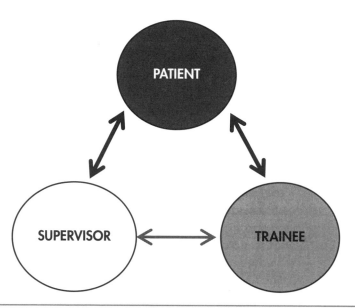

FIGURE 12–1.   The three therapeutic relationships of cotherapy.
While therapeutic relationships between patient and trainee, and between patient and supervisor, are well recognized, the therapeutic relationship between supervisor and trainee is often overlooked. This latter relationship heavily influences the others in cotherapy, distinguishing this approach from other training models.

the trainee and the patient, and between the faculty member and the trainee. In this chapter, we provide guidelines for educators on how to effectively implement cotherapy as a training model.

Key Points

- Cotherapists should share equally in the therapeutic task, despite a differential in expertise, professional training, and experience.

- The relationship between cotherapists is a crucial factor in the therapeutic change process.

- Effective cotherapists model, verbally and nonverbally, open and honest communication, active listening, and methods of problem-solving disagreements.

- Allowing time for preparation and processing after each session optimizes learning and builds the cotherapy relationship.

- Preparing for a cotherapy experience begins even before the patient enters the room. The following stages are recommended to ensure a successful experience for the trainee and the patient.

Stage 1: Developing Cotherapy Mentorship

Take the Time to Introduce the Cotherapy Model to the Trainee

Discuss the trainee's past experiences with cotherapy and other models of supervision. What was helpful about each model, and what was challenging? Invite discussion about the anxiety of working directly with a supervisor, and normalize any performance anxiety that either party might be experiencing. It is helpful to anticipate three stages of the cotherapy mentorship relationship: 1) the trainee's initial fear about starting cotherapy, along with relief that he or she is not alone; 2) risk taking by both trainee and faculty member in actively addressing disagreements; and 3) resolution, either successful or unsuccessful, of disagreements.

Learn About the Trainee as a Person

Start by inquiring about the trainee's personal and professional values and goals. Share your teaching objectives with the trainee and explore how to align your goals in the context of cotherapy.

> You discover that a junior trainee rotating with you is interested in global health and increasing access to care. How might you align your cotherapy teaching goals with hers?
>
> The World Health Organization has promoted "task-shifting," or training laypeople in specific diagnostic or treatment modalities, to improve access to mental health care in resource-poor areas. Cotherapy may serve as a powerful teaching tool to quickly train health workers in psychotherapy in such a setting. Communicate to your trainee that your cotherapy work together can add value to her training and future career.

Stage 2: Preparing for the Cotherapy Encounter

Get Patient Buy-In

Patients should be informed and agree to cotherapy at the onset. Some patients may be hesitant; clearly explain the reasons for cotherapy and the roles of the cotherapists. Attempt to start the therapy conjointly. Be explicit with patients that confidentiality rules are the same: nothing that is said during therapy will leave the room unless someone is in imminent danger.

Discuss Goals for the Upcoming Session

Week by week, evaluate your joint approach to running the session. The respective roles can be tailored to a trainee's level of experience and comfort. Early on a faculty member might take on a more active role, while the trainee does more observing. Faculty and trainee can also divide the content of the session, with, for example, one taking the lead on homework and the other focusing on new concepts in a cognitive-behavioral framework. Changing therapeutic dynamics, and gradually shifting toward more equal roles, can create more opportunities for the trainee to lead and learn.

Stage 3: Conducting Cotherapy

Address Your Trainee Directly During Therapy Sessions

Conversational interactions between the supervisor and trainee can relax the patient and the cotherapists. This can be especially valuable when a patient is overwhelmed during a difficult session and needs time to regulate. Moreover, dialogue with the trainee serves to model healthy communication to the patient and permits the cotherapists to problem-solve a therapeutic impasse in a transparent manner. Modeling psychodynamically oriented exchanges can be particularly helpful with patients who have little experience with this less concrete (and often less intuitive) therapeutic framework.

> Jean is a 19-year old patient who has been in cotherapy for 5 weeks. When talking about a recent argument with her parents, Jean begins to tear up. She puts her head down, stops talking, and disengages. The trainee cotherapist empathically states, "That sounds like it was very difficult for you." Jean remains mute. The faculty cotherapist addresses the trainee. "Jean seems very upset—her reaction appears as though she is experiencing past traumas. I recall that Jean has spoken about how she has not felt valued or understood by her parents—particularly when she felt so depressed in high school. I wonder if that is what she is experiencing now?" The trainee replies, "Yes, that does make sense. Jean has used therapy very well, but when she is overwhelmed by emotion, it may be very hard to talk about." Jean's eyes open. "You're right. I don't even like to think about that time, let alone talk about it."

Stage 4: Processing the Encounter

Process the Patient Encounter in a Self-Revealing Manner

Establish a regular time for reflection, ideally a few minutes immediately following each appointment and for a longer period of time at the end of each clinic day. Immediate processing improves recollection of the details of the session, enhancing the feedback of both you and the trainee. It is critical that you create a safe and supportive space for the trainee to candidly reflect. Self-revealing debriefs after sessions are an opportunity to humanize the learning process and reduce performance anxiety.

A delicate balance must be found between, on the one hand, promoting open feedback and communication and, on the other, adhering to the practical need for evaluation of a trainee's performance. There is a natural and potentially fruitful tension that arises within this context—one that parallels the tension that a therapist might experience with a patient—between being more permissive or questioning and being perceived as an equal or as an authority. These shifting dynamics provide an opportunity for rich discussion and deeper understanding of oneself as a tool for therapeutic intervention.

Caleb is a 16-year-old male who presents with 2 weeks of new-onset psychosis. He is accompanied by his domineering father and his soft-spoken mother. The parents are divorced at the time of the consult. Caleb and his mother appear frustrated by the father's repeated interruptions, during which he denies his son's auditory hallucinations and the diagnostic and treatment possibilities that you and your cotherapist are attempting to discuss. The father becomes increasingly dismissive and belittling throughout the sessions.

Following the session, the trainee alerts his supervisor that she was making more eye contact with the mother than she was with the father, presumably as a means of validating the mother's frustration. They explore how this may have inadvertently antagonized the father. The supervisor gains new insights and uses this feedback to more effectively work with Caleb's parents.

Specific Challenges and Strategies

- **My institution seems uncertain about adopting cotherapy as a training model.** Cotherapy requires additional resources. The institution receives decreased reimbursements because both clinicians cannot bill for the therapy hour. Faculty must devote valuable time to both developing and debriefing with their trainees. That being said, cotherapy is a highly efficient training method and a powerful recruiting tool that may also attract medical students and competitive residents to the field of psychiatry.
- **My patient seems hesitant, uncomfortable, or unengaged with cotherapy.** Despite having consented to cotherapy, the patient may seem unengaged or exclusively addresses only one member of the cotherapy team. Curiosity in the unfolding dynamic may help break the impasse. For example, one cotherapist may ask: "I notice that you are primarily talking to me during the session. I wonder how we might understand that?" Self-consciousness around two therapists or intuiting power dynamics between the cotherapists may be at play. Typically, if the issue is addressed early, the patient will become comfortable and engage more productively.
- **It's difficult to make time for debriefing.** If debriefs with the trainee cannot be scheduled after each appointment, try to structure just a few minutes between every few patients. Before beginning a cotherapy clinic, identify which patients are more complex and devote extra time to prepare for these sessions with the trainee.

Questions for the Supervisee

■ How has it been sharing patient responsibilities with me? Are there times when you wish you had more or less ownership of a session?

■ There are times when I'm uncertain, and yet I feel as though I'm supposed to have all the answers because I'm the attending. I wonder if there are times that you feel especially aware of our roles in this joint therapy?

■ How are our debrief sessions going for you? Is there anything that could make you feel more comfortable in candidly talking about our cotherapy sessions?

Additional Resources

Bernard HS, Babineau R, Schwartz AJ: Supervisor-trainee cotherapy as a method for individual psychotherapy training. Psychiatry 43(2):138–145, 1980

Hendrix CC, Fournier DG, Briggs K: Impact of co-therapy teams on client outcomes and therapist training in marriage and family therapy. Contemporary Family Therapy 23(1):63–82, 2001

Steinberg E, Gedzior, J, Mervis P, et al: Group cotherapy in a training clinic. Group 37(3):229–237, 2013

References

Romans JSC, Boswell DL, Carlozzi AF, et al: Training and supervision practices in clinical, counseling and school psychology programs. Prof Psychol Res Pr 26(4):407–412, 1995

Tanner MA, Gray JJ, Haaga DAF: Association of cotherapy supervision with client outcomes, attrition, and trainee effectiveness in a psychotherapy training clinic. J Clin Psychol 68(12):1241–1252, 2012 22899235

Chapter 13   Other Supervisory Techniques

Before, During, and After the Patient Encounter

Jessica Gold, M.D., M.S.

Jessica Bentzley, M.D.

Whether working with a supervisee on the inpatient wards or in outpatient clinics, supervisors have several effective techniques at their disposal for enhancing supervisee learning before, during, and after the patient encounter. Many techniques are particularly useful within inpatient, consultation-liaison, or psychopharmacology clinic venues, such as effective educational questioning ("pimping"), SNAPPS, and 1-minute preceptor or mini chalk talks. Others are useful across any supervisory venue, such as goal setting, modeling, pimping, talking out loud, reflecting, and self-monitoring as well as encouraging self-directed learning. In this chapter, we outline those additional evidence-based supervision methods using the following hypothetical, but typical, case example:

> A 28-year-old female graduate student from India presents to a student mental health center with 2 months of amotivation, depressed mood, insomnia, impaired concentration, low energy, and hopelessness.

Key Points

- Conceptualize supervision in three stages: before the patient encounter, during the patient encounter (workup, diagnosis, and management), and after the patient encounter (reflection).

- Use techniques that maximize learning in limited time.

- Create a safe, nonjudgmental learning environment.

- Do not assume supervisees recognize automatic thought processes. Make clinical reasoning explicit.

- Follow-up with supervisees after requesting they research specific topics.

Prior to the Patient Encounter

Patient-based supervision is time-intensive, thus preplanning roles, learning objectives, and patient selection are invaluable techniques used prior to the patient encounter (Irby and Bowen 2004). It is important to first define the roles of the supervisee and the supervisor (e.g., Will the supervisor or supervisee lead the interview?). Next, learning objectives need to be elicited from the supervisee (e.g., Is the goal of the interaction to untangle a difficult diagnosis, an interview technique, or explore symptoms?). Techniques can also be selected based on the level of knowledge of the supervisee, which can be quickly elicited by asking good questions (see subsection "Educational Questioning (Pimping)" below) and briefly observing the supervisee in a clinical setting (Irby and Wilkerson 2008). Lastly, patient selection must be carefully considered. After patients consent to participate in training, those selected often have challenging diagnoses or diagnoses that fulfill curriculum objectives (Doshi and Brown 2005).

During the Patient Encounter

Many techniques have been studied for supervision during the patient encounter that can be applicable to psychiatric supervision and supervisee learning. These include modeling, effective educational questioning ("pimping"), thinking aloud, SNAPPS, the 1-minute preceptor, and mini chalk talk.

Modeling of Clinical Skills

Modeling is a commonly employed supervision technique during a patient encounter that is largely attributable to the continued apprenticeship style in medicine. Modeling allows a supervisee to directly observe a senior clinician interact with patients and learn how an experienced clinician interviews, delivers diagnoses, and handles difficult situations (Doshi and Brown 2005). Modeling is intentional and includes not only skills and knowledge but also ethics and attitudes (Irby 1986). Reflection and feedback occur afterward to cement learning points.

Educational Questioning ("Pimping")

Although most agree that the mistreatment associated with the term "pimping" should be left in the past, educational questioning, or "good pimping," is thought to be an effective tool for educators in the clinical setting and can help with learning retention (Detsky 2009). To employ this approach effectively, supervisors might use purposeful questions. Educators should know what they intend to accomplish by asking a supervisee a question. If, when they reflect on the purpose of asking a question, any elements are intended to mistreat the learner because of their degree of difficulty, for example, the question should be changed. Categories of questions include the following (Kost and Chen 2015):

1. *Knowledge-centered questions.* These focus on facts, concepts, or skills, and their purpose is to ascertain the learner's knowledge base and/or teach or review material. For instance: "What are the other diagnostic criteria used to classify this patient as having MDD?"
2. *Learning-centered questions.* These questions encourage supervisees to modulate their own learning experiences by asking progressively harder questions to help identify areas of improvement or identify misconceptions or preconceptions about the material. An example is: "What if you uncovered that 6 months ago this patient had 1 week of decreased need for sleep?"
3. *Assessment-centered questions.* These allow supervisors to give comprehensive feedback to supervisees on their knowledge and ability to apply existing knowledge to new patient cases. One might ask a supervisee: "What other information would you absolutely need to obtain from the patient before starting her on medication" and then provide feedback on each fact that the supervisee decides is important.
4. *Community-centered questions.* These are designed to involve the entire team of learners and might include asking supervisees a question then allowing the shared knowledge drive additional teaching opportunities, such as chalk talks. For example, "Compare side effects of antidepressants and why one might be selected over another."
5. *Interpretive questions.* These questions aim to activate critical thinking skills. For example, "What role does culture play in her symptomatic description?"

All these question types have utility. Supervisors should be thoughtful in matching question selection to purpose. Furthermore, supervisors should foster a safe learning environment to retain knowledge instead of detract from its retention. This can be accomplished by discussing how questions can be intimidating yet build knowledge, praising a supervisee when he or she answers questions correctly (Detsky 2009), and modeling that there are no repercussions for stating "I don't know." The supervisor could even use a supervisee's lack of knowledge as an opportunity to provide a short lecture on the unknown information. Supervisors should attempt to be as sensitive and nonthreatening as possible and establish a noncompetitive learning environment. Remember that trainees react differently to Socratic questioning ("pimping") (Wear et al. 2005), so it is important to adjust questioning styles accordingly.

Diagnostic Decision Making: Thinking Aloud

"Thinking aloud" teaches critical reasoning skills and explicates autonomic thought processes. When supervisees think aloud with their supervisors, they can clarify and check for understanding in their reasoning and conclusions and get immediate feed-back (Pinnock et al. 2016). Examples include morning report, wherein trainees pause for discussion throughout a case and ask participants to verbally illustrate the differential thought process (Hsu et al. 2015). Alternatively, when supervisors think aloud, they not only make their own reasoning explicit but also demonstrate humility and model to supervisees that uncertainty and mistakes are common in medicine (Houchens et al. 2017).

Diagnostic Decision Making for the Experienced Trainee: SNAPPS

SNAPPS (Summarize, Narrow down, Analyze, Probe, Plan, Select) is a six-step active-learning model for experienced trainees occurring after a trainee has seen a patient (Irby and Bowen 2004; Wolpaw et al. 2003). This learner-centered technique has been shown to help supervisees express their clinical reasoning and identify areas of uncertainty (Wolpaw et al. 2009).

Stepwise, the trainee is asked to

1. *Summarize briefly the history and findings.*
2. *Narrow the differential to two or three relevant possibilities.*
3. *Analyze the differential by comparing and contrasting the possibilities.* For instance, "I am leaning toward major depressive disorder (MDD), because she has five or more diagnostic criteria for a depressive episode. However, we should also consider an adjustment disorder, because she recently moved here from India. Unlike MDD, in an adjustment disorder, there is a clear trigger and the diagnostic time frame is different. Additionally, she reports cold intolerance, fatigue, and is overweight, so we must also consider hypothyroidism."
4. *Probe the preceptor by asking questions about uncertainties, difficulties, or alternative approaches.* For example, "I do not understand how to differentiate an adjustment disorder from major depressive disorder. Do you have a general approach? Also, should I always order thyroid function tests for a patient with depressive symptoms?"
5. *Plan management for the patient's medical issues.* "Next, let's get a thyroid function test. For treatment, let's offer her an antidepressant and a psychotherapy referral."
6. *Select a case-related issue for self-directed learning.* "I will look up the incidence of hypothyroidism in patients presenting to a clinic with a chief complaint of depression and report back tomorrow before morning rounds."

One-Minute Preceptor

This model employs five "microskills" to teach a specific "clinical pearl" and has been shown to help better identify a learner's needs and knowledge base, engage the learner, teach clinical decision making, enhance feedback, and improve disease-specific teaching (Farrell et al. 2016). Both positive and constructive feedback from supervisors and supervisees may improve with this model (Salerno et al. 2002). The five "microskills" of the one-minute preceptor method (Farrell et al. 2016; Tsao 2010) are as follows:

1. *Get a verbal commitment.* After a supervisee presents a case, a supervisor can ask the supervisee to commit to a specific impression, such as, "What do you think is going

on diagnostically with this patient?" This approach provides a focus for subsequent teaching.

2. *Probe for supporting evidence.* As a follow-up, a supervisor may ask a "who, what, where, when, or why" question. For example: "What aspects of her history support your diagnosis?" Like thinking aloud, probing for evidence helps foster critical thinking skills.

3. *Reinforce what was done well.* The supervisor should provide specific positive feedback beyond general praise. For instance, a specific comment such as "Your diagnosis of MDD is well supported by the history and mental status exam" reinforces learning better than a general statement such as "You did well."

4. *Give guidance about errors and omissions.* After positive feedback, the supervisee should also be given guidance about mistakes or incorrect decisions. The supervisor should avoid words with negative connotations like "wrong," and instead say, "Your evaluation would be more complete if..." or "A more preferable approach might be...."

5. *Teach a general principle.* The supervisor should end with an educational pearl of wisdom from the case. For example, "It is important to screen patients for eating disorders when you might want to prescribe bupropion."

Mini Chalk Talk

A "peri-encounter" clinical teaching skill, the mini chalk talk, is a facilitated, mobile, and flexibly given 1- to 3-minute adaptation of the classic lecture. Some tips to consider when using this teaching method include the following:

1. *Develop "teaching scripts"* (Pitt and Orlander 2017). Scripts are topics commonly triggered by a patient case or discussion. The supervisor should generate a list of scripts by thinking about typical patients on a clinical service, prior teaching sessions, or clinical questions that come up often. The scripts can also be triggered by "prerounding" on the clinical service and preplanning teaching ideas geared toward those patients.

2. *Identify objectives for each topic.*

3. *Don't just lecture.* The supervisor should prepare memorable visuals, such as Venn diagrams or flow charts, covering common topics. For the patient described at the beginning of this chapter, one might draw a treatment algorithm or a typical clinical course for a patient treated with medication. Other ideas to engage supervisees would be to include games and encourage peer-to-peer teaching.

After the Patient Encounter

Supervision should not end when the patient encounter ends. Additional time spent with the supervisee allows for reflection and feedback and can direct future learning.

Reflection and Self-Monitoring

After the patient encounter, reflection has been shown to help physicians critically evaluate an experience within their own context, values, and beliefs as well as their patients'

(Wald et al. 2009). It has been found to lead to psychological growth, which can be stunted during clinical training (Branch 2000). Although psychiatrists are accustomed to reflecting on patient encounters, it should be taught as a skill to supervisees. For example, a supervisor could ask, "What feelings did you have about your interaction with this patient?" and then use his or her own facilitation skills to lead the group conversation. As in psychotherapy, supervisors can observe reactions of their supervisees and use this material to delve deeper. It is also important for supervisees to learn about their own reactions to a clinical situation, which can subsequently guide conversation with a patient and diagnosis. Supervisees should be encouraged to ask themselves, "How might prior experiences be affecting my emotional response to this patient? What does this tell me about the patient's condition?"

Reflection can also occur through writing and sharing narratives (Wald et al. 2009). Supervisees can do this alone by thinking about their thoughts and emotions about patient experiences. A supervisor might also provide structured feedback on narrative writing (Wald et al. 2009), suggest prompts, or encourage a team to confidentially reflect on one another's writings.

Directed Further Reading

To expand their knowledge about a clinical encounter or question, supervisees should be directed toward reliable resources, understand the rationale behind researching a specific question, and be given adequate time to discuss their findings with a supervisor. Group discussion of researched topics can promote additional questioning and reflection that can broaden a trainee's perspective and assist them in critically assessing information. Learning how to answer a question with appropriate resources and how to appraise literature are key skills for medical professionals.

Specific Challenges and Strategies

- **I don't have enough time to teach!** Maximize time by preplanning with topics based on common diagnoses and using efficient teaching methods such as the 1-minute preceptor.
- **I feel too pressured to "know everything."** Create a space where saying "I don't know" is encouraged and supervisors model their own uncertainty.
- **I have a tough time engaging supervisees.** Use interactive techniques involving patients, group learning and discussion, and reflection.

Questions for the Supervisor

■ Based on what I teach, which technique might be most helpful to my supervisee?

■ Am I comfortable reflecting with supervisees and learning from their experiences? If not, how might I go about reducing the discomfort?

■ What are some of the barriers to supervising supervisees? How might the techniques discussed in this chapter impact those barriers?

Additional Resources

Novack D, Saizow R, Ferris A, Landau B: DocCom Module 42: Effective Clinical Teaching. Academy of Communications in Healthcare and Drexel University College of Medicine. Available at: https://webcampus.drexelmed.edu/doccom/db/readDocComDemo.aspx?m=42

One Minute Preceptor (instructional video): https://vimeo.com/76305964

References

Branch WTJr: Supporting the moral development of medical students. J Gen Intern Med 15(7):503–508, 2000 10940138

Detsky AS: The art of pimping. JAMA 301(13):1379–1381, 2009 19336716

Doshi M, Brown N: Whys and hows of patient-based teaching. Adv Psychiatr Treat 11:223–231, 2005

Farrell SE, Hopson LR, Wolff M, et al: What's the evidence: a review of the one-minute preceptor model of clinical teaching and implications for teaching in the emergency department. J Emerg Med 51(3):278–283, 2016 27377967

Houchens N, Harrod M, Fowler KE, et al: How exemplary inpatient teaching physicians foster clinical reasoning. Am J Med 130(9):1113.e1–1113.e8, 2017 28454903

Hsu HC, Lee FY, Yang YY, et al: Self- and rater-assessed effectiveness of "thinking-aloud" and "regular" morning report to intensify young physicians' clinical skills. J Chin Med Assoc 78(9):545–554, 2015 25982162

Irby DM: Clinical teaching and the clinical teacher. J Med Educ 61(9 Pt 2):35–45, 1986 3746867

Irby DM, Bowen JL: Time-efficient strategies for learning and performance. Clin Teach 1:23–28, 2004

Irby DM, Wilkerson L: Teaching when time is limited. BMJ 336(7640):384–387, 2008 18276715

Kost A, Chen FM: Socrates was not a pimp: changing the paradigm of questioning in medical education. Acad Med 90(1):20–24, 2015 25099239

Pinnock R, Fisher TL, Astley J: Think aloud to learn and assess clinical reasoning. Med Educ 50(5):585–586, 2016 27072473

Pitt MB, Orlander JD: Bringing mini-chalk talks to the bedside to enhance clinical teaching. Med Educ Online 22(1):1–7, 2017 28178911

Salerno SM, O'Malley PG, Pangaro LN, et al: Faculty development seminars based on the one-minute preceptor improve feedback in the ambulatory setting. J Gen Intern Med 17(10):779–787, 2002 12390554

Tsao CI: One-Minute Preceptor model: brief description and application in psychiatric education. Acad Psychiatry 34(4):317–318, 2010 20576996

Wald HS, Davis SW, Reis SP, et al: Reflecting on reflections: enhancement of medical education curriculum with structured field notes and guided feedback. Acad Med 84(7):830–837, 2009 19550172

Wear D, Kokinova M, Keck-McNulty C, et al: Pimping: perspectives of 4th year medical students. Teach Learn Med 17(2):184–191, 2005 15833730

Wolpaw TM, Wolpaw DR, Papp KK: SNAPPS: a learner-centered model for outpatient education. Acad Med 78(9):893–898, 2003 14507619

Wolpaw T, Papp KK, Bordage G: Using SNAPPS to facilitate the expression of clinical reasoning and uncertainties: a randomized comparison group trial. Acad Med 84(4):517–524, 2009 19318792

Part 4   Clinical Supervision Venues

Chapter 14 Inpatient Psychiatry Supervision

Malathy Kuppuswamy, M.D.

William O. Faustman, Ph.D.

Stephen T. Black, Ph.D.

S. Dina Wang-Kraus, M.D.

A minority of mental health professionals work in inpatient settings. Yet, inpatient training remains a core feature of psychiatry and clinical psychology education. Why the ongoing emphasis on inpatient training? The likely reason relates to the unique supervision and training opportunities available in the inpatient setting. There are few comparable training settings that allow for such intensive, personal, and often interdisciplinary supervision. In this chapter, we offer specific suggestions for supervision of inpatient trainees and discuss how inpatient supervision affords important and unique opportunities for professional development.

Key Points

- Provide a structured and supportive orientation at the start of training that includes safety issues.
- Assess supervisee's skills to help identify training needs.

- Make maximal use of supervision techniques that are powerful and easily accessible in inpatient settings, such as modeling, live observation with feedback, integrating interdisciplinary contributions, safety debriefings and group supervision.

- Employ the above techniques to encourage professional development in key inpatient learning experiences such as differential diagnosis, psychopharmacology, forensics, healthcare maintenance, and leadership/supervision skills.

Getting Trainees Started in the Inpatient Setting

Often the most challenging times for a supervisor is the start of training, especially for early-stage trainees. Less experienced trainees start with anticipation and anxiety about expectations and role functions. Supervisors spend significant time in the first weeks teaching logistical issues, protocols, and routines—a time-consuming process that takes place concomitantly with patient care. Supervisor preparation helps ensure that this period is not excessively stressful for both parties. Helpful strategies include meeting with the trainee on the first day to welcome him or her and provide an overview of the unit routine. A handout outlining logistical and procedural details for patient care may provide a useful reference. The initial orientation should offer perspective on the inevitable stresses during training. New trainees come to inpatient training with significantly different baseline clinical skills and training needs. For many trainees the inpatient setting may be their first experience with acutely ill patients. Professional development goals may be divided into general domains (e.g., professionalism, documentation) that are shared across training experiences in addition to site-specific training competencies that are more unique to inpatient training (e.g., handling emergency situations, forensic practice).

Initial supervision sessions with trainees should focus on reviewing background experiences and identifying relative deficiencies. The development of training needs and goals remains a fluid process during training, as unique situations that arise in clinical care may add to training goals well into the course of a rotation. This process often assists trainees in becoming more self-aware of their deficiencies.

Optimizing Safety

Working with severely ill patients in acute crisis is not without significant risks. In fact, acute inpatient units are associated with a relatively high risk of personal injury to staff members (Iozzino et al. 2015). It is essential that supervisors teach trainees to optimize safety from their very first moments in inpatient care. Unlike trainees in outpatient settings, inpatient trainees need a comprehensive orientation to the physical training environment. Trainees need to be oriented to where patients should and should not be interviewed in order to optimize safety. Some settings mandate training in specific methods to manage and prevent disruptive behavior, including how to physically escape from injury while minimizing the risk of injury to patients.

Most acute psychiatry units have protocols for high-risk patients (e.g., suicide precautions). Supervisors may model how to collaborate with nursing staff in making decisions for the use of intensive observation. Whereas extensive training is typically given for the assessment of suicidality, there is often relatively less supervision and teaching given for the standardized assessment of dangerousness to others. Although predicting danger to others is fraught with difficulties, supervision can integrate the use of standardized assessment tools (e.g., Historical Clinical Risk Management–20; Douglas et al. 2014) that help ensure that known factors related to dangerousness are assessed and documented in the clinical record. In sum, assertively integrating safety training and monitoring into supervision leads to a greater sense of support and safety for trainees and thus allows them to better focus on professional development and clinical learning.

Acute inpatient care often includes supervision and teaching of procedures for handling emergency situations such as the use of restraints. Making decisions about the use of restraints involves teaching a range of skills (e.g., the proper use of de-escalation procedures, use of PRN medications, working with other staff under pressure) that are integral to providing care with the goal of avoiding use of restraints in the first place. Supervisors can provide formal instruction and role-playing in deescalation techniques that are periodically needed in inpatient settings. Supervision should include direct observation of how trainees respond to emergencies as well as debriefing, feedback, and emotional support for the trainee.

Supervision Strategies and Techniques

Modeling

As Bandura (1977) remarked, "Most human behavior is learned observationally through modeling." Teaching new behavior is difficult. For instance, an expert's verbal descriptions of how to perform a behavior often omits critical but subtle components (e.g., vocal tone, body language). The senior clinician teaching active listening may not say anything about vocal tone or body language (e.g., eye contact, leaning forward), though these behaviors may be crucial to communicating attention and sincere interest and are immediately available to an observer.

Direct modeling of the behavior provides a rich guide to performance that speeds learning by avoiding the long process of trial and error (Greer et al. 2006). The modeled event can make for a lush context to focus discussion of the delicate aspects of interacting with patients—for example, when communicating the diagnosis of mental illness or negotiating the initiation of medications.

It should be noted that taking advantage of the efficiency of modeling for the trainee requires increased effort on the part of the supervisor. The supervisor must make time to model the behavior and then provide even more time to discuss the modeled event. In sum, the supervisor should teach by example and use live observation as a core element of training.

Direct Observation and Immediate Feedback

There is a voluminous literature on the factors that enhance the effect of feedback on learning (Hattie and Timperley 2007; van de Ridder et al. 2015). Immediate and frequent feedback enhances the speed of task acquisition and performance. Inpatient supervisors often directly observe the clinical activities of trainees and can thus provide feedback when the interaction is still fresh in the minds of all parties (e.g., after each patient is interviewed in rounds with an attending observing a trainee). Feedback is often more easily received if corrective comments are integrated with positive comments. It is preferred to offer feedback in a way that minimizes threats to the self-esteem of trainees, especially in an inpatient setting, where stress levels are already elevated. A full processing of each interaction may not be possible because of workload/time pressures, but the most important points can be reviewed in further detail during formal supervision sessions.

Optimizing Teaching and Supervision Powers of Interdisciplinary Teams

Comprehensive care of acutely ill inpatients typically requires the collaborative input of professionals from multiple disciplines. Social workers are typically involved in understanding the social supports of patients, formulating discharge plans, reaching out to families, and performing therapy. Psychologists may assist in diagnostic assessment, perform psychological testing, and offer individual and group psychotherapy. In addition, in some settings psychologists may provide formal supervision to psychiatry trainees, thus supplementing and broadening the supervision provided by psychiatry staff. Supervision by psychologists in inpatient settings can include training in the latest evidence-based psychotherapies, such as cognitive-behavioral therapy for psychosis, insomnia, and depression. Psychological assessment training by psychologists can teach psychiatry trainees about the rich complexity of cognitive functioning (e.g., assessment of executive functioning, distinct types of memory functioning), thus extending the knowledge of psychiatry trainees beyond mere mental status evaluations using screening instruments.

Supervisors should educate trainees about the unique contributions of interdisciplinary colleagues. Supervisors can provide ongoing suggestions for unique interdisciplinary learning (e.g., having psychiatry trainees observe the psychological testing performed by psychology trainees). Supervisors can emphasize to trainees that teams offer a setting for the practice of leadership skills that include collaboration, consensus building, and including the unique input of all other professions into clinical practice. In sum, an inpatient supervisor can mold and shape supervision for trainees so that it includes the unique input of diverse professions, an opportunity that is likely most easily obtained in inpatient settings.

Supervising Around High-Impact Events

Acute inpatient psychiatry is often the setting in which trainees have their first experiences with high-impact events such as restraining a patient, being threatened by a patient, having a patient be assaultive to staff or other patients, and, less commonly, being confronted by and having to address a suicidal behavior by the patient while on the unit or learning of such a behavior soon after the patient has left the hospital. Helping a trainee work through these experiences can be a difficult task requiring sensitivity and perspective.

Teaching trainees the proper procedures for dealing with high-impact events is often straightforward. For instance, most inpatient units have protocols for restraints—for example, trainees do not take part in therapeutic containments ("take-downs"). High-impact-event protocols should be communicated to trainees early in their inpatient training. One should address a trainee's personal reaction to the specific events that may come in rapid succession or combination—for example, when a trainee is threatened by a patient and then participates in restraining the patient. Immediate processing with the trainee is optimal.

The following tips are supervising high-impact events:

- Seek out trainees following high-impact events and be proactive in approaching trainees.
- Do not assume the trainee is traumatized by the event; inquire about his or her reaction to the event.
- Investigate the trainee's understanding of the event. What does he or she think happened and why?
- Gently determine whether the trainee feels responsible for a negative outcome (e.g., "I should've been able to calm him down so he wouldn't be violent").
- As much as possible, use the event as a teaching opportunity. Review response protocols. Review the event to determine what alternative actions could have been taken and when to have changed the outcome. Be careful not to engage in blame placing if possible, but be honest if the trainee made a mistake, as he or she needs to know.

Opportunities for Group Supervision

Many inpatient training settings have multiple psychiatry trainees or trainees from other disciplines (e.g., psychology) concurrently training in the programs. Group supervision can take the format of designated supervision groups with multiple trainees and/or supervisors. Additionally, a significant amount of group supervision can occur during team rounds, where patients may be interviewed with an interdisciplinary team and the meeting with a patient is reviewed by the full team after each patient is seen. Doing supervision in groups has many benefits (see Bernard and Goodyear 2009 for a review), including the following:

- Trainees are afforded an opportunity for learning from a range of supervisors and other trainees rather than just a single supervisor. Thus, trainees can obtain a much broader training experience, obtaining the viewpoints and suggestions of multiple perspectives and across disciplines.
- Trainees can obtain support from other trainees and gain perspective, emotional support, and normalization of training experiences in the intensive inpatient environment
- Trainees can obtain some experience in offering supervision to others and supervision groups allow for supervisors to do supervision of other trainees providing supervision.
- Supervision in a team rounds setting allows for real-time reflection and processing/debriefing, during which the trainee can speak an ask questions openly and honestly, and should be encouraged to do so.

Key Supervision Topics in Inpatient Mental Health

There has recently been a growing interest in the delineation of specific core competencies and directing training and supervision toward the mastery of these competencies. Supervision is optimized by detailing the target competencies as training goals at the initiation of inpatient supervision. In the following subsections, we outline helpful supervision and teaching strategies for some of the major core competencies and learning goals that are common to inpatient psychiatry.

Differential Diagnosis

Inpatient care demands a thorough admission evaluation of patients with the need for rapid and accurate diagnosis. A review of past records and obtaining collateral information from others who are familiar with the patient is essential. Learning goals includes the appropriate integration of history, clinical presentation, medical data, and collateral information. Supervision of trainees typically involves feedback on the decision-making process of the trainee in developing a diagnostic formulation. Trainees often need supervision in how to conduct diagnostic interviews that are as thorough as possible while recognizing that acutely ill patients may not tolerate lengthy questioning. Workload issues may place further time pressures on the ability to complete a comprehensive assessment.

Growth in diagnostic assessment of trainees is optimally shaped and taught from live observation. Some trainees benefit from reviewing structured clinical interviews such as the Structured Clinical Interview for DSM (First et al. 2002; now available for DSM-5 [SCID-5]; First et al. 2016). SCID provides examples of how questions should be asked so that patient responses are in keeping with DSM criteria. Additionally, structured interviews are designed as decision-making tools that ask the minimum number of questions while assessing for the maximum potential diagnoses. Thus, integration of a research tool into supervision may make for an effective teaching aid, especially for trainees who are acquiring a working knowledge of the diagnostic criteria and interviews skills.

Psychopharmacology

There are numerous unique aspects of inpatient training and supervision in psychopharmacology. Patients are often admitted in an acute state of decompensation and off-treatment medications. Supervision should be focused on how to select agents for treating targeted symptoms related to acute issues (e.g., lack of sleep, agitation) as well as the primary presenting diagnosis. Supervision can focus on emergent side effects (e.g., akathisia, dystonic reactions) that are more commonly related to medication initiation. Patients who remain in the hospital long enough (e.g., 2–3 weeks) can be a focus for supervision and teaching directed toward the features and speed of symptom improvement associated with medications. Many inpatient units have strong relationships with pharmacists who specialize in psychopharmacology, and trainee supervision benefits significantly from integrating these experts into the treatment team.

Optimal supervision includes didactics regarding selecting medication, teaching trainees to recognize and treat emergent side effects, and teaching trainees to use standardized outcome measures to measure the effects of pharmacological interventions.

Forensic Practice

Forensic situations (e.g., dangerousness warnings), which are only periodically encountered during outpatient practice, occur with regularity during inpatient care. Accordingly, supervisors in inpatient settings should offer ongoing teaching and supervision of forensic practice. Inpatient supervision necessitates teaching on involuntary civil commitment laws. Trainees must be closely supervised to ensure that the civil rights of patients are protected. Continued involuntary detention beyond the initial days of hospitalization often mandates a judicial review hearing. Such hearings in many cases represent the initial opportunity for trainees to serve as an expert witness. Supervisors should offer intensive supervision and training on the basics of the local civil commitment law as well as how to enter information into testimony. One can model and shape such events by conducting mock/practice testimony, attend court hearings to directly observe the trainee, and offer feedback as soon as feasible. Finally, trainees need training and ongoing supervision on how and when to make mandated reports that are required in cases of child and elder abuse/neglect.

Health Maintenance and Wellness

Postgraduate training is a stressful period, and it is important that supervisors make every effort to facilitate well-being. This can be difficult given time constraints but is an important supervisor responsibility. Supervisors may bring up situations that affect one's psychological and physical stability at the start of the rotation. A debriefing at the end of each day or after a difficult situation is often helpful. Providing individual supervision to discuss difficult patients and offering perspective and strategies on self-care during residency is valuable. Supervision can include discussions on the prevention of burn out, mindfulness, exercise, and therapy. Thus, supervision can educate trainees about self-care and group supervision sessions on these topics may be especially useful in drawing on the experiences of multiple trainees and supervisors. In sum, a culture that encourages trainees to be proactive in their health maintenance benefits the trainees and the patients they treat.

Supervising Leadership and Supervision Skills

Inpatient units often have entry-level trainees (e.g., medical students, psychology practicum students), and supervision for these students is often provided by more senior trainees. Accordingly, supervisors may often be required to assist trainees in the "supervision of supervision." Trainees may need assistance in learning how to form a supervisory relationship, maintain appropriate boundaries, and provide feedback to other trainees for likely the first time in their careers. It is often helpful for supervisors to share with trainees their own personal reflections on experiences about when they themselves were new supervisors.

Specific Challenges and Strategies

- **My supervisee is frustrated by my desire to get a medicine consult.** The intersection between medicine and psychiatry can be a challenge for some supervisors. Some supervisors insist that all things medical need to be covered by medicine specialists, whereas others view inpatient psychiatry as a unique opportunity to teach the basics of medicine and model a holistic mind-body approach. Those who believe medical problems need to be addressed solely by a consult service are likely to encounter resistance from residents who may have completed medicine rotations and thus feel broadly skilled. Such situations can be handled with an open discussion explaining one's point of view and rationale. Often statements such as "I realize this is confusing, but I would like to explain to you the rationale behind my method of practice" are helpful to facilitate dialogue. In sum, one often needs to provide supervision on how and when to obtain consultation from other medical services.

- **My supervisee has a difficult time when I deviate from evidence-based practices.** Patients are frequently admitted on a regimen of medications that are not consistent with evidence-based practice. Some challenging patients require multiple medications to obtain behavioral control. These situations can be difficult for new psychiatry trainees. The first step for the supervising psychiatrist is to acknowledge that the situation is atypical and then develop an action plan. These supervision situations provide an opportunity to seek pharmacy consultation, thus modeling for trainees how to seek consultation from other specialists. Collaboration in patient care needs to be modelled, demonstrating to trainees that supervisors are open to consultation from others. Comments such as "I know this is confusing, I am also confused" may reassure trainees and diffuse tension. These challenging clinical situations allow a supervisor to explain the vagaries of psychiatry and clinical medicine, resulting in a rich discussion about challenges in learning.

- **My supervisee knows way more than me!** Some trainees function at a level beyond their level of training. They are efficient, learn quickly, get the job done, seem to know more than one would expect, and have a fund of knowledge from prior professional experiences. These trainees can pose a challenge for supervisors as they look for ways to make clinical training more relevant and challenging. The supervisor can sometimes feel put on the spot by the questions the resident poses not because they are trying to do so but simply because the trainee thinks deeply and is analytical in approach. The supervisor may feel unsettled with knowing less than the trainee in certain areas. Recognizing the competence and advanced status of some of trainees provides a good start for supervisors. Such trainees may benefit from the setting of unique and specific training goals from the outset, thus seeking additional resources or training opportunities in their area of interest. The supervisor needs to avoid falling into the rabbit hole of self-doubt and pressure to please. Such situations are reminders to supervisors to look inward and to take stock of one's strengths and acknowledge areas that one needs to work on—an opportunity of growth and modeling. In sum, some trainees can provide rich learning experiences for supervisors.

- **I don't know how to manage this difficult resident.** At times supervisors have the uncomfortable and difficult experience of supervising a trainee who is problematic for reasons ranging from cutting corners to not completing work, misrepresenting facts, and other problems. Such situations are difficult and need to be addressed in a balanced and fair-minded manner. It may help to consult with a colleague to see if he or she has had similar experiences with the trainee. If there is sufficient reason for concern it would be appropriate to talk with the trainee while keeping in mind that the goal is not to reprimand but to problem-solve. It is often important for the supervisor to understand the current life stressors of the trainee that may be affecting his or her functioning. Sometimes it may be sufficient to have a frank and constructive discussion about expectations. Offering support, clarifying expectations, and setting a time frame for improvement is an effective strategy. Accusations and finger pointing are rarely effective and are counter-productive.

- **I'm feeling so burned out (and my resident is too!).** Supervisors are often aware of the extended time commitments required to support and supervise trainees in addition to completing their routine responsibilities. Supervisors may experience long days and stress while trying to balance work and personal life. Supervisors may benefit from carrying out advanced planning, optimizing efficiency, and focusing on time management. Supervisors experience stress reduction from having an acceptance of an unpredictable schedule. Supervisors need an awareness that trainees are impressionable and are quick to absorb both positive and negative experiences. It is imperative that supervisor habits enhance patient care and model professionalism. The ability to help trainees be aware of their values and to understand that clinical care is not just about doing things right but about something bigger is a role that is bestowed on providers by the trusting patient.

Questions for the Supervisor

■ Has the trainee been adequately oriented on unit procedures, on safety measures, and on where and how to meet with patients?

■ Have I integrated extensive modeling for the trainee?

■ Have I demonstrated interview and assessment techniques?

■ Have I directly observed the trainee while engaged in clinical care and offered immediate and useful feedback?

■ Do I adequately process recent high-impact events (e.g., restraint use, assault, significant agitation) with the trainee, determine the impact on the trainee, and offer adequate supports and teaching around the event?

Additional Resources

Crowder MK, Jack RA: Educational opportunities and inpatient psychiatry. Psychiatr Med 4(4):417–429, 1987

Greenberg WE, Borus JF: Focused opportunities for resident education on today's inpatient psychiatric units. Harv Rev Psychiatry 22(3):201–203, 2014

Houghtalen RP, Guttmacher LB: Facilitating effective residency education on short-term inpatient units. Psychiatric Quarterly 67(2):111–124, 1996

Lim S, Rohrbaugh R: Why inpatient psychiatry training still matters (now more than ever). Acad Psychiatry 31(4):266–269, 2007

References

Bandura A: Social Learning Theory. New York, General Learning Press, 1977

Bernard JM, Goodyear RK: Fundamentals of Clinical Supervision. Colombus, OH, Merrill, 2009

Douglas KS, Hart SD, Webster CD, et al: Historical Clinical Risk Management–20, Version 3: development and overview. International Journal of Forensic Mental Health 13:93–108, 2014

First MB, Spitzer RL, Gibbon M, et al: Structured Clinical Interview for DSM-IV-TR Axis I Disorders, Research Version, Patient Edition (SCID-I/P). New York, Biometrics Research, New York State Psychiatric Institute, 2002

First MB, Williams JBW, Karg RS, Spitzer RL: Structured Clinical Interview for DSM-5— Clinician Version (SCID-5-CV). Arlington, VA, American Psychiatric Association Publishing, 2016

Greer RD, Dudek-Singer J, Gautreaux G: Observational learning. Int J Psychol 41:486–499, 2006

Hattie J, Timperley H: The power of feedback. Rev Educ Res 77:81–112, 2007

Iozzino L, Ferrari C, Large M, et al: Prevalence and risk factors of violence by psychiatric acute inpatients: a systematic review and meta-analysis. PLoS One 10(6):e0128536, 2015 26061796

van de Ridder JM, McGaghie WC, Stokking KM, et al: Variables that affect the process and outcome of feedback, relevant for medical training: a meta-review. Med Educ 49(7):658–673, 2015 26077214

Chapter 15 Night Float

Working With Supervisees Remotely

Kristin S. Raj, M.D.

Sallie G. De Golia, M.D., M.P.H.

Night float (NF) supervision is unique. Unlike in most other supervisory situations, the supervisor rarely, if ever, makes face-to-face contact with a patient and/or supervisee, and, occasionally, may never meet the supervisee during training. This supervision typically takes place by phone, texting, emailing or other digital formats and is described as "indirect" or "remote." As such, the complex process of developing trust with the supervisee and overseeing patient safety and care while also enhancing a supervisee's skill base presents unique challenges for this mode of supervision.

NF presents an important opportunity for residents to hone independent decision making and time-efficiency skills (Bricker and Markert 2010). However, the challenge of the NF supervisor is to provide enough supervision while allowing for graduated or progressive levels of autonomy so that supervisees gain skills and experience. Failing to provide enough supervision places patients at risk and leaves supervisees feeling abandoned and uncertain; too much oversight fails to offer supervisees needed opportunities to learn through practice, may generate feelings of apathy and lack of faith in their own competence, and may leave them unprepared to practice independently (Farnan et al. 2009; Kashner et al. 2010).

Bricker and Markert (2010) reported poor ratings associated with NF rotations compared with other rotations in areas of continuity of patient care, establishment of expectations between the attending and resident, amount of didactics, feedback, discussion on history and physicals, clinical decision making, and role modeling. However, with improved supervisory strategies, NF can represent a venue full of rich educational opportunities for residents (Hanson et al. 2014). Although this chapter focuses on NF, many of these strategies also apply to supervising on-call residents.

Key Points

- Clarify expectations at the beginning of the shift, including importance of communicating uncertainty and the ability to seek guidance as needed and required.

- Assess the supervisee's competence early in the rotation either through direct communication, demonstrated behaviors paired with outcomes, and/or feedback from colleagues.

- Utilize specific supervisory techniques to optimize the educational experience.

Setting Up Night Float Supervision

The supervisor might contact the supervisee at the beginning of the supervisee's shift to introduce himself or herself and find out about the supervisee's prior experience on NF. What has been most difficult? What tends to be most anxiety-provoking while working independently at night? How might the supervisor best help develop their skills? Supervisors should keep these goals in mind as they work with residents throughout the rotation. If the supervisor and supervisee work more than a few nights together, the supervisor might check in with the supervisee to see if needs are being met and how the supervisor might be more useful.

The supervisor should also clarify expectations at the start of a shift, including how cases might be presented, timing and content of documentation, and when to call (e.g., patient discharges, uncertainty about medication regimens, concern for substance withdrawal, at the end of shifts, when a patient goes in or out of restraints, and any time if needing support). The supervisor should be clear about the need to call should any concerns or uncertainty on behalf of the supervisee arise.

Assessing a New Supervisee

Supervising trainees indirectly the first time can be stress-invoking because supervisors worry about the level of supervisees' skills and clinical competence. Where on the continuum does the supervisee lie regarding ability to identify what he or she knows and does not know? How willing is the supervisee to seek supervision if needed? How accurate is the supervisee's self-assessment? Although physicians have been shown to be poor self-assessors (Davis et al. 2006), the supervisor should try to evaluate the supervisee's capacity and accuracy of self-assessment. Knowing when to seek guidance provides the greatest security to patient safety.

Other strategies to assess supervisee competency and develop a level of trust involve use of one or more of the following approaches.

Funnel Information Approach

The supervisor might ask the supervisee to begin supervisory calls by providing detailed case presentations, assessments, and plans. The supervisor can evaluate whether the supervisee has collected all pertinent information, considered an appropriate differential, and carefully thought through a plan for each problem. The supervisor assesses where the supervisee tends to omit important information and whether he or she understood the relevance of information presented and is able to appropriately ask for guidance in developing a plan. Once the supervisor has a better sense of the supervisee's level of competence, the supervisor can ask the supervisee to *funnel down* the amount of material presented in subsequent cases. However, this approach is time intensive and requires exquisite focus, particularly in the middle of the night.

Process Approach

It is important for supervisees to be aware of what they do and do not know, and to understand that seeking guidance when uncertain and/or required is critical. The supervisor should model for the supervisee how to talk through one's thought process about a case, including areas of uncertainty. If done in a nonjudgmental way, this helps the supervisee understand what the supervisor is looking for and how to express reservation and/or a knowledge deficit. The supervisor should also, if necessary, explore ways to help the supervisee decrease barriers to seeking guidance. This is particularly challenging not only because developing a "remote" alliance is difficult enough, but because helping a subordinate convey a deficiency is not easy, particularly to someone who will be an evaluator of one's performance.

Life or Death Approach

Often the goal of NF is not to perform a comprehensive psychiatric consultation but rather to conduct a semifocused evaluation in order to stabilize and/or determine immediate disposition of the patient. In this setting, the supervisor may choose to specifically hone in on the aspect of greatest importance: assuring a patient's safety. With this in mind, a supervisor could have a set of "must-address" points for a supervisee. For example, for a patient with a history of suicidal ideation who is being considered for discharge from the emergency department (ED), has access to weapons been evaluated and documented? For the admission to the psychiatric ward, has daily alcohol consumption and risk of withdrawal been assessed? Develop a list of "life or death" scenarios to ensure that critical items are considered by the supervisee in the appropriate setting. This allows the supervisor to quickly identify safety omissions, address important educational opportunities, and ultimately assuage (or intensify) any trust issues with a supervisee.

Communication

Because of the lack of a face-to-face encounter with patients *and* supervisees, clear communication is critical in describing what supervisors and supervisees expect, feel, observe, and are concerned about in the context of patient care, education, and support. Feelings, intentions, or feedback that is often communicated through nonverbal cues must be communicated as clearly, accurately, and *explicitly* as possible during NF rotations.

Practicing clear communication about how a patient presents is a useful skill for communicating with colleagues in the future. The supervisor should ask the supervisee to *paint a picture* of what the supervisor might see if he or she were present. If something seems missing in a narrative, the supervisor should encourage a supervisee to be explicit about assumptions made and to describe a mental status in greater detail, or perhaps ask for a moment-by-moment description of events in order to piece the "video" together.

Educational Techniques

Night float allows supervisees to develop autonomy in their clinical reasoning and case management. The supervisor can foster this specific educational opportunity by utilizing some of the following strategies.

Socratic Questioning

Use of Socratic questioning may help supervisees develop clinical reasoning, expand their knowledge base, and identify gaps in competencies. Although challenging in the middle of the night, supervisors should encourage supervisees to describe their plan with reasons prior to offering their own thoughts on a plan. At times, supervisees might see the attending as a "phone-a-friend" answer to any question that arises. For example, when supervisees pose questions about the starting dose of a medication or questions that might require a quick review of the literature, the supervisor should ask them how *they* might find the answer. This promotes independence as well as encourages development of life-long learning skills.

Talking Out Loud

Supervisors often worry about worse-case scenarios occurring at night. Modeling how to think through a case by talking out loud allows supervisees to observe the attendings' thought processes and how attendings prevent or mitigate potential negative outcomes. It also helps them learn how the burden of liability for potential negative outcomes can mitigate the risk one is willing to take on. This approach may also help supervisees identify gaps in their knowledge as well as in their ability to process a case.

Listening for Reasons Not to Pursue a Plan

When a supervisee presents a patient, the supervisor should listen for reasons why a proposed plan might not be appropriate. For example, a supervisee may make a case for dropping a hold on a patient who came to the ER with suicidal ideation. The supervisor should listen for stated (or not stated) reasons why this may not be an optimal plan (e.g., no collateral provided, no social support at home, no psychiatric follow-up). The supervisee should be queried about any concerns until satisfied with an agreed-on plan.

Reviewing Prior NF Cases

If supervising for more than one day in a row with the same supervisee, the supervisor can provide the supervisee with the opportunity to learn from recent patient outcomes. The supervisor should ask follow-up questions on any patient admitted together in prior days to provide learning opportunities in diagnosis, course of illness, treatment, or systems issues. If the outcome of a case was unexpected, supervisor and supervisee can explore together whether this was due to something missed at the initial evaluation, or if the diagnosis required more time to reveal itself. Were there barriers to obtaining needed information? If the day team changed an intervention or discharged a patient unexpectedly, what was the reason? Was there something overlooked, or does the case provide an opportunity to discuss alternative ways of managing cases? The process of working through these questions together with the supervisee may help NF shifts feel more collaborative and foster an excitement and curiosity about learning as well as model practice-based learning approaches.

Evaluation and Feedback

Supervisees prefer a collaborative approach to supervision that includes constructive feedback (Busari et al. 2005). The supervisor should communicate early and directly about those aspects on which the supervisee will be evaluated. This might include prioritization of patient safety, recognition and communication of risk, provision of clear presentations and accurate documentation, ability to seek attending help when needed, ability to recognize and articulate limitations while also presenting one's own conceptualized reasoning and plan, accountability, and follow-through (Table 15–1). Once evaluation of the supervisee has taken place, the supervisor should provide specific feedback on areas in which the supervisee is performing well and on areas requiring improvement. Timing of feedback presents a potential challenge during NF. Supervisees usually call supervisors with a semi-urgent question, an ED discharge, or sign out after a tiresome shift—less than ideal times to provide feedback—and, therefore, the learning opportunity may be lost. The supervisor should try providing brief and specific feedback in the moment rather than waiting until shift end. Another method is to set up a specific time in which to give feedback, such as at the end of the shift following sign out (see Chapter 1, "Elements of Supervision").

Specific Challenges and Strategies

- **Supervisees don't call when they are uncertain.** Because of a program's "culture," or hidden curriculum, supervisees might feel discouraged to ask for help despite uncertainty. Pressures to maximize productivity and efficiency can also motivate supervisees to migrate beyond boundaries of safe practice (Kennedy et al. 2009; Rotenstein et al. 2016). Reassuring a supervisee that it is okay to call is often not sufficient to create behavior change. It is more effective for a supervisor to specify scenarios in which to call (Loo et al. 2012). For example, "Feel welcome to call at any time, and especially prior to considering discharge for any patient, uncer-

TABLE 15–1.   Night float (NF) and Call skills that meet expectations

NF/Call skills	Meets expectations	Progressing	Unable to assess
Knowledge			
1. Recognizes and communicates risk			
2. Prioritizes patient safety			
3. Presents a concise, organized, and accurate case summary with patient findings and pertinent positives and negatives			
4. Presents a complete and/or relevant mental status exam			
5. Presents a reasoned, conceptualized plan for patient care			
6. Articulates an appropriate capacity assessment			
Administrative			
1. Articulates regulations and guidelines for supervision			
2. Demonstrates appropriate documentation of involuntary paperwork			
3. Provides accurate and appropriate written documentation			
4. Demonstrates how to place orders			
Process			
1. Uses active listening with supervisor			
2. Modifies interview style based upon patient presentation and need			
3. Demonstrates willingness to seek assistance			
4. Incorporates feedback and modifies performance			
5. Accurately self-assesses areas for growth or in need of greater supervision			
6. Describes comfort with performing on call tasks with indirect supervision			
7. Demonstrates an ability to recognize and articulate limitations			

tainty about an admission plan, or potential for withdrawal. I can also be of assistance with logistical or social challenges."

- **Supervisees don't want to call because they're trying to develop their independence.** Supervisees feel a pressure to work independently as they strive to lay claim to their identity as doctors. The unspoken rules of the medical community encourage supervisees to integrate the talk and practices of those more experienced before having the knowledge and skills to back them up. This can make it challenging for an attending to identify the skill level of a supervisee based on expressed confidence or self-report (Kennedy et al. 2009). Making the implicit explicit can help with this challenge. The supervisor can clarify for supervisees that they are likely striving to develop their autonomy, and explain that it is important for the supervisor to stay abreast of specific issues for liability, patient safety, and to serve as back-up for blind spots supervisees may have while learning. As a supervisor becomes more comfortable with a supervisee's skillset, the supervisor can begin to tailor aspects of oversight.

Questions for the Supervisee

■ What would you like to do for this patient and why?

■ Is there any more information you would need prior to deciding between those two options?

■ How did presenting that patient to me go for you? Anything you would make sure to keep doing next time? Change for your next presentation? Do you think I'm left with any burning questions after hearing the presentation?

■ How have you been progressing over the course of night float? Are you growing in your sense of confidence and autonomy? How can I help support and teach you?

Additional Resources

Farnan JM, Johnson JK, Meltzer DO, et al: Strategies for effective on-call supervision for internal medicine residents: the superb/safety model. J Grad Med Educ 2(1):46–52, 2010

References

Bricker DA, Markert RJ: Night float teaching and learning: perceptions of residents and faculty. J Grad Med Educ 2(2):236–241, 2010 21975627

Busari JO, Weggelaar NM, Knottnerus AC, et al: How medical residents perceive the quality of supervision provided by attending doctors in the clinical setting. Med Educ 39(7):696–703, 2005 15960790

Davis DA, Mazmanian PE, Fordis M, et al: Accuracy of physician self-assessment compared with observed measures of competence: a systematic review. JAMA 296(9):1094–1102, 2006 16954489

Farnan JM, Johnson JK, Meltzer DO, et al: On-call supervision and resident autonomy: from micromanager to absentee attending. Am J Med 122(8):784–788, 2009 19635283

Hanson JT, Pierce RG, Dhaliwal G: The new education frontier: clinical teaching at night. Acad Med 89(2):215–218, 2014 24362386

Kashner TM, Byrne JM, Henley SS, et al: Measuring progressive independence with the resident supervision index: theoretical approach. J Grad Med Educ 2(1):8–16, 2010 21975879

Kennedy TJT, Regehr G, Baker GR, et al: "It's a cultural expectation..." The pressure on medical trainees to work independently in clinical practice. Med Educ 43(7):645–653, 2009 19573187

Loo L, Puri N, Kim DI, et al: "Page me if you need me:" the hidden curriculum of attending-resident communication. J Grad Med Educ 4(3):340–345, 2012 23997879

Rotenstein LS, Ramos MA, Torre M, et al: Prevalence of depression, depressive symptoms, and suicidal ideation among medical students a systematic review and meta-analysis. JAMA 316(21):2214–2236, 2016 27923088

Chapter 16 Hospital-Based Consultation-Liaison and Emergency Department Supervision

Margaret May, M.D.

Divy Ravindranath, M.D.

Consultation-liaison (CL) psychiatry and emergency psychiatry rotations widen the practice of hospital-based psychiatric care beyond the psychiatry wards. These unique Accreditation Council for Graduate Medical Education (ACGME)–mandated clinical experiences embed supervisees in multi-disciplinary settings, working alongside emergency medicine, internal medicine, and surgical care providers (Accreditation Council for Graduate Medical Education 2017). Given that supervisees often field consultation requests and perform emergency psychiatric evaluations during their call shifts as early as intern year, the skills covered in these rotations comprise several core psychiatric competencies that warrant introduction at the outset of training followed by elaboration and reinforcement during the clinical rotations. Surveys demonstrate that, particularly during call shifts, direct supervision may not always be available; yet the importance of appropriate supervision (particularly directly available supervision early in training) is increasingly emphasized in the updated ACGME Common Program Requirements (Bennett et al. 2010).

Supervision in these settings provides opportunity to emphasize professional and clinical development in the domains of psychiatric assessment, clinical decision making based on acuity and risk assessment, and, crucially, effective cross-discipline liaison skills given the integrated nature of the services being provided. Supervisors must be especially attuned to the advancement of these skills to facilitate supervisees' ability to collaborate with, guide, and advise other members of the medical profession. For a field that struggles with the stigma of mental illness even among fellow physicians, this work remains critically important. Furthermore, at least one study has drawn a connection between the quality of emergency psychiatry training conditions and future plans to treat publicly funded patients, which represents a significant public health need (Dennis and Swartz 2015).

In addition to serving the education of psychiatry trainees, the CL and emergency department (ED) environments are ideal educational experiences for supervisees who will develop into non-mental health providers (e.g., medical students, nurse practitioner students). These supervisees benefit from learning an approach to psychiatric assessment that will be applicable for the patients they encounter in future hospital, ED, and ambulatory settings.

Key Points

- Core learning objectives in CL and ED psychiatry cover many key elements of the six ACGME core competencies.

- CL and ED psychiatry rotations are unique experiences in psychiatric assessment and decision-making in an interdisciplinary setting.

- Diversity and unpredictability of consultation questions and ED presentations can create challenges in workflow, supervision and systematic learning.

- A variety of supervision formats may be appropriate based on the training level of the resident.

- Unique challenges include managing agitated patients, ensuring safety during assessment, triaging workflow, working collaboratively between disciplines, and navigating team dynamics.

- Supervision should help provide a blueprint for the liaison role of psychiatrists in collaborative care, necessitating a focus on professionalism and interpersonal communication skills.

Core Learning Objectives in Consultation-Liaison and Emergency Department Psychiatry

Core learning objectives in CL and ED psychiatry cover many key elements of the six ACGME core competencies. Table 16–1 provides an outline of common learning objectives.

TABLE 16–1.	Common learning objectives for consultation-liaison and emergency psychiatry rotations
Patient care and medical knowledge	Identify and manage delirium
	Identify and manage agitation
	Identify and manage substance intoxication and withdrawal
	Perform dangerousness (suicide and violence) risk assessments
	Perform grave disability assessments
	Appropriately recommend admission to inpatient psychiatry units
	Assess for appropriate level of medical clearance
	Identify psychiatric versus non-psychiatric behavioral disturbances
Professionalism	Ensure timely response to requests for assistance
	Accept consultation requests in a courteous manner
	Pay attention to input from ancillary health care staff where appropriate
	Ensure respectful involvement of patients' families where appropriate
	Manage transitions in goals of care
Interpersonal and communication	Clarify the consultation question
	Ensure collegial communication of recommendations
	Attempt to understand multiple collaborator perspectives
	Maintain involvement in multidisciplinary team meetings
	Maintain involvement in family meetings
	Provide documentation for multiple audiences
	Identify areas of communication breakdown
Practice-based learning	Develop familiarity with standardized cognitive assessment instruments
	Develop familiarity with evidence base for patient care objectives
	Include clinical reasoning using evidence base in documentation
	Survey literature for relevant evidence
Systems-based practice	Call a consult
	Track consult productivity
	Develop safety protocols
	Develop delirium prevention protocols
	Ensure appropriate involvement of ancillary staff (social workers, case managers, nurses)
	Ensure appropriate involvement of consultative services (neuropsychology, bioethics, neurology)

Formats of Supervision

Many supervision formats are applicable to the CL and ED environments, each with their own benefits and drawbacks.

Direct Observation

Early supervisees may require direct observation by their supervisor. In this format, the supervisee and the supervisor engage the patient together. It can start with either party taking the lead, but the supervisee should have an opportunity to talk with the patient while the supervisor observes. This allows the supervisor to assess the supervisee's capacity for patient engagement and safety assessment skills. The supervisor can also step in to redirect a patient encounter that may be heading in the wrong direction. However, direct observation may also intimidate the learner and confuse the patient given that there are two people "in charge."

Sequential Rounding

In this format, the supervisee sees the patient first, followed by the supervisor. This allows the supervisee to take a central role in the patient encounter. The drawback of this format is that the patient is engaged at two different time points. This format can become even more cumbersome if there are multiple supervisees, and can risk confusing the patient or taking up their time unnecessarily. This format is most appropriate for intermediate-stage supervisees, who are comfortable talking with a patient alone and sufficiently skilled that they will not irritate or agitate the patient.

Asynchronous Supervision

More advanced supervisees may benefit from a format where supervision occurs asynchronously. The supervisee would see a series of patients and bank questions for processing during a prespecified supervision time. This format is common in outpatient practices. However, the supervisee would need to be sufficiently advanced such that waiting for the supervision does not interrupt patient care or lead to negative patient outcomes. This format is also sometimes used on call shifts for routine concerns; supervisees on-call may be instructed to call for any admission or discharge decisions but to save discussion of routine floor management until the end of their call shift.

Each format of supervision has a role within the CL and ED environments but needs to be selected for correct fit with the supervisee and the clinical situation. A supervisor may ask to attend all new patient encounters, especially early in a rotation, such that work is done quickly and the supervisor has a chance to assess the supervisee skill level. Supervision can then shift to a sequential format and feedback can shift from reporter/interpreter themes to interpreter/manager themes. At the end of the rotation, or for more senior supervisees, the supervisor may choose to pursue asynchronous supervision, giving the supervisee the freedom to be independent in his or her assessments and the supervisor time to pursue other activities. Feedback in this format is more in line with manager themes. However, an urgent clinical matter, such as a consult at the end of the day or a highly agitated patient in the ED, may result in reversion to a direct observation format for purposes of efficiency. In this way it is important for the supervisor to exercise flexibility to shift between formats and to communicate the fluctuating expectations to the supervisee for clarity.

Supervision must also occur at the level of the supervisee's interactions with referring providers. A beginning supervisee may need to be directly observed when communicating recommendations to the referring providers to ensure that the correct information is communicated. Interruption by the supervisor to clarify points may be considered, but doing so risks diminishing the supervisee's standing in the eyes of the referring providers, making it harder to build rapport within that dyad. An intermediate or advanced supervisee may be trusted to communicate recommendations directly to the treatment team, giving them more opportunity to develop their own collegial style.

Specific Challenges and Strategies

- **It's difficult to predict work flow!** Sequencing of a patient's psychiatric evaluation on these rotations can be more complex than on psychiatric units because of the unpredictability of requests, triaging of acuity, the number of medical teams involved, and the simultaneous management of other medical issues (Blair et al. 2017). In practice, this means that patients and referring providers may be hard to locate. The supervisor should discuss strategies with supervisees at the outset: calling the unit clerk ahead of time to discuss a patient's schedule, for example, or sharing the contact information and typical charting locations of referring providers.
- **My supervisee has a difficult time getting a good patient history on CL.** Patients with shameful, paranoid, or anxious emotions may not be forthcoming in a medical environment, which usually offers less privacy. Interviewing sessions may be disrupted by other aspects of care. These challenges can be mitigated by establishing as much privacy as possible at the outset, teaching rapid rapport-building tools, and pre-formulating the most important pieces of information to get in an interview in case time is cut short. Supervisors should be understanding that information may come in piecemeal and that some details can be clarified on follow-up.
- **My supervisees worry about their physical safety as well as that of their agitated patients.** Many patients in the CL and ED environments are agitated and/or in altered states of consciousness. Moreover, both environments contain greater access to dangerous items and contraband than is allowed on an inpatient psychiatric unit. A major challenge to supervision and clinical care in these environments is the issue of physical safety. A supervisee who is afraid for their safety may struggle to engage the patient fully. To facilitate physical safety, basic training in recognition and management of agitation should be presented at the outset, and every encounter with an agitated patient should be debriefed. A direct observation supervision format may be most helpful; supervisor modeling of de-escalation techniques or the decision to leave an interview is valuable. Attunement to "gut instincts" regarding safety should be emphasized.
- **My supervisees aren't used to patients dying on service.** This is less the case in other training environments, and it can leave the supervisee who has invested emotional energy into the patient relationship feeling numb or bereaved (Ponce Martinez et al. 2017). Patients who die by suicide can be especially challenging and

raise doubts and anxieties within supervisees about their clinical skills or malpractice actions. Thus, a core task of the supervisor is to recognize these emotional experiences and guide reflection and self-care as appropriate. Encounters that include a patient's death can be turned into opportunities to explore learning objectives associated with palliative care.

- **My supervisees struggle with patients who may present with secondary gain.** Confronting the challenge of patients who present for care because of secondary gain presents a unique learning opportunity. The term *malingering* is often used in the emergency setting, somewhat pejoratively, to insinuate a knowing manipulation of the hospital's resources, but patients' insight into such behaviors may be poor. In many cases, the patients may simply be using a limited set of coping strategies having failed to achieve various outcomes in other ways. These patients may elicit negative counter-transference; supervision provides a unique opportunity to model a compassionate approach and to reduce bias that might occur. Behavioral approaches that positively reinforce preferred behaviors should be emphasized as well as strategies to set appropriate boundaries in a professional manner.

Questions for the Supervisee

- What is the consult question being asked? Is there an unstated question underneath it?

- What do you think the consulting or referring team is most worried about?

- How do you think the emergency department doctors are thinking about this patient?

- What are the treatment decisions that need to be made at this stage and how do these interrelate with the patient's general medical treatment plan?

- What factors will you use to determine the acuity of this patient's presentation?

- What feelings did the patient, team, collaborator, and staff member bring up in you?

- Where is the communication in this situation going wrong? What parts remain confusing (and to whom)?

- How do you think the patient and/or family are experiencing this issue?

- Who are the most important people to be connecting with about the care issues?

- What are the most crucial pieces of information that we need to get right now? (in advance of starting an interview)

- What did we do well and what could we have done better to manage that patient's behavior? (for debriefing encounters where a patient becomes physically or verbally assaultive)

Additional Resources

Gitlin DF, Schindler BA, Stern TA et al: Recommended guidelines for consultation-liaison psychiatry training in psychiatry residency programs: a report from the Academy of Psychosomatic Medicine Task Force on Psychiatric Resident Training in Consultation-Liaison Psychiatry. Psychosomatics 37(1): 3–11, 1996

Husarewycz MN, Fleisher W, Skakum K: Medical training in psychiatric residency: the PGY-1 experience, 2014 update. Can J Psychiatry 60(6):1–8, 2015

Worley LLM, Levenson JL, Stern TA et al: Core competencies for fellowship training in psychosomatic medicine: a collaborative effort by the APA Council on Psychosomatic Medicine, the ABPN Psychosomatic Committee, and the Academy of Psychosomatic Medicine. Psychosomatics 50(6):557–562, 2009

References

Accreditation Council for Graduate Medical Education: Program requirements for graduate medical education in psychiatry. July 1, 2017b. Available at: https://www.acgme.org/Portals/0/PFAssets/ProgramRequirements/400_psychiatry_2017-07-01.pdf. Accessed July 28, 2017.

Bennett JI, Costin G, Khan M, et al: Postgraduate year-1 residency training in emergency psychiatry: an acute care psychiatric clinic at a community mental health center. J Grad Med Educ 2(3):462–466, 2010 21976099

Blair T, Wiener Z, Seroussi A, et al: resident workflow and psychiatric emergency consultation: identifying factors for quality improvement in a training environment. Acad Psychiatry 41(3):377–380, 2017 27928767

Dennis NM, Swartz MS: Emergency psychiatry experience, resident burnout, and future plans to treat publicly funded patients. Psychiatr Serv 66(8):892–895, 2015 25873026

Ponce Martinez C, Suratt CE, Chen DT: cases that haunt us: the rashomon effect and moral distress on the consult service. Psychosomatics 58(2):191–196, 2017 27979603

Chapter 17

Psychopharmacology Clinic Supervision

G. Mark Freeman Jr., M.D., Ph.D.

Sixty minutes can feel like an eternity when you are stuck inside a full-capacity airliner that is grounded on the tarmac; however, for even the most experienced psychiatrists, 60 minutes (the time frequently allotted for an initial psychopharmacology intake) can feel very brief. Patients are complex and often walk into psychiatrists' offices burdened by decades of ill health, psychosocial hurdles, trauma, and possibly less-than-satisfactory patient-doctor relationships. Within these contexts, how do psychiatrists learn to effectively and efficiently assess and treat patients while also developing strong therapeutic alliances? Effective supervision during training can prove essential in this regard.

Yet despite the fundamental importance of clinical supervision, trainees often experience widely varying types and degrees of such supervision. Secondary to the structure of many training programs, ambulatory care is often pushed toward the latter half of training when supervising physicians may assume that trainees already have internalized much of what they need to know. However, outpatient psychiatry has its own unique set of challenges to which trainees are frequently unaware. For example, trainees often have difficulty dealing with the sense of powerlessness that can be felt when a patient at elevated risk walks out the office door. Supervision is essential both to help trainees properly contextualize these experiences and to provide the fundamental academic and logistical knowledge necessary for them to operate later as independent practitioners.

Key Points

- Always use an overarching biopsychosocial formulation to guide clinical care.

- Emphasize the importance of therapeutic alliance.

- Be explicit about goals and expectations of supervision.

- Know the "stage" of your trainee, and work to advance him or her to the next stage.

- Use measurement-based care to enhance supervision.

It's Not All About the Medications: The Formulation

The mere label of "psychopharmacology clinic" often suggests to trainees that these clinics are where they learn outpatient medication management. In fact, these clinics are where they learn outpatient psychiatric *care*. This is not a subtle distinction, and supervisors should emphasize this point from the first day onward. When patients first visit a psychiatry office, they may or may not believe that medications will be prescribed; what they will most certainly believe is that the doctor will carefully assess their concerns and offer informed recommendations. Recommendations may include medications; however, they may also emphasize psychotherapy, social work services, work/volunteerism, or many other nonpharmacological interventions. It is crucial to ensure that trainees learn to think about mental health treatment holistically, especially if they hope to aid their patients in maximal recovery.

Action Item

Routinely ask trainees to provide an oral biopsychosocial formulation of their patients (even for frequently seen patients) and have them routinely address both pharmacological and nonpharmacological interventions (even if the recommendation is "no change").

It's Not All About the Medications: The Alliance

An oft-cited analysis of the Treatment of Depression Collaborative Research Program indicates that prescriber attributes can greatly affect clinical outcomes (McKay et al. 2006; see also the article by Mintz and Flynn [2012] in "Additional Resources" near end of this chapter). In brief, even under controlled clinical trial conditions, some psychiatrists can repeatedly achieve better results with placebo than others do with active drug. While it was not possible to flesh out the specific prescriber attributes in this particular study, accumulating evidence points to the *therapeutic alliance* as being crucial (Figure 17–1).

Action Item

Have trainees ask their patients during the first visit, "What has been the most important part of your previous encounters with doctors?" Not only does the question help trainees to know what their individual patients value, but it can also signal to patients that their doctor cares about their experiences, and it will naturally start the therapeutic relationship out on the right track. Asking questions such as "Have you had any experiences with doctors that were less positive? If so, what was it that made it difficult?" can help doctors understand possible areas of difficulty in alliance building.

Be Explicit About Goals and Expectations of Supervision

Caring isn't reserved just for patients. A great way to let your trainee know that you care about their education and performance is to sit down with him or her at the very beginning and talk about your and his or her goals and expectations. This holds true for even one-time supervision.

While setting expectations is important, routinely following up on expectations is crucial. If trainees are required to write progress notes, read them and give constructive feedback. If trainees are expected to perform specific administrative tasks (i.e., filing conservator paperwork), follow up to see if they completed the task, have questions, or need guidance. Modeling good clinical care is a powerful way both to educate and to reinforce professional traits, including compassion, competence, and conscientiousness.

A recently developed 26-item inventory, the Psychopharmacotherapy–Structured Clinical Observation (P-SCO) Tool, provides a nicely consolidated checklist that can be readily used by supervisors to monitor these clinical interactions over time (Young et al. 2018).

Know the "Stage" of Your Trainee…and Work to Advance Him or Her to the Next Stage

Literature specific to supervision in outpatient psychiatry settings is surprisingly limited; however, Newman et al. (2016) utilized the Dreyfus model of skill acquisition to provide a framework for how psychiatry supervisors might conceptualize the skill level of trainees and work to advance their practice (Table 17–1).

Measurement-Based Care Is Here

Trainees are likely aware of the wide array of screening and diagnostic inventories that form the basis for outcome measures in clinical trials. Following a recent report from The Kennedy Forum entitled "Fixing Mental Health Care in America: A National Call for Measurement Based Care in Behavioral Health and Primary Care," the Joint Commission has now begun requiring health care organizations to use these standardized

Effective Communication

Shared decision making

Therapeutic alliance   =   Improved outcome

Positivity

FIGURE 17–1.   If a patient could write a prescription for a good doctor-patient relationship.

instruments to monitor patient progress and inform treatment goals and strategies (Fortney et al. 2017). Although the initiative is laudable in many respects, it raises several questions for supervisors and trainees to consider together, including: What instrument(s) should be chosen for each patient? Do we talk about the findings together? If so, how do we do this and how frequently?" "How does the trainee routinely fit these measurement tools into their busy workflow?"

Action Item

Create a list of all the measurement instruments that the trainee might use while in clinic. Then, go over these instruments with the trainee so that he or she is familiar with the questions and scoring. A more advanced step would then be to talk about how specific scores might affect treatment planning, or how specific scores relate to those referenced in clinic trials (see Chapter 42, "Integrating Measurement-Based Care Into Supervision").

Action Item

Make the instruments easily accessible. For questionnaires, encourage trainees to integrate them into electronic medical record flowsheets or note templates. For paper-and-pencil tests, have trainees keep copies in file folders in their offices.

Specific Challenges and Strategies

- **There is not enough time to supervise in a full psychopharmacology clinic.** Yes, there is! Effective supervision can take on many forms. Supervision techniques can (and should) be adjusted on the basis of the time constraints and goals of the supervisor and trainee (Table 17–2).
- **It's difficult to supervise multiple trainees simultaneously.** Often in psychopharmacology clinics, several trainees see their respective patients in the same time block. In some practice sites, supervisors are required to meet with each patient and trainee briefly to approve the plan or answer questions of the trainee, amplifying significant constraints on time and physical presence. Preparation and time management are of the utmost importance. Several approaches may be used to supervise (Table 17–2). Because there is rarely time to fully discuss a case, consider identify-

TABLE 17–1.   Applying the Dreyfus model of skill acquisition to psychiatric training

Stage	Characteristic	Relevant example	Approach to supervision
Novice	Adheres rigidly to rules with little situational perception	Medical student uses a standardized template to interview patient and does not recognize patient-specific factors	Provide immediate feedback on structure and content of interview
Advanced beginner	Continues to demonstrate limited situational perception, and uses rules to guide actions	Intern performs a full review of systems for mania on a patient who presents with severe depressive symptoms	Help resident to attend to and utilize the patient's affect to guide interview
Competent	Uses standardized and routinized procedures, but now actions are seen at least partly in terms of longer-term goals	Resident performs psychiatric intake in a fluid manner which involves good mix of open and close-ended questions to obtain pertinent information	Ensure that resident is creating a full biopsychosocial formulation that addresses the chief complaint from all perspectives
Proficient	Views situations holistically, and sees what is most important in a situation	Senior resident begins to build a therapeutic alliance in the first interview and adeptly navigates the clinical interview to obtain a timely formulation	Help trainee to begin thinking about possible treatment strategies while the interview is in progress
Expert	Has intuitive grasp of situations based on deep understanding	Psychiatrist builds therapeutic alliance, understands biopsychosocial aspects of patient's concerns, and develops patient-centered strategy for treatment	Appreciate the utility of clinical experience and "pattern-matching" to expedite diagnosis and formulation; however, also remember to emphasize the uniqueness of each patient's life history

Source.   Adapted from Newman et al. 2016.

ing additional time to meet with all trainees together. Crucially, frequently reassess the supervision approach for effectiveness and make changes as needed to maximize its utility.

- **My trainee feels undermined when I come in the room and change the treatment plan.** The power differential inherent within the supervisor-trainee relationship can frequently prevent a trainee from even expressing this type of concern; therefore, it requires significant *attunement* on the part of the supervisor to both recognize that a trainee feels undermined and be able to respond appropriately. Although multiple factors modulate a trainee's receptivity to in-session feedback and correction, supervisors can minimize the chance of trainees feeling undermined by incorporating the following: active listening, constructive feedback, shared decision

TABLE 17–2.	**Approaches to supervision**
Types of supervision	Individual (single trainee)
	Sequential individual (multiple trainees)
	Group (multiple trainees)
Methods of supervision	Face-to-face (in-session, preclinic, postclinic)
	Instant messaging (in-session; ideally coupled with face-to-face supervision)
Timing of supervision	**In-session**
	Pros: Provides real-time feedback for trainee; increased patient-supervisor contact to support continuity of care across trainees; supervisor can model advanced techniques/skills for the trainee; supervisor can independently assess patient and compare his or her impression to that of the trainee; complex decision making can be easier in this setting.
	Cons: Patient may see supervisor as "the doctor"; trainee may feel disempowered if supervisor's role is too prominent; trainee may feel uncomfortable with potential for being "corrected" or "educated" in front of their patient (most of these negatives can be mitigated if the supervisor is mindful of their possible presence); this method can be more difficult to utilize if supervising multiple trainees simultaneously.
	Preclinic
	Pros: Is conducive to multidisciplinary team approach (i.e., input from social work, psychology, etc.); supervisor may help the trainee frame and prepare for likely concerns/issues that will arise in-session; easier for supervising multiple trainees simultaneously.
	Cons: Allows little opportunity to anticipate and provide counsel on unexpected topics/issues that may arise in-session; benefits of in-session feedback are not met (see above).
	Postclinic
	Pros: Maximizes autonomy of the trainee (feedback is only retrospective); good method for group supervision where multiple trainees can present and learn from each other; more time might be available for in-depth discussion.
	Cons: Benefits of in-session feedback are not met (see above); if clinics run late, supervision may be truncated as trainees must move on to other obligations.

making, and postsession instruction and feedback. As previously stated, trainees are more receptive to feedback when they feel that their supervisors "care" about their education and performance. Finally, and very importantly, whether the supervisor revises the ultimate treatment plan or not, they should *always* ask the trainee to explain the plan's rationale. Even if the ultimate plan seems appropriate, the underlying rationale may be flawed. Education is more than learning *what* to think—it is learning *how* to think.

Questions for the Supervisee

- ■ As we set an agenda for today's supervision, which patients are you seeing, and can you begin with a brief biopsychosocial formulation of each one?

- ■ Have you encountered any administrative or logistical issues you want to discuss?

- ■ What medications would you consider prescribing at this point given your overall clinical formulation?

Additional Resources

Fortney J, Sladek R, Unutzer J: Fixing mental health care in American: a national call for measurement-based care in behavioral health and primary care (issue Brief). June 2017. Available at: http://thekennedyforum-dot-org.s3.amazonaws.com/documents/KennedyForum-BehavioralHealth_FINAL_3.pdf.

Mintz DL, Flynn DF: How (not what) to prescribe: nonpharmacologic aspects of psychopharmacology. Psychiatr Clin North Am 35(1):143–163, 2012

References

Fortney J, Sladek R, Unutzer J: Fixing mental health care in American: a national call for measurement-based care in behavioral health and primary care (issue brief). June 2017. Available at: https://thekennedyforum.org/wp-content/uploads/2017/06/Issue-Brief-A-National-Call-for-Measurement-Based-Care-in-Behavioral-Health-and-Primary-Care.pdf. Accessed August 9, 2018.

McKay KM, Imel ZE, Wampold BE: Psychiatrist effects in the psychopharmacological treatment of depression. J Affect Disord 92(2–3):287–290, 2006 16503356

Newman M, Ravindranath D, Figueroa S, et al: Perceptions of supervision in an outpatient psychiatry clinic. Acad Psychiatry 40(1):153–156, 2016 25085500

Young JQ, Irby DM, Kusz M, et al: Performance assessment of pharmacotherapy: results from a content validity survey of the Psychopharmacotherapy–Structured Clincal Observation (P-SCO) tool. Acad Psychiatry 42(6):765–772, 2018 29380145

Chapter 18   Supportive Psychotherapy Supervision

Randon S. Welton, M.D.

Marie E. Rueve, M.D.

Supportive psychotherapy (SP) carries the sobriquet "the Cinderella of psychotherapy" because it does a lot of arduous clinical work but garners very little recognition or appreciation. This ubiquitous intervention can be neglected during training. A survey of psychiatry residency training directors found that 70% of psychiatry residencies had 30 or more hours of training in psychodynamic psychotherapy, but only 15% had that much training in SP. Almost half of the programs had less than 30 hours of supervised, clinical experiences in SP over the course of the 4-year residency (Sudak and Goldberg 2012).

Supportive psychotherapy's utility stems from its flexibility. Modifying the goals and interventions of SP enables its use in even the most intense and fast-paced practice. When trainees are being prepared to care for the seriously ill, SP's emphasis on a thorough assessment and management of psychosocial factors promotes comprehensive treatment and, when added to a biomedical approach, represents a return to the biopsychosocial model (Margison 2005). Supervisors can enhance the SP provided by our trainees by emphasizing its specific foci and interventions.

Key Points

- Supervisors should help supervisees identify when to use SP.

- Supervisors should teach how to collaborate on goals.

- SP supervision emphasizes the common elements of psychotherapy such as empathy and the therapeutic alliance.

- Developing strategies to alleviate the patient's current distress and optimize their functioning is a vital feature of SP supervision.

- SP supervision helps the supervisee identify and utilize the patient's strengths and existing support systems.

- The SP supervisor should help the supervisee enhance the patient's cognitive functioning.

- Discussions about the importance of treatment adherence should be a regular feature of SP supervision. Supervisees should be guided to regularly assess obstacles to care.

- Supervision should be used to assist in teaching the principles of SP.

Help Identify When to Use Supportive Psychotherapy

Trainees should consider providing SP in all patients with severe psychiatric symptoms, those having problems with daily functioning, those in severe distress, or those who are currently overwhelmed by their circumstances. These patients often present with problems in affective control and self-esteem and/or have ineffective coping strategies. In these cases, SP may be the most helpful psychotherapy because it addresses modifiable factors in these patients' lives and can lead to dramatic improvements in quality of life.

Teach How to Collaborate on Goals

Supportive psychotherapy supervisors guide supervisees in collaborating with patients to establish and work toward therapy goals. Such goals might include 1) developing and maintaining supportive relationships; 2) increasing healthy coping skills (e.g., assertiveness) and healthy behaviors (e.g., exercise, sleep hygiene, not misusing substances); 3) working on reality testing, problem-solving, or decision-making strategies; 4) using simple strategies (e.g., relaxation techniques) to increase tolerance of anxiety and affect; and/or 5) developing healthy self-esteem (Winston et al. 2012). In general, these will be SMART Goals (i.e., Specific, Measurable, Achievable, Relevant, and Time-limited). Supervisors should periodically inquire as to the progress being made toward these goals to keep them the central focus of therapy.

Practice Empathy, Acceptance, and Validation

Empathy, acceptance, and validation are some of the most efficacious components of psychotherapy and should be emphasized with SP patients. During treatment and supervision, the supervisee can learn to appropriately express an understanding of patients' emotions and choices. Supervisors can role-play specific situations with the trainee, alternating between the roles of therapist and patient. Supervision can examine and improve the supervisee's use of verbal and nonverbal communication in these role-plays. Supervisor and supervisee can watch the trainee's facial expressions and body language during video-recorded interactions, or the supervisor can comment on these factors during supervision. Supervisors can point out the different messages that can be conveyed by altering the tone, pace, or emphasis of speech. Trainees can practice making empathic or validating comments when the supervisor asks them to summarize what the patient is feeling at specific moments of a videoed interaction. The supervisor might even show clips from other therapy sessions or even from popular media and ask the trainee to make empathic statements regarding emotionally intense moments.

Focus on the Therapeutic Alliance

The therapeutic alliance significantly impacts the efficacy of any therapy. This is especially true with the seriously ill patients who are receiving SP. The supervisor may help the supervisee recognize that an alliance is fostered through discussions of the roles and expectations of both therapist and patient, through the collaborative development of immediate and long-term goals, and by the therapist's purposeful attention to displaying respect, warmth, and a positive regard toward the patient while maintaining proper boundaries. Supervisees can be encouraged to periodically assess the strength of the therapeutic alliance through discussion or standardized measures, such as the Working Alliance Inventory (Horvath and Greenberg 1989).

Attend to Acute Distress and Promote Adaptive Coping Strategies

Supportive psychotherapy will focus on the immediate emotional and functional concerns of the patient. Therapeutic interventions should directly target these issues and can be summarized as providing HOPE for the patient (Crocker 2017):

- **H**ear, understand, and reflect the patient's feelings and emotions.
- **O**rganize the patient's narrative and experience.
- **P**romote adaptive psychological functioning, including coping and self-esteem.
- **E**ffect changes in collaboration with the patient to reduce stressors and increase support.

Patients with mental illness often find themselves bewildered by their intense emotions and loss of control. Therapists can help patients consolidate their experiences into a cohesive narrative. By helping patients describe the course of their illness, clarify ambiguous situations, and reframe experiences in a more accurate manner, the therapist can make patients' lives more understandable and less unpredictable and frightening. Supervision can be an opportunity for the supervisee to try out summarizing statements and to practice offering a narrative that the patient can understand. Supervisors can identify and fill in gaps in the trainee's understanding of the patient by asking for a comprehensive biopsychosocial formulation. Psychoeducation about the nature, manifestation, and prognosis of a patient's mental illness can aid the patient's understanding of his or her life story. This too can be practiced in supervision. The supervisor can help the trainee identify the patient's productive and maladaptive coping strategies and develop strategies to optimize functioning. While respecting patient autonomy, therapists can offer advice on how to improve functioning (e.g., sleep hygiene, taking their medications as prescribed) in ways acceptable to the patient. Healthy activities (e.g., exercise) are encouraged, while unhealthy ones (e.g., substance abuse) are discouraged. Therapists can encourage patients to break self-destructive or self-limiting patterns of behavior. Supervisors will need to help trainees set the boundary between giving sound therapeutic suggestions and being overly directive and controlling. Supervisors can further encourage the alleviation of patient's immediate distress by practicing interventions such as relaxation training, reframing pessimistic assessments, or supplying reasonable hopefulness.

Help Supervisees Identify Strengths and Support Systems

Patients with serious mental illnesses often emphasize their failures, faults, and weaknesses. Supportive psychotherapists can be taught to help the patient identify past successes, positive qualities, and accomplishments. Both supervisees and patients may come to appreciate their struggles and efforts at self-improvement. The supervisor will emphasize the positive moments and successes the patient experiences during therapy and discuss how the trainee can appropriately praise the patient based on the patient's changing behavior. These interventions help patients develop a healthy self-esteem. The supervisor can stress the importance of exploring the patient's network of relationships and the adequacy of his or her social support. Supervision should help focus attention on the positive and negative aspects of the patient's existing relationships with friends and relatives. The supervisee and patient may then choose to explore options for minimizing unhealthy interactions, optimizing healthy ones, or seeking new relationships.

Help Supervisee Enhance the Patient's Cognitive Functioning

Patients who are feeling overwhelmed or are experiencing profound or prolonged psychiatric symptoms may demonstrate a number of ineffective cognitive strategies. They are prone to pessimism, self-fulfilling prophecies, confirmation bias, and disqualifying evidence that is positive or hopeful. The supervisor can assist the trainee in identifying these patterns and can practice challenging them via role-playing exercises. Supervisors will focus attention on the patient's limited problem-solving skills. SP can help patients explore options when faced with choices and develop strategies for decision-making (e.g., listing pros and cons). Patients can be taught to consider all realistic options and outcomes before deciding on a course of action and to balance negativistic thinking with more realistic assessments. Enhancing reality testing may need to be a focus for patients experiencing hallucinations or delusions. Without active supervision, trainees may neglect these vital tasks.

Guide Supervisees to Regularly Assess Obstacles to Care

Keeping patients engaged in treatment is the primary means of decreasing their emotional distress. Predicting and addressing potential obstacles to treatment becomes a primary focus of SP. Numerous factors limit treatment adherence in patients with serious mental illnesses. Supervisees need to recognize that the severity of the patient's illness, limited insight, past treatment experiences, and practical issues such as transportation and ability to afford treatment might adversely affect a patient's alliance with the therapist and his or her adherence to the treatment regimen. The supervisor can prompt the supervisee to regularly assess and target these factors as they change over time. Predictable obstacles can often be avoided by proactively addressing them in supervision and then with the patient, which increases the chance of a successful outcome for the patient and a positive experience for the trainee.

Use Supervision to Assist in Teaching the Principles of Supportive Psychotherapy

Supervision often incorporates many techniques used in SP. The supervisor's use of techniques adopted from SP, and the subsequent discussion of such use, enliven the supervision. The supervisor should work with the supervisee to set clear goals for supervision and review these goals periodically. The goals of supervision often reflect the goals of SP: 1) to help the supervisee develop a trusting alliance with the supervisor; 2) to optimize the supervisee's technical skills; 3) to help the supervisee develop effective coping when complex moments arise in the session; 4) to model and help the supervisee learn affective control in the session; and 5) to help the supervisee develop confidence and professional self-esteem. The supervisor should actively seek feedback about the effectiveness of supervision and make adjustments accordingly. Challenges in the supervision should be identified and problem-solving techniques employed just as the supervisee helps patients work through the problems in their lives. Didactic education, modeling, and role-playing can play a part in both supervision and SP. The supervisor seeks to help the trainee feel heard and understood and consolidate therapy experiences, promote the trainee's self-esteem as a therapist, assuage a new therapist's distress while learning the ropes, and improve the trainee's decision making as a developing therapist. This multidimensional aspect of supervision adds depth and vitality to the supervisee's learning as he or she experiences the efficacy of SP-like techniques (McNeill and Worthen 1989).

Specific Challenges and Strategies

- **My supervisee believes that SP is just having a good relationship with the patient.** Although SP prioritizes the formation and maintenance of a solid therapeutic alliance, SP also involves specific goals and techniques that differentiate it from being vaguely supportive of a patient. Creating and maintaining a stable therapeutic environment where patients can safely experience and express emotions and develop an awareness of their illness is often an independent goal of SP, but it also permits therapists and patients to do more specific work. Supervisors can emphasize that SP seeks to purposefully optimize the patient's overall functioning, self-esteem, affective control, cognitive functioning, and coping strategies (Brenner 2012; Meaden and Van Marle 2008; Novalis et al. 1993; Winston and Roberts 2019). The supervisee should come to equate SP with developing a strong therapeutic alliance and providing active interventions to achieve short-term and long-term goals created collaboratively by the patient and therapist.
- **I can't differentiate SP supervision from supervising CBT or psychodynamic psychotherapy.** Some SP interventions, including forming a therapeutic alliance, displaying empathy, and maintaining appropriate boundaries, are common to most psychotherapies (Plakun et al. 2009). These common elements alone often provide significant therapeutic benefit (Lambert and Barley 2001). Practitioners of SP might also borrow specific cognitive, behavioral, interpersonal, or psychodynamic techniques, but these are in addition to an overarching emphasis on targeting the patient's deficits and reaching the patient's immediate goals (Crocker 2017; Novalis et al. 1993). The SP supervisor helps the trainee keep a constant focus on interventions that have been shown to directly minimize distress, improve functioning, enhance self-esteem, and increase social support.
- **My supervisee's patient does not feel understood.** Patients with chronic or severe mental illness often feel isolated or excluded from the mainstream of society. Impersonal or perfunctory encounters with previous mental health providers amplify the belief that no one understands or cares for them. The SP therapist can undermine this mindset by encouraging the patient to relate their experiences at length. The supervisor can teach methods to encourage patients to elaborate on topics. These can vary from restating their last sentence to simply asking, "Can you tell me more about that." Trainees should practice paraphrasing or restating their patients' communications with their supervisor. Supervisors can work to increase the supervisee's ability to accurately and appropriately express empathy and validation via verbal and nonverbal expressions.
- **Our program doesn't offer didactics in SP, so I can't teach it in supervision.** Although a lack of formal training in SP is a considerable challenge, it may not be an insurmountable one. By modeling the provision of SP within supervision, you will help your supervisee learn about SP experientially. At the commencement of

supervision, a supervisor can explore the trainee's existing knowledge and inventory of skills in order to identify goals and objectives for the supervision. As these goals are elucidated, the supervisor can denote how similar the process is to establishing goals for SP with the patient. In both cases, existing strengths, skills, and deficits are acknowledged and plans to improve them are formulated. By exploiting this parallel processing, adept clinicians can translate their supervisory activities into teaching opportunities.

Questions for the Supervisee

■ Why is supportive psychotherapy the best choice for this patient?

■ What challenges will there be in maintaining a positive therapeutic alliance with this patient?

■ Which maladaptive coping strategies and psychological defenses does the patient regularly use?

■ Which strengths and resources does this patient have?

■ How might you enhance this patient's functioning?

■ What are your specific goals in treating this patient?

■ Which techniques and interventions might you use to help the patient achieve these goals?

Additional Resources

Winston A, Pinsker H, Rosenthal RN: Learning Supportive Psychotherapy: An Illustrated Guide. Washington, DC, American Psychiatric Publishing, 2012 [This succinct text contains a thorough discussion of SP as well as video examples and an assessment of competency in SP.]

References

Brenner AM: Teaching supportive psychotherapy in the twenty-first century. Harv Rev Psychiatry 20(5):259–267, 2012 23030214

Crocker EM: Supportive psychotherapy. Scientific American Psychiatry. Edited by Black DW. Decker Intellectual properties, September 2017. Available at https://www.deckerip.com/products/scientific-american-psychiatry/table-of-contents. Accessed August 9, 2018.

Horvath AO, Greenberg LS: Development and validation of the Working Alliance Inventory. J Couns Psychol 36:223–233, 1989

Lambert MJ, Barley DE: Research summary on the therapeutic relationship and psychotherapy outcome. Psychotherapy 38:357–361, 2001

Margison F: Integrating approaches to psychotherapy in psychosis. Aust N Z J Psychiatry 39(11–12):972–981, 2005 16343297

McNeill BW, Worthen V: The Parallel Process in Psychotherapy Supervision. Prof Psychol Res Pr 20(5):329–333, 1989

Meaden A, Van Marle S: When the going gets tougher: the importance of long-term supportive psychotherapy in psychosis. Adv Psychiatr Treat 14:42–49, 2008

Novalis PN, Rojcewicz SJJ, Peele R: Clinical Manual of Supportive Psychotherapy. Washington, DC, American Psychiatric Press, 1993

Plakun EM, Sudak DM, Goldberg D: The Y model: an integrated, evidence-based approach to teaching psychotherapy competencies. J Psychiatr Pract 15(1):5–11, 2009 19182560

Sudak DM, Goldberg DA: Trends in psychotherapy training: a national survey of psychiatry residency training. Acad Psychiatry 36(5):369–373, 2012 22983467

Winston A, Roberts LW: Supportive psychotherapy, in The American Psychiatric Association Publishing Textbook of Psychiatry, 7th Edition. Edited by Roberts LW. Washington, DC, American Psychiatric Association Publishing, 2019

Winston A, Rosenthal RN, Pinsker H: Learning Supportive Psychotherapy: An Illustrated Guide. Washington, DC, American Psychiatric Publishing, 2012

Chapter 19 Cognitive-Behavioral Therapy Supervision

Enhancing Learning and Promoting Expertise

Donna M. Sudak, M.D.

Cognitive-behavioral therapy (CBT), like most psychotherapeutic approaches, has a long-standing tradition of educating novice therapists in supervisory relationships. Guidelines, descriptions, expert consensus statements, and reviews of the supervisory process in CBT provide a framework for the supervisor. In this chapter, I provide a review of evidence available supporting CBT supervision and its components, describe differences between CBT supervision and other types of psychotherapy supervision, and detail the component processes of CBT supervision.

Key Points

- The supervisory relationship in CBT mirrors that of therapy in structure and in the emphasis on guided discovery and self-practice.

- Rating work samples, reviewing written case conceptualizations, and examining data about patient progress provide the central focus for supervision sessions.

- Active and experiential learning, along with specific action plans that facilitate supervisee growth, is an essential component of CBT supervision.

Evidence Regarding CBT Supervision

As described by Milne and Reiser (2015), a variety of publication types exist regarding CBT supervision, including research studies (e.g., Bambling et al. 2006; Breese et al. 2012; Milne et al. 2011; Townend et al. 2002), expert consensus statements (e.g., Milne and Dunkerley 2010; Roth and Pilling 2008), narrative reviews (e.g., Gordon 2012; Milne et al. 2010; Reiser 2014; Reiser and Milne 2012) and systematic reviews (e.g., Reiser and Milne 2014). The actual empirical basis for CBT supervision and its component parts remains limited, and further study is needed.

Understanding the Supervision Process in CBT

The foundation of CBT supervision is the supervisory relationship. Forming a strong bond, setting well-defined specific goals, and establishing clearly the tasks to achieve these goals are vital to the process. Because supervision frequently entails an evaluative component, the supervisor must explicitly review expectations regarding supervisee performance and review evaluation methods. Facilitating trust and self-disclosure by the supervisor about his or her own struggles (Ladany et al. 1999) are key to forming a strong alliance.

Performing a Needs Assessment

Performing a needs assessment increases learner engagement and models the practice of self-reflection that produces life-long learning. The supervisee is asked to identify goals and problem areas along with specifying strengths in CBT or in more general therapeutic skills by means of questions that stimulate reflection regarding knowledge and skills, patient types, and patient care issues that pose challenges. Rating a work sample with the Cognitive Therapy Scale (Young and Beck 1980) or the Assessment of Core CBT Skills (Muse et al. 2017) is an excellent way to assess basic competencies.

Setting Learning Goals

Parallels between CBT as a therapeutic approach and CBT supervision include setting collaborative learning goals. Such goals should be specific and measurable, lead to desired changes in the supervisee's approach, and be revisited and revised frequently. An overarching goal for the supervisor is to help the supervisee attain the capacity to competently employ CBT in patient care, with smaller subgoals determined by the specific strengths and learning needs of the supervisee. For example, beginning CBT practitioners must learn generic CBT techniques and strategies, such as how to prepare a case formulation and plan treatment. More experienced CBT therapists may have knowledge deficits about specific applications of CBT to a diagnosis (e.g., CBT for eating disorders) or goals that relate to specific techniques (e.g., "I am not comfortable implementing exposure").

Establishing Supervision Contracts

A formal agreement that exists between the supervisor and supervisee specifying the salient aspects of the relationship and the learning goals increases transparency and safety for the supervisee, provides a tangible reminder of the seriousness of supervision, and makes explicit a commitment to learning. This document should specify the framework (e.g., establishing cancellation and lateness policies, emergency contact numbers, duration, time, and fee structure) and expectations of the relationship (including those regarding work sample submission), indicate learning goals and evaluation methods to be employed, and include provisions regarding disclosure of the supervisory relationship to patients.

Conceptualizing the Supervisee

Supervision is enhanced when the supervisor arrives at a conceptualization of the trainee. Similar to therapy, more tailored and precise educational interventions may occur when the supervisor develops a framework that incorporates the cultural and educational background of the supervisee, the supervisee's experience in managing patients and conducting psychotherapy, the training environment and responsibilities of the supervisee, and the beliefs the supervisee has about CBT or therapy in general.

Evaluating Competency

Similar to CBT therapy, CBT supervision incorporates rating scales as a critical metric of progress. Rating scales have two purposes. The first is to assess patient progress, which teaches the supervisee the value of monitoring patient outcomes and allows the supervisor to ensure quality care. The second is to assess the supervisee's competence in CBT. The most commonly used scale of CBT competency in adults is the Cognitive Therapy Scale (Young and Beck 1980). The Assessment of Core CBT Skills (Muse et al. 2017) is a newer empirically validated competence scale. Both can be used as educational tools. Supervisees should rate their own work samples and the samples of expert therapists (for further discussion, see the 2015 book by Sudak et al. in "Additional Resources" near the end of this chapter).

Establishing an Agenda in Supervision

The structure of supervision typically parallels the structure of a CBT session, which enhances learning and efficiency (Liese and Beck 1997; Padesky 1996). When supervisees know what a typical session will entail, there is less anxiety and a greater degree of preparedness. Sessions include a check-in, agenda setting, review of items assigned after the last session, work on each agenda item, periodic summaries, development of an action plan, final summary, and bidirectional feedback. Each of these has a specific purpose in the supervisory process. Setting an agenda allows for specific items of greatest concern to the supervisee to be addressed and ensures that the learning goals are monitored. There is a focus on goal attainment in the work assigned, and the relationship is attended to with feedback.

The supervisor must establish a focused and targeted agenda that leads to work on learning goals. This agenda may be derived from a supervision question brought by the supervisee, the work sample reviewed for the session, or patient care issues. Supervisees must be oriented to the process of supervision and taught to formulate a supervision question. If the supervisee has demonstrated proficiency in assessment and case presentation, the time spent while he or she presents the patient is of limited value.

Working on Agenda Items in Supervision

Generally, CBT supervision reviews a recorded work sample, after the supervisee provides a patient conceptualization and history in advance. Regular review of work samples is essential. Nondisclosure is a significant problem in supervision (Ladany 1996); even if the supervisee is clear about what has transpired, poor recall of the nuances regarding the execution of therapy will certainly exist. Other work products reviewed, in addition to recordings, include case conceptualizations, patient problem and goal lists, and thought records. Written case conceptualizations and treatment plans are particularly useful to understanding the supervisee's thought process, gauging his or her understanding of the cognitive-behavioral model, and guiding the planned implementation of CBT for a particular patient.

There is a genuine tension involved in supervision; one overarching goal is to allow the supervisee to struggle and learn *how* to proceed independently when there is an impasse. However, the welfare of the patient and efficiency of supervision must be considered. If therapy skills are not present, no amount of struggle on the part of the supervisee will be effective. For example, a therapist treating a severely depressed patient with no training in behavioral activation will not be able to effectively proceed.

The supervisor should attempt to determine an emotionally charged issue for the supervisee—for example, something that engenders anxiety about the patient—and address it with more than one method of instruction. Milne (2008) highlights how supervisors who employ multiple methods of instruction engage and promote learning more effectively. Experiential learning is vital, either with role-play, self-practice, or experiential exercises that illustrate concepts.

Developing Action Plans

Supervision must provide the supervisee with assignments to do outside of session. Doing assigned readings, reviewing taped samples with an instrument such as the Cognitive Therapy Scale (Young and Beck 1980), watching tapes of expert therapists, practicing self-reflection, and incorporating self-practice of CBT tools like automatic thought records are all examples of interventions that augment knowledge and skills. Practice outside of session is critical, because continual improvement and growth as a therapist requires such a commitment.

Providing Feedback

Two types of feedback are important in supervision: formative and summative. Formative feedback is consistently employed in CBT supervision. The supervisor should take detailed notes when reviewing work samples so as to refer to the specific words used by the supervisee. Explicit feedback about how to improve can be powerfully enhanced by such detail. Rating scales teach the critical elements of the treatment approach, provide an opportunity for feedback, and help the supervisor monitor trainee progress. Praise and specific direction about skill deployment, conceptualization, selection of interventions, and management of the relationship with the patient are critical areas to attend to in providing feedback.

Specific Challenges and Strategies

- **I'm not sure what skill and capability deficits exist in the supervisee.** Determine if a skill deficit or a capability deficit is the reason for the supervisee's difficulty by using role-play, observation, and targeted questioning. Beliefs therapists hold often prevent them from using particular therapy approaches even when skills are available.
- **My supervisee mistakes diagnostic criteria for problem lists.** A limited problem list leads to inadequate or vague treatment goals, so teach the supervisee to find a focus and determine a list of patient problems.
- **There are no "ideal patients" for CBT.** Although there is literature regarding "ideal patients" for supervision (having an acute problem, no severe or chronic illness) (see Sokol and Fox 2015), in this author's experience, it is unusual to have such patients predictably available. Mental health professionals are regularly tasked to treat multiply diagnosed, chronically ill patients, with daunting psychosocial challenges, particularly in training settings. Supervisors must identify ways the supervisee can employ CBT interventions to help the patient and learn the treatment. Adherence to medications, affect regulation, problem solving, distress tolerance, exposure, and behavioral activation can be used in a conceptually driven way in difficult patients with good results. In addition, the therapist must be able to forge a treatment bond with such complicated patients. Skills to help patients with consistent attendance and promptness, and to use therapy tools outside of session, are of significant importance in such work. Supervision must also help the therapist maintain a sense of optimism and morale, by delineating realistic expectations, maintaining a sense of perspective ("the long view") and highlighting the tools of CBT that the therapist is employing.
- **My supervisee wants to "blend" treatments.** Frequently, therapists learning more than one type of therapy or who have a previous grounding in another type of therapy express the desire to "blend" CBT with another school of thought. This practice is inadvisable—there are no data regarding the outcome of such work, and it is far more confusing to learn therapy in such a fashion.
- **I always seem to be telling the supervisee what to do with the patient.** Resist the initial impulse to directly tell the supervisee alternative strategies to manage a clinical situation. Instead, role-play and reverse role-play to facilitate supervisee reflection. Guided Socratic questioning may lead to a new understanding as well.

Questions for the Supervisee

- What is your supervision question?

- Do you know the cognitive model and have the skills to treat this patient?

- Are you following a plan? Does the plan make sense?

- Do you have clear conceptualizations?

- What obstacles exist in the treatment, and what are your contributions to these obstacles?

Questions for the Supervisor

- What were my presession goals?

- Did they get met? What topics emerged?

- What interventions did I use? What experiential learning techniques?

- How strong is my relationship with the supervisee? What strengths did I observe?

- What new learning goals do I have?

Additional Resources

Milne DL, Reiser RP: A Manual for Evidence-Based CBT Supervision. Hoboken, NJ, Wiley, 2017

Sudak DM, Codd RT 3rd, Ludgate JW, et al: Teaching and Supervising Cognitive Behavioral Therapy. New York, Wiley, 2015

References

Bambling M, King R, Raue P, et al: Clinical supervision: its influence on client-rated working alliance and client symptom reduction in the brief treatment of major depression. Psychother Res 16(3):317–331, 2006

Breese L, Boon A, Milne DL: Detecting excellent episodes in clinical supervision. A case-study, comparing two approaches. Clin Supervisor 31:121–137, 2012

Gordon PK: Ten steps to cognitive behavioral supervision. Cogn Behav Ther 5:71–82, 2012

Ladany N: Nature, extent, and importance of what psychotherapy trainees do not disclose to their supervisors. J Couns Psychol 43(1):10–24, 1996

Ladany N, Lehrman-Watreman D, Molinaro M, et al: Psychotherapy supervisor ethical practices adherence to guidelines, the supervisory working alliance, and supervisee satisfaction. Couns Psychol 27(3):443–475, 1999

Liese BS, Beck JS: Cognitive therapy supervision, in Handbook of Psychotherapy Supervision. Edited by Watkins CE. New York, Wiley, 1997, pp 114–133

Milne DL: CBT supervision: from reflexivity to specialization. Behavioural and Cognitive Therapy 36:779–786, 2008

Milne DL, Dunkerley C: Towards evidence-based clinical supervision: The development and evaluation of four CBT guidelines. Cogn Behav Ther 3:43–57, 2010

Milne DL, Reiser RP: Evidence-based supervisory practices in CBT, in Teaching and Supervising Cognitive Behavioral Therapy. Edited by Sudak DM, Codd RT, Ludgate J, et al. New York, Wiley, 2015, pp 208–209

Milne DL, Reiser RP, Aylott H, et al: The systematic review as an empirical approach to improving CBT supervision. Int J Cogn Ther 3:278–294, 2010

Milne DL, Reiser RP, Cliffe T, et al: SAGE: Preliminary evaluation of an instrument for observing competence in CBT supervision. Cogn Behav Ther 4:123–138, 2011

Muse K, McManus F, Rakovshik S, et al: Development and psychometric evaluation of the Assessment of Core CBT Skills (ACCS): An observation-based tool for assessing cognitive behavioral therapy competence. Psychol Assess 29(5):542–555, 2017 27668487

Padesky CA: Developing cognitive therapist competency: teaching and supervision models, in Frontiers of Cognitive Therapy. Edited by Salkovskis PM. New York, Guilford, 1996, pp 266–293

Reiser RP: Supervising cognitive and behavioral therapies, in The Wiley International Handbook of Clinical Supervision. Edited by Watkins CE, Milne DL. Chichester, UK, Wiley, 2014, pp 493–517

Reiser RP, Milne DL: Supervising cognitive behavioural psychotherapy: pressing needs, impressing possibilities. J Contemp Psychother 42:161–171, 2012

Reiser RP, Milne DL: A reconceptualization of outcome evaluation in clinical supervision. Train Educ Prof Psychol 8:149–157, 2014

Roth AD, Pilling S: A competence framework for the supervision of psychological therapies. 2008. Available at: https://www.ucl.ac.uk/pals/research/clinical-educational-and-health-psychology/research-groups/core. Accessed on August 9, 2018.

Sokol L, Fox M: Training CBT survivors, in Teaching and Supervising Cognitive Behavioral Therapy. Edited by Sudak DM, Codd RT, Ludgate J, et al. New York, Wiley, 2015, pp 230 231

Sudak DM, Codd RT, Ludgate J, et al: Teaching and Supervising Cognitive Behavioral Therapy. New York, Wiley, 2015, pp 67–83

Townend M, Iannetta L, Freeston M: Clinical supervision in practice: a survey of UK cognitive behavioural psychotherapists accredited by the BABCP. Behav Cogn Psychother 30:485–500, 2002

Young J, Beck AT: Cognitive Therapy Scale: Rating Manual. Unpublished manuscript, University of Pennsylvania, Philadelphia, PA, 1980

Chapter 20 Psychodynamic Supervision

Deborah L. Cabaniss, M.D.

Psychodynamic psychotherapy is a psychosocial intervention based on the premise that unconscious factors affect our conscious thoughts, feelings, and behaviors. It can be long-term or short-term, individual or group; but, in any form, it uses free association, confrontation, and interpretation to help uncover unconscious material. Psychodynamic psychotherapy sessions are generally open-ended, allowing patients to "say whatever comes to mind" to gain access to thoughts and feelings beneath the surface. Too often, however, psychodynamic therapists transpose these same techniques to supervision, using an open-ended approach that leaves supervisees wondering what they are supposed to be learning (Jacobs et al. 1997). Thinking about psychodynamic supervision as a teaching activity like any other turns psychodynamic supervision into a clear, productive learning experience designed to help supervisees master this important therapeutic skill set.

Key Points

- Psychodynamic psychotherapy supervision should
  - Be conducted in the context of a strong supervisory alliance.
  - Be based on clear, operationalized learning objectives.
  - Address common factors and careful assessment of patients.
  - Be synergistic with supervisees' didactic instruction.
  - Attend to both microprocess and macroprocess.
  - Be operationalized in order to clearly convey concepts.

Important Aspects to Remember

It's Supervision, Not Treatment

To feel free to talk about countertransference, reveal mistakes, admit uncertainty, ask questions, and try out hypotheses, supervisees have to feel confident that their supervisors are interested in them, able to contain their anxiety, tolerant of differences of opinion, and available during emergencies. That means establishing an alliance. In doing this, it is important to remember that establishing an alliance with a psychodynamic psychotherapy supervisee is different from establishing an alliance with a psychodynamic psychotherapy patient. For example, although psychodynamic psychotherapists who are trying to foster the transference do not generally self-disclose, psychodynamic supervisors can often profitably share their feelings and experiences with supervisees. Sharing one's clinical experiences (provided the focus predominantly remains on the supervisee) can be extraordinarily helpful to supervisees who imagine that they are the only ones who are uncertain in clinical situations or who get angry with patients. This kind of self-disclosure can help forge the supervisory alliance and model therapeutic self-reflection. It is also key to discussing parallel process—that is, the way that the patient's split-off experiences are enacted by supervisor and supervisee. Discussion of parallel process is generally initiated by supervisors who are willing to be open about their experience in the supervision and tuned into the way that this discussion can further understanding of the patient.

Don't Forget Common Factors!

Studies indicate that common factors such as alliance, empathy, and instilling hope are directly related to outcome in all types of psychotherapy, including psychodynamic psychotherapy (Martin et al. 2000). Thus, carefully teaching these skills is an important part of psychodynamic psychotherapy supervision. Although the temptation in psychodynamic supervision may be to focus on techniques that are classically linked to psychodynamic psychotherapy, such as interpreting resistance or transference, it is equally, if not more, important for supervisees to learn how to listen empathically, convey understanding, set the frame and instill hope. Supervisors should include explicit instruction about how to do this in their psychodynamic supervision. In fact, psychodynamic supervision with junior supervisees may fruitfully focus almost exclusively on common factors.

Be Explicit About Assessment of Patients

Similarly, supervision should always include practice in conducting an assessment for treatment. Just because a supervisee is "sent" a patient for psychodynamic psychotherapy by their program or clinic does not mean that the patient is in fact appropriate for this modality. Supervisors will do well to start every new supervision by meeting the patient, working with the supervisee to make a careful DSM diagnosis, and carefully reviewing the patient's function, including their dominant patterns of self-experience and self-esteem, relationships with others, adapting to stress, cognition, and work and play. This type of diagnostic rigor is essential for psychodynamic psychotherapy supervision and models the importance of always conducting one's own assessment.

Link Supervision and Didactics

Psychodynamic psychotherapy is generally taught using both didactic seminars and individual supervision. Thus, psychodynamic supervisors need to be familiar with the didactics in which their supervisees are participating. Supervisors are, in effect, the lab instructors of the psychodynamic curriculum (Cabaniss and Arbuckle 2011). Supervisees learn something in class and then apply it with their patients under supervision. Think of it this way: if this were an undergraduate chemistry curriculum, the lab instructors would coordinate their lab activities with what their students learned in class earlier that day. The practicum augments the classroom learning. The same is true for supervision. Supervisors need to coordinate what they are doing in supervision with what their supervisees are learning in class. If supervision is not coordinated with didactic classroom learning, contradictory experiences in class and supervision can lead to confusion and loss of interest. Supervisors should ask supervisees about their didactic seminars and should be in touch with the didactic instructors to obtain syllabi and reading materials. Reading along with supervisees helps to frame supervision in the language and developmental trajectory used in class, again optimizing the way that supervision and didactic learning synergistically augment each other.

Microprocess and Macroprocess

Microprocess is the moment-to-moment activity of therapy. Examining microprocess in supervision is essential for teaching technique. It means helping supervisees understand what they heard, how they processed it to decide on a therapeutic strategy, and how and why they intervened (Cabaniss et al. 2017). *Macroprocess* is the overall trajectory of the treatment. It is the big picture. Examining macroprocess is essential for teaching formulation. It means helping supervisees understand how things evolved in the treatment and how both therapist and patient participated in the process. As a supervisor, it is important to toggle between microprocess and macroprocess, sometimes focusing on a moment in the treatment and sometimes looking at the big picture. Having a supervisee do short writing exercises in which he or she details both microprocess and macroprocess can help teach both technique and formulation in supervision (Cabaniss and Graver 2008; Cabaniss et al. 2017).

Learning Objectives for Supervision

Learning objectives are what educators hope that learners will take away from a teaching activity. Ideally, learning objectives for psychodynamic supervision should be developmental, with junior learners focusing on common factors such as alliance and listening for meaning, and senior learners focusing on independently formulating and interpreting. Although several psychodynamic educators have suggested universal learning objectives for clinical learning in psychodynamics (Moga and Cabaniss 2014), training programs will do best to use these suggestions as jumping off points for creating objectives that make sense for their supervisors and supervisees. Both supervisor and supervisee should make sure to ask about the learning objectives that will guide the supervisory experience. Talking about the goals of the supervision up front will help focus the supervision and will make evaluation a natural, expected, helpful, and transparent exercise.

Supervising by Operationalizing

Conducting psychodynamic psychotherapy is a skill, and skills can be taught in several ways. In the apprenticeship method, supervisees learn by watching experienced therapists. This is widely applied in individual supervision; when a supervisor says, "Good, but here's what I would have said…," they are using this method. Although this approach allows the supervisor to give information, it does not help the supervisee know why the supervisor decided to make the intervention, and thus may not be helpful for building skills. Psychodynamic psychotherapy can also be taught through reading, which may lead to increased knowledge but may not translate into skill building. In contrast, operationalizing helps to build skills by breaking down psychodynamic technique into clear steps that can be taught, mastered, and evaluated. This helps supervisees understand what makes up the skills, and how to decide when and how to apply them in clinical situations.

One way of operationalizing psychodynamic psychotherapy is the Listen/Reflect/Intervene model (Cabaniss et al. 2016). This three-step approach, outlined below,[1] can be used to teach psychodynamic psychotherapy clearly, both in class and in supervision. Each step can be actively taught in supervision. It is very helpful to be very specific about what supervisees should listen for, how they should use what they hear to form a therapeutic strategy (reflecting), and the interventions to use in this treatment.

- **Listening**—Supervisees are taught to listen above and beneath the surface for affect, resistance, transference, countertransference, and major unconscious themes, including conflicts, dreams, and fantasies.
- **Reflecting**—Three sets of reflecting principles help supervisees decide how and when to intervene:
  - *The three choosing principles:* Supervisees can use the following to help them choose where to intervene:
    - Following the affect
    - Going from surface to depth
    - Listening to countertransference

    These help therapists know what to focus on from among the material they hear.

  - *The three readiness principles:* Supervisees can use the following to determine whether a patient is ready to use an intervention:
    - State of the alliance
    - Phase of the treatment
    - Patient's current function

---

[1]This outline of the Listen/Reflect/Intervene model is adapted from Cabaniss DL, Cherry S, Douglas CJ, et al.: *Psychodynamic Psychotherapy: A Clinical Manual.* New York, Wiley, 2016.

- *The three organizing sources:* The following help supervisees organize what they hear from the patient:
  - Their working formulation
  - Their knowledge of theory and technique
  - Their own personal/clinical experience
- **Intervening.** Both supporting and uncovering interventions are used in psychodynamic psychotherapy. Supporting interventions support function (Cabaniss et al. 2016); uncovering interventions (confrontation, clarification, interpretation) help make people aware of unconscious thoughts and feelings.

Supervisors should be very explicit early in supervision that learning these techniques, along with how to use the common factors, is the major learning objective of the supervision. They should also clarify that the supervisee's progress will be evaluated.

Using Video

Although it is sometimes called the "talking cure," psychodynamic psychotherapy is about much more than words. Silence, body language, laughter, facial expressions—supervisors need to see and hear these as much or even more than the words themselves. In addition, supervisees' notes rarely accurately capture what the patient or they say. Using video for psychodynamic supervision helps with all of these issues. Once patients sign written consent for video recording, all sessions can be taped and watched in supervision. Supervisors need to be mindful of the fact that (at least at first) being watched on video makes supervisees very anxious and should address this overtly in supervision as part of establishing the supervisory alliance.

Once video is being used, supervisees no longer need to take verbatim notes and can simply note the timing of moments they particularly want to watch in supervision (e.g., "minute 22–transference interpretation" or "minute 32–help!"). Supervisees do not have the time to review all of their video before supervision, but they can look over problematic moments they would like to review. Supervisors can encourage their supervisees to begin by summarizing the most recent sessions, noting the dominant affect, resistance, transference, countertransference, and themes in those sessions. This encourages the reflective process and diminishes a supervisee's reliance on the supervisor to be the arbiter or metabolizer of the week's material. Using a "drop the needle" method, in which supervisees show any short (5- to 7-minute) segment to the supervisor, presumes that learning can happen after watching any part of the session. If a supervisee never shows a beginning or an ending, the supervisor will do well to ask to see this from time to time. For the sake of confidentiality, videos should be purged directly after supervision, and confidential videos should not be carried around on flash drives (see Chapter 9, "Video Recordings: Learning Through Facilitated Observation and Feedback").

Incorporating Writing Exercises

Short writing exercises can also help the supervisory process. The "microprocess moment" (Cabaniss et al. 2017) asks supervisees to write about how they listened, reflected, and intervened during a short episode in the treatment. Asking for a brief formulation helps supervisees to shape their ideas about the way that the patient's development shaped his or her current function. Writing a treatment summary (Cabaniss and Graver 2008) can help clarify where the therapy has been and where it is going. Supervisors should help their supervisees to work on these and should discuss them when completed. Writing exercises will help supervisees to learn technique and will help supervisors to evaluate their students—and their own supervision.

A Typical Supervisory Hour

As discussed earlier in this chapter, a typical supervisory hour fruitfully begins with the resident summarizing the dominant affect, resistance, transference, countertransference, and themes of the intervening sessions. Supervisees can begin by writing this down prior to supervision, but they will gradually be able to report this spontaneously. It might sound something like this:

> SUPERVISEE: Mr. A was very angry this week-although he was superficially bright and joking about his wife's apparent insensitivity. I really felt that there was anger beneath the surface. He was late to both sessions-this is unusual—and I felt that he was avoiding having to talk about how angry he was. He also got a little bit angry with me—perhaps displacing some of the anger on to me for things like my not remembering that he was going away next week. Forgetting that might have been part of my countertransference—I felt frustrated this week that after all this time he still has such difficulty talking about his feelings. So the major theme this week is clearly the difficulty he has feeling and expressing difficult emotions.

Supervisors should check in with the supervisee to gauge any major issues related to the patient *or* to the supervisee since the last supervisory session. Then, right to the video. Again, it's useful to ask the supervisee to choose the material to watch, since the learning objectives for the developmental phase of training can be taught from almost any part of the session. After watching a 5- to 10-minute segment in which both supervisee and patient speak, the supervisor can stop the video and begin to teach microprocess using the listen/reflect/intervene method. This exchange might sound something like this:

> SUPERVISOR: OK—let's stop there. Great. So let's start with *listening*. What did you hear in that segment?
> SUPERVISEE: Well, I wanted to show this segment to you that because I thought that that was one of those jokes about his wife that wasn't really a joke—he was laughing but saying, "What can I expect? Her mother never listened to her father either? It's a family trait-like brown eyes." So I heard anger, but I also heard his typical defense against strong feelings—humor and avoidance. I guess that's a resistance in the sessions too.
> SUPERVISOR: What about the transference and countertransference?
> SUPERVISEE: I felt like he was trying to treat me like "one of the boys"—like we were talking at a bar rather than in a therapy office. I felt irritated—like he wasn't thinking of me as a professional, like he wasn't trying.
> SUPERVISOR: We know that that's one of the ways that he deals with anger—he reduces people—and he was doing that with you, too. So how did you *reflect* on what you heard to come up with your therapeutic strategy?

SUPERVISEE: I used the choosing principles and followed the affect—I felt that the most important thing was that he was so angry but wasn't saying it, so my strategy was to try to help him understand how he felt.

SUPERVISOR: Great—so that's why you said, "You're laughing at that joke, but it actually sounds like something you're upset about." How would you label that *intervention*, and do you think that it was uncovering or supporting?

SUPERVISEE: I was trying to uncover the unconscious affect—I guess I'd call it a confrontation—because I was trying to get him interested in the discrepancy between the content and the affect.

SUPERVISOR: Terrific. What might it have sounded like if it had been an interpretation?

SUPERVISEE: Something like, "You're laughing at the joke because it's too upsetting to feel how angry you are at your wife."

SUPERVISOR: Exactly—it would include an hypothesis about why he was using the defense.

This gives an idea of the kind of guided reflection that really helps supervisees learn skills in an operationalized way in supervision. When done in a structured way, it can serve as the basis for periodic evaluation, either in a one-on-one practicum or as a discussion of a written microprocess moment (Cabaniss and Arbuckle 2011). The same thing can be done for formulation: actively asking regularly about how the supervisees understand why patients are thinking, feeling and behaving in a particular way is key to helping them learn to formulate on their own (Cabaniss et al. 2013).

Promoting Lifelong Learning

Over time, supervision requires less actively guided teaching and becomes more of a collegial conversation. Offering supervisees the opportunity to have "check-ins," even after formal supervision ends, is a nice segue from the weekly supervision of their traineeship to the internally motivated peer learning of their independent practice. Modeling that this kind of conversation should happen for the rest of their career promotes the idea of lifelong learning as a psychodynamic psychotherapist.

Specific Challenges and Strategies

- **My supervisees never have good psychodynamic patients!** There's no such thing as a "good" psychodynamic patient. Supervisees can learn about psychodynamic psychotherapy from any patient. They might learn more supporting or more uncovering, or they might learn an enormous amount about confronting resistance. Plus, psychodynamic patients are made not born—so much is in how we help patients to use this type of psychotherapy. Helping supervisees help patients to use psychodynamic psychotherapy is an incredibly important part of psychodynamic supervision.
- **You can't really know what's going on in the treatment without process notes.** Many supervisors learned to conduct psychodynamic psychotherapy with process notes and are uncomfortable using video. While it may be uncomfortable to switch modalities, the information on the video is so rich, most supervisors never want to turn back. The supervisee can take notes after supervision to retain a sense of the arc of the treatment. Give it a try!

- **I'm not analytically trained—can I supervise psychodynamic psychotherapy?** Yes! In fact, providers who work on inpatient units, in psychiatric emergency rooms, and on consultation-liaison services who are not analytically trained are very important psychodynamic supervisors, particularly of supportive interventions.

Questions for the Supervisor

■ What are my learning objectives for this supervision? Are they appropriate for the supervisee's level of training?

■ Am I familiar with the supervisee's current didactics in psychodynamics?

■ How am I going to measure my supervisee's progress? What does the supervisee do well? What are some challenges?

■ How can I communicate these strengths and challenges to the supervisee in an operationalized way during the course of the supervision?

Additional Resources

Cabaniss DL, Cherry S, Douglas CJ, et al: Psychodynamic Formulation. New York, Wiley, 2013
Cabaniss DL, Cherry S, Douglas CJ, et al: Psychodynamic Psychotherapy: A Clinical Manual, 2nd Edition, New York, Wiley, 2016
Jacobs D, David P, Meyer DJ: The Supervisory Encounter. New Haven, CT, Yale University Press, 1997
Mackinnon RA, Glick RA, Neutzel E: Teaching psychoanalytic psychotherapy: the use of the treatment summary. Journal of Psychiatric Education 10(3):170–177, 1986

References

Cabaniss DL, Arbuckle MR: Course and lab: a new model for supervision. Acad Psychiatry 35(4):220–225, 2011 21804039
Cabaniss DL, Graver R: Mapping the macroprocess. J Am Psychoanal Assoc 56(4):1249–1260, 2008 19037125
Cabaniss DL, Cherry S, Douglas CJ, et al: Psychodynamic Formulation. New York, Wiley, 2013
Cabaniss DL, Cherry S, Douglas CJ, et al: Psychodynamic Psychotherapy: A Clinical Manual. New York, Wiley, 2016
Cabaniss DL, Havel LK, Berger S, et al: The microprocess moment: a tool for evaluating skills in psychodynamic psychotherapy. Acad Psychiatry 41(1):51–54, 2017 26646408
Jacobs D, David P, Meyer DJ: The Supervisory Encounter. New Haven, CT, Yale University Press, 1997
Martin DJ, Garske JP, Davis MK: Relation of the therapeutic alliance with outcome and other variables: a meta-analytic review. J Consult Clin Psychol 68(3):438–450, 2000 10883561
Moga DE, Cabaniss DL: Learning objectives for supervision: benefits for candidates and beyond. Psychoanal Inq 34(6):528–537, 2014

Chapter 21

Time-Limited Dynamic Psychotherapy Supervision

A Therapy-Driven and Competency-Based Model

Hanna Levenson, Ph.D.

Time-limited dynamic psychotherapy (TLDP) is a fourth-generation brief dynamic approach assimilating concepts and techniques from a variety of clinical sources and emphasizing experiential-affective factors and cyclical maladaptive patterns (CMPs) as critical in the therapeutic process (Levenson 2017).

Training in TLDP for beginning therapists (usually third-year psychiatry residents and predoctoral psychology interns who are doing a 6-month outpatient psychiatry rotation) ideally consists of a 1-hour didactic seminar and a 2-hour group supervision per week. Each supervisee videos one patient for an entire therapy (up to 20 sessions) and selects portions of that week's video to show in the next group supervision. Supervisees receive supervisory input from the supervisor, participate in formulating one another's cases, and put forth possible intervention strategies as they watch their colleagues' videos. In this way they get feedback on their specific cases, have the chance to practice clinically relevant behaviors, and get to see the process of a brief therapy unfold with different patient-therapist dyads.

Key Points

- TLDP is a psychodynamic, experiential, attachment-based therapy.

- Supervision in TLDP is therapy-driven (i.e., parallels the practice of TLDP) and competency-based.

- Supervision makes extensive use of videos for demonstrations of what to do and assessments of the supervisee's (hopefully growing) competence.

- Resistances to working within a time-limited attitude need to be worked through.

- Supervisee's countertransferential reactions to patients provide useful data regarding formulation and intervention.

- Group supervision affords ample opportunity to learn by observing and contributing to therapeutic process and outcome as manifested with different therapist-patient dyads.

Supervision in TLDP is guided by two fundamental models that cover implicit (therapy-driven) and explicit (competency-based) modes of training. Thus, supervisees learn by being immersed in an integrative, attachment-based supervision privileging experiential, reflective, and relational aspects as well as being instructed in how to acquire specific knowledge and skills.

Therapy-Driven Supervision

The assumptions made about TLDP supervision parallel those of the therapy. TLDP as a brief therapy is based on an integrative, attachment-based framework incorporating psychodynamic, relational, experiential, emotion-focused, and systems approaches with cognitive and behavioral elements (Levenson 1995). Thus, to a large extent, supervision in TLDP mirrors the same *assumptive world* as therapy using TLDP (Friedlander and Ward 1984). There are nine parallels between the clinical practice of TLDP and supervision in TLDP, as discussed below.

Basis in Attachment Theory

Both TLDP therapy and TLDP supervision rest on an attachment theory base. In both, people (patients, supervisors, supervisees) are seen as innately motivated to search for and maintain human relatedness. When people feel safe and secure, they explore, take calculated risks to learn more about their intrapsychic and interpersonal world, and are able to learn from a more regulated intrapsychic place (Obegi and Berant 2008). In TLDP supervision, the supervisor and supervisee work best when they can co-create a positive supervisory alliance, which engenders an atmosphere of a connected bond, leading to an agreement on the supervisory tasks and goals (Watkins and Scaturo 2013). The supervisor's attuning to the supervisee's needs, learning style, culture, and so forth encourages the supervisee to experience "felt security" (Bowlby 1988) in the supervisory space in which "mistakes" are viewed as learning opportunities. For example, in TLDP therapy the therapist's countertransference is considered a form of empathy and a way of experientially understanding the patient's relational dynamics (Levenson 1995, 2017). Furthermore, from the perspective of attachment theory, supervisors consider how their interpersonal styles and those of their supervisees intertwine and affect each other, and they encourage supervisees to reflect on how their own attachment patterns may affect treatment.

Avoidance of Focus on Pathology

TLDP does not focus on pathology but rather assumes that patients are doing the best they can given their internal working models of self and other. Therefore, patients are seen as stuck, not sick (Levenson 2017). Similarly from a TLDP perspective, supervisors hold the attitude that supervisees are seen as always trying to do their best (even when they are withholding important information about their patients). So many supervisees enter supervision having been shamed in previous learning environments (Yourman 2003) and having experienced inadequate and even harmful supervision (Ellis et al. 2017). As a consequence, they have learned to withhold vital information about themselves and their patients to avoid academic or political suicide (Ladany 2017). Open learning cannot take place because they are so constricted by performance anxiety.

Length of Time

The length of the therapy and duration of the supervision are about the same (20 and 21 weeks, respectively). Most brief dynamic therapies are defined by a 20-session limit, so complete therapies are possible within an outpatient rotation. The topics for the didactic seminar (which runs for 21 weeks) parallel the expected trajectory of TLDP from the beginning (e.g., forming a therapeutic alliance, case formulation), through the middle (e.g., transference-countertransference, resistance), to the end (e.g., how to evaluate if more therapy is warranted).

Active and Focused Approach

The supervisee, as therapist, and supervisor should not shrink back from intervening directly in ways designed to accomplish the supervisory/treatment goals.

Use of Videos

Supervisors show snippets from videos of their work with patients to supervisees (as supervisees are expected to show videos of their work to supervisors). Supervisors do not need to select outstanding examples of brilliant interventions to wow supervisees, or to set a benchmark; rather, they should show places where supervisees are struggling with common TLDP issues (e.g., transferential-countertransferential reenactments). A supervisor's willingness to be vulnerable undermines (somewhat) the implicit/explicit hierarchy that exists when one is in a position of power (whether as a supervisor or as a therapist). Trying to do therapeutic work is truly a humbling experience. In addition, supervisors might try to video record their supervision sessions from time to time. Getting supervision of supervision is an important part of the learning.

Participant-Observer Duality

At times therapists (supervisees-in-training) are the *experts* observing the action and being able to make conscious decisions about where to go in the hour; at other times they are *participants* fully immersed in the co-created interpersonal interaction. TLDP supervisors are also participant-observers. What gets focused on and how the supervisory process goes are co-created, with supervisors getting pushed and pulled in the interaction with supervisees in helpful and sometimes not so helpful ways. Learning how to assess the nature of the supervisory alliance (as with the therapeutic alliance) and how to make repairs when there are ruptures (Safran and Muran 2000) is as necessary in supervision as in therapy—perhaps even more so, in that supervisees' options to choose new supervisors are limited.

Goals

There are two goals in TLDP—to provide new experiential learning and to foster new understandings. Similarly, the goals in supervision are not only to help trainees achieve an intellectual understanding (e.g., concrete knowledge) but also to have a series of new affective-action experiences (e.g., sense of competency, meaningfulness of the work). *In both therapy and supervision, experiential learning is privileged over insight.* It is assumed much of what occurs in therapy and supervision is implicit (and then needs to be made explicit, if possible).

Resistances to Termination

Supervisees stop working with their patients concurrent with ending supervision. Helping them reflect on their conflicts about ending is an important part of brief therapy training. The mixed feelings the trainees are having at ending the therapy (e.g., Will our patients be okay? Have they had enough therapy?) parallel those that they might be feeling as the training ends (e.g., Have we had enough supervision? Will we be able to do this work?).

Brief Therapy Attitudes

The attitude of the brief therapist is that the therapy will continue after the sessions end—that patients will be able to continue growing once they are on a new path. This parallels the assumption that supervisees will continue to incorporate and integrate what they have learned after the training rotation is over. Furthermore, the model of TLDP in therapy and supervision emphasizes lifelong learning—recognizing that professional growth is an ongoing process.

Competency-Based Supervision

The second model that frames TLDP supervision is a competency-based approach (Falender and Shafranske 2017). From this perspective TLDP supervision focuses explicitly on the acquisition and implementation of a certain body of knowledge (Binder 2004), specific skills (Anderson et al. 2016), and values (Levenson and Bolter 1988) congruent with TLDP supervision. These competencies are built on best practices derived from available empirical studies, supervisorial wisdom, and supervisee/patient preferences (including cultural competence).

As an example of TLDP group supervision from a competency-based perspective, consider the following example. When a supervisee shows his or her video from a recent therapy session in group supervision, the supervisor can stop the video at a place that he or she thinks provides a particular learning opportunity (e.g., when the supervisee is unwittingly replicating a dysfunctional relational pattern with the patient). The other supervisees are asked to access their felt experience watching the vignette (*competence in self-reflection*), to opine what is going on in the vignette and what led up to this point (*competence in case formulation*), to propose interventions the presenting supervisee might use (*competence in intervention strategies*), to justify their choices, and to anticipate the behavior of the patient in the ensuing moments (*competency in process analysis*). This learning approach is consistent with the teaching format of "anchored instruction" (Binder 2004) and deliberate practice (Rousmaniere et al. 2017), in which clear guidelines for expected performance are outlined and rehearsed (see Levenson 2017 for more on competencies and guidelines; see also Chapter 10, "Deliberate Practice for Clinical Supervision and Training").

Specific Challenges and Strategies

- **Supervisees say their patients don't want to be video recorded.** Have the supervisees explore the reasons for this reluctance. Sometimes patients have erroneous ideas of what will happen to the videos (e.g., they will appear on YouTube). See if they might give permission for the video to be shown once in supervision and then erased and/or ask if patients will allow just the therapist to be on video. However, sometimes the underlying issue for patient reluctance is that supervisees are afraid to expose their work on camera. If this is the case, you need to reevaluate how safe you as the supervisor are making the learning experience.
- **Supervisees have difficulty focusing on process instead of content.** You can use the cyclical maladaptive pattern method of formulating and make sure this pattern is stated free of content. A song metaphor can be used, with the "process" being the melody and the "content" being the lyrics. Lyrics can change, but the melody lingers on.
- **Supervisees are more used to giving interpretations than providing new experiences.** One strategy is to focus on a place where the supervisee has made an interpretation and examine it for how much it reenacts the cyclical maladaptive pattern versus providing an opportunity for the patient to have a new experience in accordance with the goals of treatment. (Role-playing the patient adds an experiential component.)
- **Supervisees are always coming up with reasons why the patient needs more sessions.** Quite often supervisees feel uncomfortable limiting the number of sessions for a variety of reasons. While in some of these cases this has to do with the welfare of the patients, quite often it has to do with the supervisees' own conflicts around endings. Talking about these "good reasons" for continuing the therapy helps raise the supervisee's consciousness about these issues and underscores their ubiquitous nature. Also, taking a nondefensive stance and agreeing that in most cases

therapy is good and more of it is better (Seligman 1995) allows for a fuller discussion about how change occurs, on what bases can we make decisions about what constitutes "enough therapy," and the stresses of working under today's economic pressures (Levenson and Burg 2000) as well as many other relevant topics.

Questions for the Supervisee

■ What are your "resistances" to thinking meaningful change can happen quickly?

■ When you have made enduring changes in your life, have they come about by experiences you have had or information you have acquired?

■ Are you familiar with your own cyclical maladaptive pattern?

■ Are you aware of your own feelings as you interact with patients?

■ How do you know when someone else is having a feeling?

Additional Resources

Books

Binder J: Key Competencies in Brief Dynamic Psychotherapy. New York, Guilford, 2004 [Outlines the areas of competency in TLDP.]

Levenson H: Time-Limited Dynamic Psychotherapy: A Guide to Clinical Practice. New York, Basic Books, 1995 [A practical and pragmatic casebook approach with actual transcripts of supervisors and supervisees discussing cases.]

Levenson H: Brief Dynamic Therapy, 2nd Edition. Washington, DC, American Psychological Association, 2017 [Presents explicit formulation and intervention strategies, and reviews empirical studies on training/supervisory processes and effectiveness.]

Videos

Brief Dynamic Therapy Over Time (with Hanna Levenson, Ph.D.). American Psychological Association, 2010. Available at: http://www.apa.org/pubs/videos/4310871.aspx.

Critical Events in Psychotherapy Supervision (with Nicholas Ladany, Ph.D.; hosted by Hanna Levenson, Ph.D.). American Psychological Association, 2016. Available at: http://www.apa.org/pubs/videos/4310956.aspx.

Time-Limited Dynamic Psychotherapy (with Hanna Levenson, Ph.D.). American Psychological Association, 2008. Available at: http://www.apa.org/pubs/videos/4310844.aspx.

Time-Limited Dynamic Psychotherapy (with Hanna Levenson, Ph.D.). psychotherapy.net, 2008. Available at: http://www.psychotherapy.net/video/time-limited-dynamic-psychotherapy.

[Four instructional TLDP videos with subtitles and voiceovers letting the viewer know what was going on in the therapeutic process and in the therapist's mind.]

References

Anderson T, McClintock AS, Himawan L, et al: A prospective study of therapist facilitative interpersonal skills as a predictor of treatment outcome. J Consult Clin Psychol 84(1):57–66, 2016 26594945

Binder J: Key Competencies in Brief Dynamic Psychotherapy. New York, Guilford, 2004

Bowlby J: A Secure Base: Clinical Applications of Attachment Theory. London, Routledge, 1988

Ellis MV, Taylor EJ, Corp DA, et al: Narratives of harmful clinical supervision: introduction to the special issue. Clin Supervisor 36:1–5, 2017

Falender CA, Shafranske EP: Supervision Essentials for the Practice of Competency-Based Supervision. Washington, DC, American Psychological Association, 2017

Friedlander ML, Ward LG: Development and validation of the Supervisory Styles Inventory. J Couns Psychol 31:542–558, 1984

Ladany N: Supervision Essentials for the Critical Events in Psychotherapy Supervision Model. Washington, DC, American Psychological Association, 2017

Levenson H: Time-Limited Dynamic Psychotherapy: A Guide to Clinical Practice. New York, Basic Books, 1995

Levenson H: Brief Dynamic Therapy. Washington, DC, American Psychological Association, 2017

Levenson H, Bolter K: Short-term psychotherapy values and attitudes: changes with training. Paper presented at the annual meeting of the American Psychological Association Convention, Atlanta, GA, August 1988

Levenson H, Burg J: Training psychologists in the era of managed care, in A Psychologist's Proactive Guide to Managed Mental Health Care. Edited by Hersen KS, Hersen M. Mahwah, NJ, Erlbaum, 2000, pp 113–140

Obegi JH, Berant E (eds): Attachment Theory and Research in Clinical Work With Adults. New York, Guilford, 2008

Rousmaniere T, Goodyear RK, Miller SD, et al: The Cycle of Excellence: Using Deliberate Practice to Improve Supervision and Training. Hoboken, NJ, Wiley, 2017

Safran JD, Muran JC: Negotiating the Therapeutic Alliance: A Relational Treatment Guide. New York, Guilford, 2000

Seligman ME: The effectiveness of psychotherapy. The Consumer Reports study. Am Psychol 50(12):965–974, 1995 8561380

Watkins CE, Scaturo DJ: Toward an integrative, learning-based model of psychotherapy supervision: supervisory alliance, educational interventions, and supervisee learning/relearning. Journal of Psychiatric Integration 23(1):75–95, 2013

Yourman DB: Trainee disclosure in psychotherapy supervision: the impact of shame. J Clin Psychol 59(5):601–609, 2003 12696135

Chapter 22 Group Psychotherapy Supervision

Working at Multiple Levels

Jan Malat, M.D.

The supervision of group therapy draws on many principles from the general literature on psychotherapy supervision, including developing a supervisory alliance, transmitting the values of the profession through the creation of a safe space for learning and feedback, paying close attention to the supervisee's stage of development and learning needs, identifying potential barriers to learning early in the supervision, reducing the power differential between supervisor and trainee (through the supervisor's self-disclosures about struggles in one's own clinical work), and helping the trainee develop self-reflective capacity and the ability to make use of countertransference (Leszcz 2011).

Although there is a rich variety of group therapies being delivered in diverse settings with different modalities and patient populations, certain core principles of group therapy supervision can be applied in most situations. In addition, there are several aspects about the supervision of group therapy that are unique to groups.

Key Points

- Address and explore the supervisee's anxiety about running groups early in the supervision.

- Demonstrate the value of direct observation by allowing the supervisee to observe your work.

- Demonstrate the value of judicious self-disclosure and warmth in supervision and help the supervisee model this in the group.

- Help the supervisee set realistic goals and expectations for the type of group and population being treated.

- Frequently illustrate the multiplicity of views and interventions that can occur in any group session.

- Help the supervisee appreciate and utilize therapeutic properties inherent in all groups.

- Help the supervisee identify and facilitate therapeutic group norms and group dynamics (especially increasing cohesion) early in the life of the group. Help him or her appreciate the balance of control in every group session—when to be more active and directive to create safety versus when to encourage spontaneous, emotional interactions among group members to enhance cohesion and engagement.

- Discuss the impact of isomorphy on the group—that is, how the system in which the group therapy is embedded impacts the group itself.

- Set up a weekly time to provide supervision (ideally during the postgroup debriefing), and discourage the supervisee from taking detailed clinical notes during the group.

Address Supervisee Anxiety

Groups have several unique features that can increase anxiety and feelings of incompetence in the supervisee. Because of the large volume of interactions and amount of clinical data that occurs in any group session, supervisees can get overwhelmed and become too focused on the content of what each individual said in the group versus the nonverbal process in the group (Zaslav 1988). In addition, there is much more public exposure in group therapy than in individual therapy. Supervisees often have fears that are important to explore (e.g., fears that the group will become out of control). Some supervisees may cope with their anxiety by trying to be overly controlling of the group, running it like a series of individual therapy sessions or like a classroom (Zaslav 1988) (i.e., running it as a setting for the delivery of psychotherapeutic interventions vs. an agent of change in its own right). They may not be aware that the group provides unique therapeutic opportunities. One of the first tasks of the group supervisor is to explore and normalize the supervisee's anxiety about running groups. Demonstrating confidence in the effectiveness of group therapy and resilience of groups, along with a tolerance and acceptance for mistakes (with self-disclosures of one's own errors), can significantly reduce the supervisee's level of anxiety.

Promote a Culture of Direct Observation

It is very important for the supervisee to observe the supervisor running a group (Yalom and Leszcz 2005). The public setting of group therapy provides a unique opportunity to have supervisors observed in action. Observing the supervisor can provide rich opportunities for the supervisor to model and normalize clinical fallibility and the unpredictability and imperfection inherent in all therapy groups. Similarly, it is very important for the supervisor to be able to observe the supervisee and the group by video or live observation, even if it is only for short periods of time.

Model Judicious Self-Disclosure

As part of the transmission of values of the profession, the supervisor ideally models warmth and judicious self-disclosure in the supervision (i.e., disclosure for the supervisee's and treatment's benefit), sharing his or her own struggles as a clinician and speaking authentically about emotional reactions to the group. These are important values that can in turn be modelled by the supervisee within the group to help the group members feel safe and welcomed (Leszcz 2011).

Set Realistic Goals

It is very important for the group to be a success experience for patients, many of whom arrive discouraged and demoralized. Helping the supervisee develop realistic goals and expectations for the group aids the process of selection and pregroup preparation during which consensus on goals and group guidelines can begin (Bernard et al. 2008; Yalom and Leszcz 2005). For example, the goals for an inpatient group with a lifespan of only one session (e.g., goal is for each patient to have a positive interaction with the leader or another copatient) will be significantly different from those for a long-term interpersonal group (i.e., goal is to change patterns of relating). The supervisee should be encouraged during the pregroup preparation meeting to carefully explore patient expectations and hopes for the group and try to ensure that these expectations align with what is possible to achieve in the group.

Demonstrate the Value of Common Group Therapeutic Factors

The supervisor needs to highlight the therapeutic value of spontaneous, authentic feedback among group members that harnesses several unique group therapeutic factors: universality (reduction of shame through appreciation of commonalities), altruism (increased self-esteem by helping others), instillation of hope (by seeing other members make progress), sharing of valuable information among group members, and cohesion (Bernard et al. 2008; Yalom and Leszcz 2005). Cohesion can be increased by helping supervisees facilitate member-to-member interactions during opportune moments in the group (i.e., member to member cohesion) (Burlingame et al. 2011). This is a skill that often needs to be explicitly demonstrated and reviewed in supervision. Supervisees should be encouraged to make bridging comments that help connect disclosures between different group members. Sometimes asking simple questions such as "Can anyone else relate to what was just said?" can help cultivate this process in the group. There are also member-to-leader and member-to-group bonds that also contribute to cohesion. Group cohesion is analogous to the therapeutic alliance in individual therapy and correlates with outcomes in all types of groups (Burlingame et al. 2011). Although certain types of groups and modalities do not focus explicitly on interactions between members (e.g., psychoeducation, cognitive-behavioral therapy groups), meaningful interactions between members can help increase cohesion in all types of groups, even if they occur for only brief moments. The supervisee can be encouraged to highlight and validate when this occurs in the group by making comments such as "It sounds like the two of you have a lot in common here; I am glad you can support each other."

Supervisees also need to be reminded about the value of vicarious learning in the group (i.e., less active members are still participating in one way or another and may be benefitting by observing interventions or interactions with other members) (Rutan et al. 2014) to reduce their anxiety about each member having "equal air time." This also challenges the misconception that group therapy works mainly through one-on-one interactions. It also models acceptance from the supervisor of not having total control over a group and being flexible and open to unanticipated therapeutic opportunities that arise within each session.

Help the Supervisee Address Group Norms and Group Dynamics

It is important for supervisees to be comfortable with a more active leadership style during the early stages of a group, when they help facilitate the development of positive group norms (e.g., group being a welcoming place, regular attendance, sharing openly, mutual respect, confidentiality, doing the group work), and in situations when the group's safety or cohesion is being compromised (e.g., managing excessive disclosures early in a group's life, challenging anti-therapeutic group norms, containing monopolizing or scapegoating) (Bernard et al. 2008; Yalom and Leszcz 2005). It is important to help supervisees appreciate that group process occurs at multiple levels: individuals may adopt certain roles in the group, specific interactions may occur between members, and group dynamics can operate at the group-as-a-whole level (Bernard et al. 2008; Rutan et al. 2014; Yalom and Leszcz 2005). The supervisor should strive to outline and model many different possible interventions that address the different elements of the group operating at any given moment. For example, after a significant emotional disclosure by an individual, the therapist may focus on the content of the individual's disclosure or on the reactions of the other members or the overall climate of the group in which people now feel safe to be vulnerable. The type of intervention will also be influenced by the type of group and theoretical model. For example, in some types of groups, the focus is more on individual issues (cognitive-behavioral therapy groups, psychoanalytic groups) than on interactions between members in other groups (interpersonal psychotherapy groups, support groups). However, it is important to be aware of group dynamics and group process in all groups regardless of modality, because group dynamics have an impact on the success of the group (Bernard et al. 2008).

Demonstrate the Value of Isomorphy

The supervisor can help demonstrate the value of a group perspective on a large scale by paying close attention to how the group interconnects with other "groups" and systems at different levels, a concept known as *isomorphy* (Yalom and Leszcz 2005). This includes focusing on how the group is perceived within the wider system and among colleagues and patients (e.g., Is it valued as a modality in the clinic and the teaching institution? Are there pressures to see higher volumes that impact the group?). Helping the supervisee articulate this in supervision can help him or her make sense of implicit pressures arising from the system that affect the group. For example, if group therapy is less valued either by patients or by one's colleagues and leadership, this can contribute to the therapist having diminished confidence in his of her clinical skills along with a reduced appreciation for the effectiveness of groups. Awareness of these outside perspectives can sometimes lead to opportunities for advocacy about the value of group to one's colleagues or leaders in the organization. In addition, understanding groups and systems demonstrates the generalizability and applicability of group training in a variety of other settings, including non-clinical roles such as teaching and administrative functions (Counselman 2008). Another aspect of isomorphy involves paying close attention to the relationship between the cotherapists, since tensions in this relationship can significantly impact the group through "leakage," whereby these tensions get enacted within the group sessions (e.g., cotherapists undermining each other in the group sessions).

Set Up Supervision

In addition to setting up times for observation, supervision of the group should occur weekly. If the supervisor co-leads the group with the supervisee, then supervision would ideally occur during the debrief period (usually 30–45 minutes) at the end of the group. Also, it is usually helpful to meet for at least 10–15 minutes before the group starts to address any issues that may have come up during the week and to help plan for the upcoming group session. If the cotherapists are both supervisees, the supervisor can either join their postgroup debriefing or meet with them at another time during the week. Supervisees are discouraged from taking detailed clinical notes in the group because it increases the risk of missing important clinical material. It is optimal to complete the notes right after group due to the large volume of clinical data that needs to be captured. Supervisees should be encouraged to take the lead in the supervision.

Specific Challenges and Strategies

- **Group members challenge or question me.** Although being challenged or questioned by group members may be very stressful for the supervisee, this can be an important part of the group's healthy development and may indicate that members feel safe enough to question the therapist (otherwise conflict may get redirected between members). The supervisee should be encouraged to welcome the feedback and address the concerns of the members (Yalom and Leszcz 2005).

- **There is conflict between members in the group.** This can be a very stressful experience for the supervisee. It is a good opportunity for the supervisor to normalize this occurrence in groups and to provide specific feedback on how this can be managed with concrete examples and scenarios. For example, if the interaction becomes too intense, the supervisee can encourage the members to step back and reflect on what is being triggered for them by the other member and to only discuss the impact the member is having on them emotionally rather than directly criticizing the other member (i.e., using "I feel" statements) (Yalom and Leszcz 2005). This can sometimes provide helpful therapeutic opportunities. Even if it is not possible to resolve differences, helping members to learn to tolerate differences can be very valuable. It may be helpful to remind the supervisee about the importance of group being a safe place. Also, the supervisee may find it helpful to be coached on how to actively discourage any expressions of hostility (overt or covert).

- **A group member is being scapegoated.** Supervisees are sometimes at risk of not responding quickly enough, especially if the scapegoating is subtle. Supervisees may need to be reminded about the seriousness and the need for an immediate response. The supervisor will probably have to take a more active role and provide clear guidance about possible interventions. The supervisee should be encouraged to openly name what is occurring and try to share an empathic formulation with the group that helps explain the person's behavior (e.g., "I wonder if he is pushing us away because he is afraid of rejection from the group?"). Also, the supervisee can ask other members to reflect on their own emotional reactions to redirect their focus. The group needs to be reminded that the patient who is being scapegoated often has a valuable function in the group since he/she may represent aspects that other members don't want to address in themselves (Rutan et al. 2014). However, in rare circumstances it may become necessary to remove a group member if he or she is unable to successfully participate in the group's tasks. The supervisee will probably require additional guidance about clear communication with the group since this can be quite disruptive to the stability of the group. In addition, the supervisee should be encouraged to have several subsequent individual meetings with the patient who has been removed from the group to address shame and self-blame—the message should be very clear that this is not the patient's fault and that this group was not the right fit at this time.

- **Group members are too quiet or too monopolizing.** Supervisees sometimes struggle addressing these situations which often arise in a group. Although equal levels of participation is neither realistic nor necessary, the supervisee should be encouraged to address this since members often get stuck in these roles and their behavior impact the entire group. It may be helpful if the supervisor describes several examples of how this could be addressed either during the group or during an individual meeting. It is probably less risky for the supervisee to address this during an individual meeting where the member's difficulties in the group can be explored in more depth. The supervisee should strive to collaborate with the patient on a plan to shift these behaviors in the group if possible.

- **The group has developed antitherapeutic norms (e.g., poor attendance, boundary crossings, subgrouping, members not doing work of the group).**

Supervisees need to be encouraged to address the group-as-a-whole if it seems that antitherapeutic group norms are covertly operating within the group. This should be done in a collaborative, nonthreatening manner—for example, "It feels like the group is stuck, I wonder what is going on? How have I contributed to this problem? How can we get unstuck here?"

- **I'm having strong negative feelings about the group or members in the group.** This is a very important opportunity for the supervisor to emphasize the value of emotional reactions in the therapist and to demonstrate how it can help guide therapeutic interventions (Leszcz 2011). The therapist should be guided on how to discuss this in a respectful, nonblaming manner in the group. It also allows the therapist to model how to give effective interpersonal feedback in the group. For example, "I appreciate that you felt safe enough to share with the group so openly last week, but I am worried that when you shared your plan to kill yourself 5 minutes before the group ended it made me anxious and unable to respond in the most helpful manner. I am hopeful that in the ongoing group work we can help you learn to express your needs in a manner that allows you to receive more helpful responses."

- **There is friction between the cotherapist and me.** This is a serious problem that can significantly affect the training experience for the supervisee and impact the group. The supervisor needs to address this carefully but directly, normalizing this is a common challenge in group therapy. Where possible, cotherapists should be encouraged to try to resolve (or at least accept) their differences in a way that allows them to effectively co-lead the group. However, if this is not possible, it may be best if one of the cotherapists leaves the group. If tension occurs when the supervisor co leads with the supervisee, again it should be carefully addressed. The supervisee should be encouraged to express differences of opinions in a safe manner—this becomes an important opportunity to model how working on the cotherapy relationship is an important part of group work.

Questions for the Supervisee

■ What were your emotional reactions to the group? (What did you like and not like about the group? What did you like and not like about your interventions?)

■ What was the overall climate/atmosphere in the group? How was the level of cohesion?

■ Are there any interactions in the group that stood out for you (positive or negative)?

■ Can you give me a brief summary of what each member said or did in the group?

■ Are there covert group norms that may be hindering the group's progress? For example, are members coming consistently late, are members avoiding certain topics?

■ Are there any members who are struggling or who seem stuck in certain roles (e.g., the quiet one, the cautious one, the monopolizer, the helper)?

■ How did you find working with your cotherapist? What is going well? Where are you struggling together?

Additional Resources

American Group Psychotherapy Association (AGPA): www.agpa.org (The AGPA website offers a variety of helpful resources for running groups, including a transtheoretical guide to developing and running groups.)

References

Bernard H, Burlingame G, Flores P, et al; Science to Service Task Force, American Group Psychotherapy Association: Clinical practice guidelines for group psychotherapy. Int J Group Psychother 58(4):455–542, 2008 18837662

Burlingame GM, McClendon DT, Alonso J: Cohesion in group therapy. Psychotherapy (Chic) 48(1):34–42, 2011 21401272

Counselman EF: Why study group therapy? Int J Group Psychother 58(2):265–272, 2008 18399741

Leszcz M: Psychotherapy supervision and the development of the therapist, in On Becoming a Psychotherapist: The Personal and Professional Journey. Edited by Klein RH, Bernard HS, Schermer VL. New York, Oxford University Press, 2011, pp 114–143

Rutan JS, Stone WN, Shay JJ: Psychodynamic Group Psychotherapy, 5th Edition. New York, Guilford, 2014

Yalom ID, Leszcz M: The Theory and Practice of Group Psychotherapy, 5th Edition. New York, Basic Books, 2005

Zaslav MR: A model of group therapist development. Int J Group Psychother 38(4):511–519, 1988 3182146

Chapter 23 Couples and Family Therapy Supervision

Learning to Work Systemically

Douglas S. Rait, Ph.D.

Training in family therapy is still the exception rather than the rule in psychiatry residency and clinical psychology training programs, despite the fact that couples and family therapies have been found to be effective in treating patients with a broad range of presenting problems, including most psychiatric disorders (Rait and Glick 2008). The capacity to effectively work with couples and families requires joining, recognizing the relational patterns that connect family members in both healthy and unhealthy ways, and intervening with a systemic model of change. Like all clinical supervision, the supervision of couples and family therapy draws on every dimension of both the supervisor's and learning clinician's domains of expertise and experience, including theoretical commitments, prior supervisory experiences, technical proficiency, learning style, emotional resonance, personal flexibility, family of origin experiences, and personal strengths and constraints.

Key Points

- Couples and family therapy supervision teaches supervisees how to
  - Join with the couple or family.
  - Understand the couple or family's developmental tasks, history and culture.
  - Identify systemic patterns and complementarity.
  - Work with a systemic model of change.

Structuring Supervision

Couples and family therapy supervision can be conducted through both video review and live supervision, and meetings typically focus on case formulation and hypothesizing, supporting the development of creative interventions and broadening the supervisee's style. Although individual meetings with supervisees are the norm, there are clear advantages to working with supervisees in pairs or small groups. The rationale for doing so is the same as that in treating patients in the context of their couple or family relationships: lasting individual change is often produced and reinforced by the important relationships that help encourage and maintain those changes. Additionally, changes are not limited to the individual patient, but frequently extend to others in the family. Pair or small-group supervision allows for the development of a clinical team (alliance formation), the chance to share cases (mutual learning), and opportunities to role-play clinical impasses and model therapeutic technique (enactments and in vivo learning).

The atmosphere of the supervision group tends to be lively, and supervisees value the opportunity to observe one another and learn from peers' experiences. In observing one another's work on a weekly basis, the group has the opportunity to learn as the supervisor addresses and discusses both generic clinical issues (e.g., handling "resistance") and more specific issues (e.g., understanding how a couple's particular pattern of interaction is common with mood disorders). At the same time, the goal of the supervisor is to find a way to create a safe enough place where supervisees' personal responses to cases can be identified and discussed.

Preparing for Supervision
Develop Knowledge Base

Supervision generally works best when supervisees have been introduced to systemic family therapy concepts, basic approaches to couples and family assessment, and at least a single model of couples or family treatment prior to seeing their first case. Ideally, supervisees meet weekly in small groups of two or three and present their cases, most often by showing clips from video-recorded sessions. When possible, each supervisee also receives live supervision, with the supervisor and team observing behind a one-way mirror, periodically throughout the clinical rotation.

Establish Goals

For most beginning supervisees, the most achievable outcome of training is exposure—that is, developing greater comfort sitting in the room with a couple of family, collecting a detailed history, seeing systemic patterns, and experimenting with systemic interventions. For more experienced supervisees, the goals are to help them link theory to practice, sharpen observational and interventional skills, develop a clear rationale for selecting a clinical strategy, and work with a broader range of couples and families that present a more challenging range of symptoms and problems.

Supervisors are encouraged to define and discuss clinical competencies at the outset of each rotation. Such competencies include, but are not limited to, joining with the couple or family; understanding the couple or family's developmental tasks, history, and culture; identifying systemic patterns and complementarity; and working with a systemic model of change. Idiosyncratic personal goals that each supervisee might identify, such as wanting to learn more about working with couples engaged in long-standing patterns of conflict-avoidance or how to treat a family dealing with an oppositional adolescent, would be added to the more generic supervisory goals listed above.

Addressing Key Goals of Supervision

An important part of clinical supervision is seeing it all come alive during the clinical encounter and helping the supervisee understand how to assess systemic patterns, collect a multigenerational history, devise thoughtful interventions, and create change experiences that free the couple or family from entrenched, dysfunctional interactions. The role of the supervisor is to create a trusted setting in which skills can be defined, described, demonstrated, and used effectively with couples and families. Supervisors provide specific feedback on supervisees' progress in the areas of conceptual skills and systemic thinking, assessment and engagement, planning and conducting interventions, and professional conduct.

Join With Couple or Family

Minuchin and Fishman (1981) view the family and clinician as forming a time-limited partnership that will support the process of exploration and transformation in therapy. Joining is considered to be the glue that holds together the therapeutic system, and virtually every model of family therapy highlights the importance of developing a strong initial bond and alliance with the couple or family and its members. While most supervisees are natural "joiners" and have a general idea of how to develop and maintain a strong relationship with their patients, doing so when working with a couple or family is more complex, as the clinician must form those ties with everyone in the family. As any clinician walking the tightrope between battling family members or competing coalitions knows, the most formidable clinical task involves not simply building these alliances, but sustaining them over the course of therapy (Rait 2000).

TABLE 23–1.	Developmental stages
Centripetal	Marriage
	Birth of children
	Young children
	Birth of grandchildren
	End of life
Centrifugal	Beginning school in childhood
	Adolescence
	Leaving home
	Death

Recognize Family Developmental Tasks, History, and Culture

As in individual treatment, supervisees must recognize the normal developmental tasks and transitions, beginning with couple formation and ending with death, that individuals, couples, and families routinely encounter (Table 23–1).

At the same time, each member of a couple or family brings with them an idiosyncratic history that serves as a blueprint against which current situations are appraised. The supervisor might ask supervisees to construct three-generational genograms, or family trees, that identify family patterns and themes as well as highlight connections between present family events and prior experiences (Figure 23–1). Finally, supervisors help supervisees explore and appreciate the important roles of gender, sexual and gender identity, culture, ethnicity, and class in their work with couples and families. By learning about how each family member's distinctive sociocultural background provides context and meaning for a family's traditions, choices, and preference, both through collecting detailed genogram information and learning to ask precise questions, supervisees can tailor both clinical formulations and strategies for change.

Understand Complementarity

In each case, individual "problems" are re-viewed in the context of couple and family interactions, and supervisees are encouraged to see the reciprocal relationships between family members' behaviors and individual symptoms and difficulties. In the context of working with couples, Minuchin and Nichols (1993, p. 63) observe, "In any couple, one person's behavior is yoked to the other's…it means that a couple's actions are not independent but codetermined, reciprocal forces." While reviewing video or watching sessions live from behind a one-way mirror, supervisees come to appreciate how complementarity, the linchpin of systemic thinking, functions as a defining principle in every relationship. In turn, they are asked to identify patterns of complementarity (e.g., overfunctioning/underfunctioning, teacher/student, pursuer/distancer) and recognize how these patterns organize and provide a frame for understanding couple and family interactions.

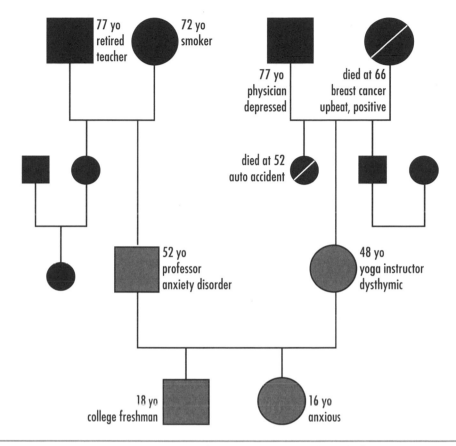

FIGURE 23–1. Genogram constructed by supervisee to identify family patterns and themes as well as highlight connections between present family events and prior experiences.

See Systemic Patterns and Identify Family Structure/Organization

At the same time, redundant patterns characterize most couple and family relationships, and supervisees learn to see the couple or family in terms of its structure and organization; instead of seeing only individuals, they begin to notice hierarchical imbalances in couples, coalitions and alliances, relationship triangles, cycles of pursuit and distancing. In doing so, they begin to prioritize process while still paying close attention to content.

Work With a Systemic Model of Change

Rather than targeting problematic individual behaviors, the systemic model of change recognizes that intervening in relationships that support and maintain these behaviors can be quite powerful. By disrupting and changing dysfunctional patterns and introducing alternatives, supervisees begin to recognize the significant difference between "first-order," or technical, change, such as improving communication skills, and "second-order," or systemic, change, in which relationship premises and patterns are modified. In doing so, the supervisee may expand the family's range by challenging constraining family patterns, promoting direct communication and successful conflict-resolution, and supporting the change process by helping family members integrate emerging patterns into new, reliable patterns of interaction (Rait and Glick 2008).

Specific Challenges and Strategies

- **My supervisee continues to work as an individual therapist within the context of couples or family therapy.** Because most supervisees have considerably more experience and comfort in working with individuals, they can respond to the anxiety and unfamiliarity of couples and family treatment by doing what they know best; that is, working with each individual person, as if in individual psychotherapy, in the presence of other family members. The reflex to think systemically rarely comes naturally, especially early on in the training experience, so the supervisor needs to help the supervisee to see individual behavior as part of a larger relational pattern while also helping the supervisee to identify ways to intervene systemically (e.g., helping one person to change by encouraging changes on the part of other family members). In every instance, the supervisor will be most successful by paying careful attention to the process and content of the supervisee's sessions, allying with the supervisee's strengths, and creating a comfortable setting where risks can be taken, feedback is genuine, and learning is valued.

- **My supervisee overidentifies with one family member.** Couples and family therapy often activates unexamined issues in the supervisee's own family or relationship experiences. For example, a supervisee may ally with one member's feelings of hopelessness when confronted with his or her depriving or hostile family member. An exploration of what feelings are being evoked by a particular couple or family interaction can be beneficial, and supervisees may also be encouraged to construct their own genograms to develop a stronger grasp of their own strengths and sensitivities that may be highlighted in their work with couples and families. When a supervisee has difficulty joining with or connecting with a family member, the supervisor might help the supervisee find something likeable about that person to help reduce the barrier to forming a therapeutic alliance.

- **My supervisee is anxious about the supervision.** Although initially anxious, most supervisees find observing themselves on video, receiving supervisory feedback in a small group, and going through the experience of live supervision to be supportive, authentic, constructive, and enjoyable. At the same time, it is important to continually assess the learning climate. Does the supervisee feel safe within the supervision context? If not, the supervisor might ask the supervisee, as well as team members, to offer ideas about what might help reduce self-consciousness and anxiety. Most supervisees readily see the benefits of observing each other's work in that they learn about the struggles of learning through their peers' experiences while also noticing their own potentially valuable contributions to their peers' cases. Live supervision can be especially helpful when cases have reached an impasse and when the supervisee can no longer find a new way to interact with and make progress with the couple or family. With direct observation, supervisees can hear the supervisor "think out loud" about case formulation, identify therapeutic choice points, challenge the thinking behind a clinical strategy, support the invention of particular interventions, and encourage authenticity, rigor, and spontaneity in the supervisee's approach (Rait and Glick 2008).

Questions for the Supervisee

■ What has been your prior clinical experience with couples and families?

■ What are your theoretical commitments in psychotherapy and in couples and family therapy, and why are those most resonant for you?

■ How would you describe previous supervisory experiences that went well or did not go so well for you? Why?

■ What are your personal goals for couples/family supervision? What part of working with families/couples do you think you will be less comfortable with?

■ What do you think your greatest areas of strength will be in terms of your work with families/couples?

■ What do you think will be the specific challenges you might encounter in working in this context?

■ Where would you like to be, with regard to working with couples and families, at the end of this rotation?

Additional Resources

Liddle H, Breunlin D, Schwartz R (eds): Handbook of Family Therapy Training and Supervision. New York, Guilford, 1988

References

Minuchin S, Fishman C: Techniques of Family Therapy. Cambridge, MA, Harvard University Press, 1981

Minuchin S, Nichols M: Family Healing: Tales of Hope and Renewal From Family Therapy. New York, Free Press, 1993

Rait DS: The therapeutic alliance in couples and family therapy. J Clin Psychol 56(2):211–224, 2000 10718604

Rait D, Glick I: A model for reintegrating couples and family therapy training in psychiatric residency programs. Acad Psychiatry 32(2):81–86, 2008 18349325

Chapter 24

Child and Adolescent Psychiatry Supervision

A Developmental Focus for the Patient and Trainee

Michelle Goldsmith, M.D.

Natalie Pon, M.D.

> Every night is a separation and every morning a reunion.
>
> —Thomas F. Anders

The ritual of night-time separation for children and their caregivers applies, in a developmentally specific way, to the supervisory relationship. Weekly, each concatenation or departure offers a rapprochement for the pair. The supervisor provides a secure base from which the supervisee explores the world of child mental health. Supervision in child and adolescent psychiatry/psychology (CAP) invites a remarkable opportunity for the adult learner to pursue his or her own professional and personal developmental milestones. Many supervisees navigate tasks related to intimacy versus isolation including possible parenthood. Working with pediatric patients allows for a didactic and experiential journey through development with a new point of vantage. Adult learners, with varying degrees of child experience, revisit the landscape of childhood to support struggling patients and families. Depending on the quality of training, and their own psychological and personal development, some supervisees may find that their new role stirs anxiety related to their own prior challenges, rescue fantasies, or feelings of insecurity (Benedek 1959). The supervising clinicians serve as guides along a reconceived path of childhood. In this chapter, we highlight skills for the supervisee caring for youth and families and underscore key principles for successful supervision.

The training and supervision of clinicians who care for the mental health of children boasts its own body of literature. Therefore, this overview showcases selected topics relevant to CAP that may differ from other types of clinical supervision; these concepts apply to psychotherapy, psychopharmacology, consultation, general case management, and other permutations of care. We highlight here the following areas as they relate to CAP supervision in the care of children and families: a developmentally informed approach, therapeutic alliance building and countertransference, and ethical principles.

Key Points

- Supervision incorporates its own developmental process for the learner.

- A stakeholder analysis is a technique for understanding the ecology of a child's life and learning to balance a patient's autonomy in the context of their age, developmental stage, and best interest.

- Prior experience with children, and knowledge of developmental milestones and theory, facilitate realistic goal setting and identification of areas for learning in supervision.

- Supervisors should teach about typical ethical dilemmas that arise with preschool age, latency age, and adolescent patients.

Developmentally Informed Supervision

The developmental consideration of a child's presenting symptoms represents a sine qua non for understanding all that follows in care. A developmentally informed assessment, diagnosis, formulation, and treatment plan fosters best practices for ideal therapeutic intervention(s) and optimization of patient and parent understanding (Winters et al. 2007). For CAP clinicians, knowledge of cognitive, motor, emotional, and social tasks forms a matrix within which key milestones can be anticipated. The supervisor will teach the novice clinician to gauge which presenting signs and symptoms suggest a neurotypical presentation versus neuroatypicality or psychopathology.

In preparing for a case, the supervisor guides the supervisee regarding the assessment format, the child's ability to describe symptoms based not only on the child's chronological age but also on his or her developmental stage. The learner's prior experience with children, relevant knowledge base, and prior clinical care of children should be examined by direct inquiry. Didactic coursework offered concurrently with clinical care complements supervision. Expecting supervisees to build and refresh their fund of knowledge regarding developmental milestones and theory is appropriate. High-yield supervision for child cases often includes cotherapy, role-playing, session recordings, and/or a "bug-in-the-ear" (microphone) (see Part 3: "Supervision Techniques," in this volume). An important skill is to teach the supervisee to use developmentally appropriate, nonpathologizing language when communicating with the patient.

Preschool-age patients typically struggle verbally to convey internal states, preferring play as a medium of communication. Therefore, a supervisor directs a supervisee toward sociodramatic and symbolic play. The supervisor prepares the supervisee for the work with young children with a selection of toys to engage the patient in fantasy or representational play to evoke expression. The weekly supervision includes interpretation of the play content and process, such as linking repetitive themes to an experience of crisis or trauma for the child, similar to flashbacks (Benham and Slotnick 2006). Supervisors may allow use of their toys in a designated space, but lending them out may lead to loss of inventory; toys are difficult to label and always should be cleaned after each use. Exploring how each supervisee may want to build and manage his or her own toy collection is an important topic.

School-age children, with increasing ability to mentalize and to engage in reality-based reasoning, share a larger role in decision making during treatment. Supervisors model tasks of development, such as industry versus inferiority, by highlighting opportunities for the supervisee (and the patient) to exercise agency. One technique for supervisors may be to incorporate discussion questions that allow the supervisee to reinforce his or her knowledge of developmental theory. For example, "How did your patient demonstrate competency and overcome inertia during play?" (Erikson, industry vs. inferiority). Alternatively, "What theorist and stage of development was observed when your 8-year-old patient kept score while playing?" (Piaget, concrete operations). Supervisees most often remember the details of developmental tasks when applied to a patient; the supervisor can review case material and supplement with charts comparing, contrasting, and linking major developmental theories.

Adolescent patients may present as more advanced in one developmental domain, such as cognitive or intellectual abilities, and lagging in other areas like social-emotional development; such discrepancies often contribute to the chief complaint. Additionally, as is consistent with the adolescent task of balancing dependence and self-determination, supervisees frequently encounter resistance on the part of the teenage patient. This is an opportunity for the supervisor to help the supervisee in connecting creatively with teens, which may be via music or art, and recruit techniques from motivational interviewing. The supervisor should urge the supervisee to consider the patient from the perspective of all current developmental tasks, and possible earlier derailments, emphasizing that adolescence is a critical factor in character formation.

The supervisor utilizes the developmental perspective to help the supervisee distinguish between diagnosis and case formulation (Jellinek and McDermott 2004). As Winters and colleagues (2007) note, "The case formulation speculates on the child's strengths, challenges, stressors, family legacy, social and cultural influences; developmental contextualization of symptoms creates meaning and suggests prognosis....A well-rounded understanding of development and developmental insults serve as a vehicle with a path marked out initially by the supervisor, for converting a diagnosis to a plan for treatment, timing and intervention" (p.114). All strong child supervision should include some opportunity to write an initial case formulation and then later review the document during successive treatment plans.

Supervision in child and adolescent psychiatry involves a parallel process of the supervisee's development and the patient's clinical trajectory; just as the patient grows, supervision is a core developmental process for the supervisee. Supervisors model how to remain flexible and develop the capability to expand technical skills as well as how to thoughtfully utilize oneself as a clinical tool (Harrison 1978). In doing so, supervisors guide their supervisees to be cognizant of their own needs, capabilities, and limitations, just as CAP does for the patient, marking and metering his or her own developmental trajectory.

Therapeutic Engagement With Children and Families and Exploration of Countertransference

Mental health care for children, unlike for adults, predictably involves multiple stakeholders, including the supervisor. Although teen youth can initiate their own treatment without parent consent (as mandated by local statutes), typically a parent(s) seeks clinical care on behalf of the "identified patient." For those new to pediatric work, prior experience with reluctant or uncooperative patients stems from situations such as capacity evaluations, involuntary commitments, and court-mandated care of adults. Techniques of active listening and empathy acquired in prior training aid the supervisee, but the experienced supervisor should prepare the supervisee to anticipate varying degrees of initial engagement and to practice flexibility with gathering information. For example, a neutral, reserved stance is often the default starting affect with adult patients; however, pediatric patients frequently need more warmth from the therapist for initial engagement. Supervisory input about the complex triangulated nature of the treatment among clinician, caregiver, and patient deserves specific attention and discussion, and the supervisory working alliance infuses yet another layer to the stakeholder analysis.

A strategy designed with multiple stakeholders in mind anticipates that each party may bear different opinions about why they present, the level of motivation to engage, what the presenting problems are, how they should be solved, and who actually needs clinical care. Conducting a stakeholder analysis to identify important individuals and entities with influence in the child's life is a useful exercise for the supervisor to teach the supervisee. Supporting parents and including them in treatment is essential; additionally, less obvious individuals, such as babysitters, grandparents, siblings, teachers, coaches, and clergy, may all play a significant role in the patient's life. How these various constituents could act as sources of collateral information (with guardian's consent and patient's assent), and how each may help the patient reach clinical goals, should be explored in supervision. Acknowledging disparate beliefs helps to establish a *dual alliance* with parent(s) and patient (Joshi 2006). This recognition extends to the supervisor and supervisee as well; some of the best learning experiences arise over disagreement on diagnosis and treatment. As mentioned earlier, the supervisee also works to attain developmental tasks such as confidence, competence, autonomy, identify formation, separation, and individuation. Thoughtful and supportive dialogue about clinical decision making within the supervisory dyad will promote the formation of these developmental milestones, paralleling how the therapist and family move closer to a working alliance.

Devoting time in supervision to create a detailed and concise narrative about the child's world supports the therapeutic alliance. The supervisor serves as an audience and poses questions about significance and relationship between points of information, and in doing so may identify crucial missing data. This narrative process should also be introduced to the patient and guardian so they too can author a story from their own perspective. The effort devoted to creating meaning in an age-appropriate manner supports a therapeutic alliance by ensuring that the family knows and experiences that the clinician practices active listening and conceptualizes the family's needs in a broad and detailed manner.

As with adult work, clinical care with children and their parents engenders varying degrees of both positive and negative countertransference, and it is the supervisor's role to navigate this territory with the supervisee. While the concept of countertransference pervades earlier training, overlapping configurations of multiple countertransferential relationships within a single case necessitate close examination in supervision. Inherently, a child psychiatric patient bears, at a minimum, a triangle of relationships (i.e., the identified patient, the caregiver/guardian, and the therapist); however, in most cases, the structure is far more complicated and expands to additional family members, the family as a unit, and other individuals (e.g., extended family, sitters, teachers), offering new challenges to building and maintaining a therapeutic alliance. For the purposes of discussing countertransference/transference, the term "parent" is used here but embodies the primary caretaker, guardian, or other main point of contact who presents with the patient.

In helping supervisees manage countertransference, supervisors navigate the frequently blurred line between supervision and therapy. CAP cases in particular may reactivate buried issues from childhood; there may be a parallel dynamic process occurring between the supervisee/supervisor and the child/parent. The supervisee's own childhood must be acknowledged and attended to without the supervision morphing into the supervisee's personal therapy/analysis. The supervisor may focus on the supervisee's here-and-now responses to patients and refrain from drawing conclusions based on what he or she knows about the supervisee personally. The supervisor can address countertransference by focusing on the supervisee's feelings generated by the patient and parent (or other stakeholders) and steering clear of how the supervisee's past plays a role (Gabbard 2017). For example, a supervisor may know some details—such as culture or ethnic background—about a supervisee's family of origin but would not derive parallels, even if they exist, between a case and the supervisee's family or make assumptions that the supervisee understands the family dynamics at play.

A common scenario that supervisees encounter is one of competing emotions toward the patient and the parent that may arise from various etiologies. Frequently, these manifest as positive, protective feelings toward the child, regarded as a product of the parental environment (e.g., depriving, chaotic), and contrasting negative feelings toward the parents, or in some cases, the "imagined" or absent parent who has "abandoned" the child (Harrison 1978). Children, drawing on rescue fantasies or rousing significant anxiety in the supervisee, may stir strong desires in the supervisee to become the "surrogate" or "perfect parent" for the child that can undermine one leg of the working alliance: the parent. The supervisor serves as a mirror for the supervisee to examine the latter's possibly exaggerated compassion and empathy toward the patient, and then shifts the focus for the supervisee to consider the parent's own underlying feelings, possibly guilt and shame. When the supervisee increases the empathic response toward the parents and presents himself or herself as an ally, progress in care often ensues. When the patient's treatment gains stall and the parent expresses dissatisfaction, this complaint often activates feelings of inadequacy, helplessness, or frustration in the supervisee—notably similar to how the parent may feel, presenting an opportunity for expressing empathy. Essentially, the supervisee cannot treat the patient without the parent's support; identifying the parent's emotional needs strategically positions the supervisee as an agent of positive change.

Self-disclosure with children represents another delicate area when therapeutic engagement is being considered. For example, an innocently posed question by the pediatric patient like "Do you have a dog?" (the type of inquiry frequently sidestepped with an adult by inserting another question, e.g., "What makes you ask?" or "I'm wondering why you're asking me?"), when unanswered by the supervisee, may confuse a child or be interpreted as a rejection. This exchange becomes a missed opportunity to bond with the patient at his or her developmental stage. Reminding the supervisee that he or she may be asked more questions by children, who are often more spontaneous and less filtered than adults, will prepare the supervisee. The supervisor should discuss with the supervisee the potential therapeutic benefit and harm of indirectly disclosing personal information. Forethought about how to establish boundaries with the pediatric patient and parents allows for customizing treatment—for example, when cultural factors are at play or a prior mental health experience influences the family. Professional conduct and clarity defining the therapeutic frame is not intended to distance the clinician; situations arise when self-disclosure is therapeutic. The supervisory relationship affords fertile ground to explore how to respond to such circumstances. The degree of self-disclosure within the supervisory dyad serves as a litmus test and deserves consideration because it too necessitates thoughtfully placed limitations. As Gutheil and Gabbard (2003, p. 410) remind us, "*External* boundaries are established so that *psychological* boundaries can be crossed through a variety of mechanisms common to psychotherapy, including empathy, projection, introjection, identification, projective identification, and the interpretation of transference."

Ethics and CAP Supervision

It is the supervisor's obligation to explore and optimize the supervisee's understanding of ethics with regard to children, discovering anew how these seemingly familiar principles (e.g.,consent and confidentiality) apply to children and families. The supervisor should teach the supervisee how to balance a patient's autonomy in the context of age, developmental stage, and best interest and educate about typical ethical dilemmas that arise with preschool, latency, and adolescent patients. Supervisors at times unwittingly impart their own principles, setting the preliminary structure from which supervisees draw their own ethical style as a clinician. Several national organizations outline ethical clinical practice and principles for working with children and adolescents to guide practitioners (see "Additional Resources" near the end of this chapter). Although each clinical scenario poses ethical points of interest, this discussion limits key ethics topics for supervision to a focus on 1) confidentiality, 2) autonomy and assent/informed consent, and 3) emerging issues related to technology.

Confidentiality

Issues of trust and confidentiality are more complex for the CAP clinician who interacts with the parent as well as the patient; the parental right to know information may or may not coincide with the patient's best interest. Such complexities position the supervisor to lead and educate the supervisee, facilitating a well-designed conversation with the patient and parent/guardian at the first clinical contact about the limits of confidentiality to protect ethical practice and ensure preservation of the therapeutic relationship. This conversation, which also happens with adults and is revisited throughout treatment in various forms, differs with children in several ways and should be preemptively discussed in supervision. Of note, as the limits of confidentiality are discussed, the supervisor may remind the supervisee that the supervisor is a member of the treatment; both the parent and the patient should be aware that the case content is discussed with all members of their clinical care team, including the supervisor. Supervisors should recommend that supervisees document that this conversation has occurred. The supervisor may role-play conversations with ethical principles in mind and explore the application of subjective beliefs when the choice is being made to break confidentiality.

The threshold for breaching confidentiality with an adolescent versus an adult is often lower given their status as minors. For youth, the natural drive for independence invites risky behavior such as experimenting with substances or sex. For example, a nearly 18-year-old patient discloses binge drinking at a party followed by an amnestic blackout that she has not shared with her parents. The supervisee, who is now triangulated with the patient and parent, risks a "secret keeping" role that poses many challenges. This dynamic of information sharing and safekeeping necessitates a conversation between supervisee and supervisor about unintended collusion with the patient and avoidance of "parentification," perhaps in support of the therapeutic "bond." When alerted, the supervisor should offer ethical approaches and psychotherapeutic options as well as advice on how to discuss the need to breach confidentiality in light of dangerous behavior. To complicate the aforementioned scenario, if the patient shared such information after her 18th birthday, the "magic threshold" into legal adulthood, then a different set of ethical rules would apply; these situations showcase the nuances of autonomy and beneficence in CAP and the need for a strong supervision experience.

Assent and Informed Consent

Minors should be involved in treatment decision making, and assent should be attained. Most general psychiatry residents lack experience with assent unless they have cared for an incapacitated or incompetent patient. For CAP, the concept of assent emerges daily in treatment planning and engagement. Legal guardians or parents must always consent to treatment; however, providers should communicate fully with the patient in the most developmentally appropriate manner to obtain patient assent. These clinical conversations should be documented for the medical record and reviewed in supervision. Particular care should be taken when the patient and parent(s) disagree— for example, with divorced parents who do not agree with treatment planning. A typical complicating factor in care is when the parent initiates evaluation and care and then the minor patient balks or refuses. This dilemma may rouse feelings in the supervisee reminiscent of internal conflicts experienced with involuntary commitment, forced medication, and coercion in general. First, the supervisor should reflect on his or her own biases regarding conflicts around consent and assent. This insight will allow for cognitive separation from the supervisee, who will naturally entertain his or her own questions and countertransference around medicating and treating reluctant minor patients.

Technology in the CAP Population

Ongoing advances in technology and unavoidable social media have a dramatic impact on the practice of child mental health. In fact, patients may access social media to investigate a clinician necessitating that the provider think about how to construct (or deconstruct) his or her own social media presence. Additionally, use of technology can be a powerful way to build rapport and reinforce a provider's presence and accessibility, and should not automatically be discouraged. Advances in technology, such as emailing, texting, and using internal patient record communication systems, should be discussed in supervision regarding optimization of clinical care, HIPAA (Health Insurance Portability and Accountability Act) compliance, and setting of limits and boundaries with patients and especially their parents. Supervisors must help supervisees consider what degree and type of information, and accessibility, they want to share. Younger supervisees educated in a pervasive digital age may be apt to approach the use of technology much differently than more senior providers; millennial-age supervisors may possess greater familiarity with current technology compared with supervisors of prior generations. The supervisory relationship is a forum for both parties to examine their own practices and beliefs as well as the many benefits and drawbacks of technology use in treatment.

Specific Challenges and Strategies

- **My supervisee is anxious because the patient is so young and he is unfamiliar with children.** Inquire about the nature of the anxiety and what it relates to without assuming that you understand it, and ask directly about the supervisee's past experience with children. Encourage the supervisee to familiarize himself with normally developing children, via videos and in vivo observations (e.g., preschool visits), and identify typical developmental milestones.

- **My supervisee needs support related to individuation and separation while simultaneously needing to foster the same for her patient.** Remind the CAP supervisee that she has completed general training and obtained confidence and competence working with adults. Draw parallels for the supervisee as she struggles with being a novice, as do adolescents when acquiring new social, emotional, and cognitive skills. By remaining cognizant of the strengths and capabilities of the supervisee, even in spite of limited experience with children, you can by extension bring this experience of self-empowerment of the supervisee to the treatment of the child. Connecting and comparing the two in vivo processes of supervisee and patient developmental tasks is a unique opportunity in CAP supervision.

- **My supervisee is having difficulty balancing the needs of the child, the caretaker, the family as a unit, and other stakeholders.** Model case formulation and discussion from the point of view of all stakeholders. Support the supervisee in developing clinical flexibility, and define the supervisee's role and professional boundaries as a consultant, family therapist, individual therapist, psychopharmacologist, and so forth.

- **My supervisee is anxious working with parents and their inquiries about supervisee competence and parental status.** Anticipate and prepare the supervisee with a scripted response: "Can you share with me why you are asking?" Discuss disclosure of one's own status as a parent in supervision, because this has significant ramifications in the patient's treatment and the impact of disclosure on therapeutic tasks, bonds, and goals. Explore the potential conflicts and/or benefits of the supervisee's sharing whether he himself is a parent.

- **My supervisee has minimal interest in child work.** For the sake of minimizing resentment and disappointment, a supervisor may first wish to identify his or her own frustration with such a supervisee because this may feel like a missed opportunity. Remind the supervisee that the clinical care of children will enhance his or her skills as a mental health clinician. Ask the supervisee to present a case formulation for an adult patient and demonstrate the utility of understanding childhood developmental milestones, strengths/protective factors, and losses.

Questions for the Supervisee

- Would you share with me your prior experiences with children including jobs, prior clinical training, and family or friend interactions? What were some of your more meaningful experiences and why?

- What is your understanding of our current patient's developmental tasks?

- How did you experience the patient? The parent?

- What barriers to the building a therapeutic alliance do you foresee?

- What defenses were employed by the patient or parent? With you? With each other? How did these affect your countertransference?

- What dynamics are you experiencing with this case?

- At the beginning of care, how will you approach reviewing confidentiality with minor patients of different age groups?

- If a patient were engaging in self-harming behavior, how would you decide to inform parents/caregivers and what ethical principles would apply?

- How would you approach informed consent with a child who is too young to cognitively understand the risks, benefits, alternatives of pharmacotherapy or psychotherapy?

- How accessible will you make yourself via technology? How will you manage boundaries both for yourself and for the patient?

Additional Resources

Pediatric Case Formulation and Development

Fox G, Katz DA, Eddins-Folensbee FF, et al: Teaching development in undergraduate and graduate medical education. Child Adolesc Psychiatr Clin N Am 16(1):67–94, 2007

Winters N, Hanson G, Stoyanova V: The case formulation in child and adolescent psychiatry. Child Adolesc Psychiatric Clin N Am 16(1):111–132, 2007

Therapeutic Alliance Building and Psychotherapy

Gabbard GO: Long-Term Psychodynamic Psychotherapy: A Basic Text, 3rd Edition. Washington, DC, American Psychiatric Association Publishing, 2017

Kernberg PF, Ritvo R, Keable H: The American Academy of Child and Adolescent Psychiatry Committee on Quality Issues: practice parameter for psychodynamic psychotherapy with children. J Am Acad Child Adolesc Psychiatry 51(5):541–557, 2012

Ethics and Boundary Issues

American Academy of Child and Adolescent Psychiatry: Code of Ethics, September 16, 2014. Available at: https://www.aacap.org/App_Themes/AACAP/docs/about_us/transparency_portal/aacap_code_of_ethics_2012.pdf.

American Academy of Child and Adolescent Psychiatry: Ethics and Child and Adolescent Psychiatry. Available at: https://www.aacap.org/AACAP/Member_Resources/Ethics/Ethics_Committee/Home.aspx?WebsiteKey=a2785385-0ccf-4047-b76a-64b4094ae07f&hkey=bf4cb017-4d6e-4b41-b342-f2aed97c4efa.

DeJong SM, Gorrindo T: To text or not to text: applying clinical and professionalism principles to decisions about text messaging with patients. J Am Acad Child Adolesc Psychiatry 53(7):713–5, 2014

References

Benedek T: Parenthood as a developmental phase; a contribution to the libido theory. J Am Psychoanal Assoc 7(3):389–417, 1959 13672860

Benham AL, Slotnick CF: Play therapy: integrating clinical and developmental perspectives, in Handbook of Preschool Mental Health Development, Disorders, and Treatment. Edited by Luby J. New York, Guilford, 2006, pp 331–371

Gabbard GO: Long-Term Psychodynamic Psychotherapy. Arlington, VA, American Psychiatric Association Publishing, 2017

Gutheil TG, Gabbard GO: Misuses and misunderstandings of boundary theory in clinical and regulatory settings. Focus 1(4):415–421, 2003

Harrison SI: Expanding the role of supervision in child psychiatric education. Child Psychiatry Hum Dev 9(1):40–55, 1978 720154

Jellinek MS, McDermott JF: Formulation: putting the diagnosis into a therapeutic context and treatment plan. J Am Acad Child Adolesc Psychiatry 43(7):913–916, 2004 15213593

Joshi SV: Teamwork: the therapeutic alliance in pediatric pharmacotherapy. Child Adolesc Psychiatr Clin N Am 15(1):239–262, 2006 16321733

Winters NC, Hanson G, Stoyanova V: The case formulation in child and adolescent psychiatry. Child Adolesc Psychiatr Clin N Am 16(1):111–132, ix, 2007 17141121

Chapter 25   Integrated Psychiatric Care Supervision

Robert M. McCarron, D.O.

Matthew Reed, M.D., M.S.P.H.

Anna Ratzliff, M.D., Ph.D.

Michelle Burke Parish, Ph.D., M.A.

Shannon Suo, M.D.

Rachel Robitz, M.D.

Jaesu Han, M.D.

Peter Yellowlees, M.B.B.S., M.D.

Key Points

- The goals of supervision differ depending on which of the four distinct models of care is used: collaborative care, embedded consultation, telepsychiatry, and preventative medicine in psychiatry.

- Collaborative care supervision must align with five core principles: patient-centered care, measurement-based treatment to target, population-based care, evidence-based care, and accountable care.

- Embedded consultation supervision is similar to traditional outpatient psychiatric care but with some key differences, including a focus on effective communication with other medical providers and an emphasis on psychiatrist role definition.

- Telemedicine supervision should focus on the appropriate use of in-person versus digital communication when establishing care coordination teams.

- Preventative medicine in psychiatry supervision goals include developing the supervisee's knowledge of preventative medicine interventions appropriate for the psychiatry clinic and verifying that intervention goals are being met (through electronic medical record metrics).

Collaborative Care

The collaborative care model uses a population health approach to provide mental health care to a large population using limited resources. The evidence base for collaborative care shows it to be both effective at improving patient outcomes and cost-effective (Archer et al. 2012; Unützer et al. 2008). Supervision of trainees is based on the five core principles that underlie the collaborative care model: patient-centered care, evidence-based care, measurement-based treatment to target, population-based care, and accountable care (University of Washington 2017). Supervisors should understand that the skills trainees will need to work on in collaborative care teams are not traditionally taught in psychiatric training programs. Supervisors must demonstrate for trainees how to function as a clinical consultant, care team educator, and team leader (Ratzliff et al. 2015). The five core principles of collaborative care are used to describe considerations when supervising trainees to work in collaborative care teams.

Patient-Centered Care

As supervisors demonstrate how to function as a clinical consultant, care team educator, and team leader, the key principle of patient-centered care cannot be lost. In primary care settings, the pace is much faster, there tend to be more interruptions, and some of the boundaries are looser. For some trainees, this faster pace may not appear patient centered. Supervisors must demonstrate the increased flexibility required for psychiatrists to have an impact in the primary care environment. Trainees should become adept at providing consultation "on the fly" and must develop skills in providing succinct and specific guidance to primary care providers (Reardon et al. 2015).

Evidence-Based Care

Working within this model requires an expanded base of clinical knowledge from what is typically seen in outpatient psychiatric settings (Ratzliff et al. 2015). Trainees should have a firm grasp of the following clinical topics: attention-deficit/hyperactivity disorder, anxiety disorders, suicide/violence risk assessment, major depressive disorder, chronic pain, psychiatric issues in pediatric populations, psychiatric issues in pregnancy, somatic symptoms, substance use disorder, and eating disorders (Ratzliff et al. 2015). Supervision of trainees should also provide training in brief psychosocial interventions, including motivational interviewing and cognitive-behavioral therapy (Reardon et al. 2015) (see Chapter 19, Cognitive-Behavioral Therapy Supervision").

Measurement-Based Treatment to Target

Trainees must become familiar with evidence-based measurement tools, and how to interpret their results (see Chapter 42, "Integrating Measurement-Based Care Into Supervision"). Supervisors can assist trainees by teaching skills for evaluating a registry to find outliers and use a targeted step-wise approach to provide both indirect and direct consultation. For example, Patient Health Questionnaire–9 scores are now often entered into electronic medical records (EMRs) in a similar manner to entering vital signs. These scores can be trended over time and compared with those of other depressed patients in a panel. Those patients not showing improvement—the outliers—can be evaluated for any common deficiencies in evidence-based treatment for depression. When such deficiencies are found, recommendations can be made to the primary care provider and care manager for treatment adjustments. After teaching this process, supervisors should directly observe trainees performing the analysis to ensure adequate data gathering and interpretation. Providing supervision to those conducting indirect consultations may require that trainees be assisted in knowing how to listen to information shared by the other team members, how to form a differential diagnosis and treatment plan with limited information, and what questions to ask to assist in developing an appropriate treatment plan (Raney 2015; Ratzliff et al. 2015)

Population-Based Care

Thinking about a population of patients as opposed to individual patients requires a different approach to care. Along with understanding how to use registries to care for populations of patients as mentioned above, supervision should provide trainees with a framework for systems thinking. Systems thinking allows them to understand the system that they're functioning in and how best to apply the collaborative care model to their system (Ratzliff et al. 2015).

Accountable Care

Trainees functioning within these systems should understand quality metrics and care reimbursement, including the way in which collaborative care programs are typically funded (e.g., more transparency in how training settings are funded). Supervision is important for helping trainees understand that the team is reimbursed for clinical outcomes and higher quality care.

Embedded Psychiatric Consultation

Embedded psychiatric consultation in outpatient settings includes psychiatric work in tandem with a patient's primary care provider. Consults are requested by medical providers as in the traditional model; however, instead of the patient seeing a psychiatrist outside of the medical provider's office as is done traditionally, the psychiatrist is physically located in the primary care or medical setting office. The consulting psychiatrist is able to see the patient in the same clinical space that is used to see the patient for his or her medical needs (Reardon et al. 2015).

The characteristics of this model are similar to those of traditional outpatient psychiatric care. Embedded care does differ from traditional models in that psychiatrists have more interaction with primary care and medical providers. Also, they may be asked to provide support to the providers in a "curbside" fashion if a patient who they mutually see presents for a primary care visit with an acute psychiatric need. When one is providing supervision for trainees working within this model, it is most important to highlight skills in communicating with and educating primary care and other medical providers, similar to inpatient consultation-liaison roles. Demonstrating the kind of succinct and targeted communication needed is essential before the trainee will be able to mirror this communication style. Trainees should have a firm understanding of their role in the embedded practice setting. In some embedded psychiatric consultation settings, psychiatric consultants provide direct consultation for a limited time (i.e., they may only see the patient for six sessions to stabilize them before re-referring them back to their primary care provider), but in other settings, once the patient has been referred to a psychiatric consultant, he or she follows with the consultant indefinitely.

Telepsychiatry

Technological changes—nano, genomic, digital, or cloud based, or some combination of these—are one of the most obvious trends currently transforming the U.S. health and education markets (Yellowlees and Shore 2018). Communication technologies are ubiquitous and are already widely used for all types of clinical work. Digital communication is likely to become the standard of practice for many clinical relationships, especially for collaborative care in which one psychiatrist may coordinate care teams at multiple sites in the same day. Digital supervision in collaborative care settings should focus on appropriate use of communication technologies both for direct patient care and for care coordination and team building (online and in-person). For example, a supervisor should help trainees understand that an in-person site visit may be preferable to videoconferencing when establishing a new care coordination team (see Chapter 4, "Virtual or Hybrid Supervision").

Preventative Medicine in Psychiatry

Preventative medicine in psychiatry refers to primary and secondary prevention of general medical conditions that disproportionately affect patients with mental illness rather than comprehensive management. This is consistent with the goal of equipping psychiatry trainees with tools to help patients successfully navigate the primary care setting. Supervision of trainees in this area may take place in general psychiatry clinics or in collaborative care settings. Supervision goals in the psychiatry clinic include developing a trainee's knowledge of appropriate preventative medicine interventions and verifying that intervention goals are being met (through EMR metrics). An example of an appropriate preventative medicine intervention for a psychiatry clinic might include screening for diabetes and hyperlipidemia and initiation of lifestyle modifications should screening return positive results.

Specific Challenges and Strategies

- **The primary care provider working with my supervisee doesn't feel that our treatment recommendations are realistic.** Often supervisees are unaware of the significant time constraints primary care physicians face. Average visit lengths may only be 15 minutes, during which multiple medical issues in addition to a given psychiatric issue must be addressed. It is essential that your supervisee understand the time constraints and competing demands before they provide clinical recommendations. One helpful method to teach this is to encourage your supervisee to "shadow" the primary care provider for one or two half-days. Instruct the supervisee to pay attention to the clinic workflow. Then discuss what the supervisee observed and what interventions he or she now believes are feasible. Doing this can have a significant impact on the quality of recommendations your supervisee provides to the primary care physician.

- **My supervisee is frequently frustrated with the care coordinator.** At times supervisees may become so focused on panel "outcomes" and "metrics" that they neglect key relationships. Their relationship with the care coordinator is essential. When this relationship suffers, communication with the primary care clinic and implementation of treatment recommendations may be compromised. You can prevent deterioration of this key relationship by demonstrating the kind of respectful and collaborative relationship you want the supervisee to develop. Emphasize the importance of this relationship by asking about it during each of your supervision sessions. Any issues that arise can then be addressed early on before any impasses develop.

Questions for the Supervisor

- Does my supervisee have a sound understanding of the primary care clinics patient workflow?

- Does my supervisee have a collaborative relationship with his or her care coordinator?

- Does my supervisee understand his or her role on the team?

- Are my supervisee's recommendations implemented by the primary care provider? If not, why?

Additional Resources

Integrative Care

Cowley D et al: Teaching psychiatry residents to work at the interface of mental health and primary care. Acad Psychiatry 38(4):398–404, 2014

Raney LE (ed): Integrated Care: Working at the Interface of Primary Care and Behavioral Health. Arlington, VA, American Psychiatric Association Publishing, 2015

Preventive Medicine in Psychiatry

McCarron RM, Xiong GL, Keenan CR, et al: Preventive Medical Care in Psychiatry: A Practical Guide for Clinicians. Arlington, VA, American Psychiatric Publishing, 2014

McCarron RM, Bourgeois JA, Chwastiak LA, et al: Integrated medicine and psychiatry curriculum for psychiatry residency training: a model designed to meet growing mental health workforce needs. Acad Psychiatry 39(4):461–465, 2015

McCarron RM, Xiong G, Keenan C, et al: Preventive Medical Care in Psychiatry: A Practical Guide for Clinicians: Study Guide. Arlington, VA, American Psychiatric Association Publishing, 2016

Psychiatric Consultation

Desan PH et al: Proactive psychiatric consultation services reduce length of stay for admissions to an inpatient medical team. Psychosomatics 52(6):513–520, 2011

Telepsychiatry

American Telemedicine Association: www.americantelemed.org

Yellowlees P, Shore JH: Telepsychiatry and Health Technologies: A Guide for Mental Health Professionals. Arlington, VA, American Psychiatric Association Publishing, 2018

References

Archer J, Bower P, Gilbody S, et al: Collaborative care for depression and anxiety problems. Cochrane Database Syst Rev 10:CD006525, 2012 23076925

Crowley RA, Kirschner N; Health and Public Policy Committee of the American College of Physicians: The integration of care for mental health, substance abuse, and other behavioral health conditions into primary care: executive summary of an American College of Physicians position paper. Ann Intern Med 163(4):298–299, 2015 26121401

Lund C, De Silva M, Plagerson S, et al: Poverty and mental disorders: breaking the cycle in low-income and middle-income countries. Lancet 378(9801):1502–1514, 2011 22008425

Mark TL, Levit KR, Buck JA: Datapoints: psychotropic drug prescriptions by medical specialty. Psychiatr Serv 60(9):1167–1167, 2009 19723729

Mercier A, Benichou J, Auger-Aubin I, et al: How do GP practices and patient characteristics influence the prescription of antidepressants? A cross-sectional study. Ann Gen Psychiatry 14(1):3, 2015 25632295

Raney LE (ed): Integrated care: Working at the Interface of Primary Care and Behavioral Health. Arlington, VA, American Psychiatric Association Publisher, 2015

Ratzliff A, Norfleet K, Chan YF, et al: Perceived educational needs of the integrated care psychiatric consultant. Acad Psychiatry 39(4):448–456, 2015 26122347

Reardon CL, Bentman A, Cowley DS, et al: General and child and adolescent psychiatry resident training in integrated care: a survey of program directors. Acad Psychiatry 39(4):442–447, 2015 25778670

University of Washington: Principles of Collaborative Care. Collaborative Care Principles. Seattle, University of Washington AIMS Center, 2017

Unützer J, Katon WJ, Fan MY, et al: Long-term cost effects of collaborative care for late-life depression. Am J Manag Care 14(2):95–100, 2008 18269305

Yellowlees P, Shore JH: Telepsychiatry and Health Technologies: A Guide for Mental Health Professionals. Arlington, VA, American Psychiatric Association Publishing, 2018

Chapter 26 Community Mental Health Supervision

Serving the Underserved

Ripal Shah, M.D., M.P.H.

Lawrence M. McGlynn, M.D., M.S.

Community mental health care—the focus on those with persistent and chronic illness, often publicly insured—falls within many competencies. One way of accomplishing the training of multiple competencies is by placing supervisees into clinical rotations serving the community, allowing for the supervision of complicated patient care with varying access to resources. Since many in psychiatry feel they have been marginalized to function as medication managers (LeMelle et al. 2013), and insurance companies may dictate the execution of only time-limited behavioral therapies, community supervisors have a rare opportunity to train supervisees in adjusting to the changing landscape of the mental health care system in the United States.

The delivery of services to varying geographic or demographic catchment areas can be challenging. Examples of demographically focused community programs include clinics for victims of torture, refugees, undocumented immigrants, those who are living with HIV, and/or members of a specific racial, ethnic, or sexual orientation group. In addition to providing services based on a primary mission, these clinics oftentimes work with patients who may not otherwise have the means or coverage to receive treatment for their medical, behavioral, or substance use disorders. The supervision, then, becomes complicated by the varying psychosocial issues the patients may be facing, while trying to fit treatment planning into the limitations of a publicly insured system (e.g., limited to no coverage of psychotherapy sessions). Community mental health centers are sometimes multidisciplinary, as comorbid conditions (i.e., homelessness, poverty, medical illnesses, mental illnesses, addiction) must be addressed in order to achieve recovery; as such, many of these facilities attempt to provide the co-location of medical and behavioral healthcare, social services, and pharmacy. Recently, mobile units have begun to provide medical, psychiatric and dental care to the homeless and other underserved communities (e.g., neighborhoods struggling with poverty or poor access to public transportation). In some clinical rotations, the supervisee is encouraged to participate in these mobile clinics or in-home visits with attending providers or outreach workers, and it is not uncommon for supervisees to request closer observation or supervision for these, due to limited training in this setting.

Community mental health clinics provide supervisees with an understanding of the challenges and stressors facing the underserved, and the local, state, and federal regulations protecting, or limiting, patients' ability to receive essential services. This improves the ability of supervisees to feel prepared for ultimately working independently, by treating or caring for a diverse group of patients with unique psychosocial stressors.

Key Points

- Supervisors must develop and maintain a working knowledge of the social, political, demographic, and economic factors affecting the community.

- Supervision in a community setting often involves advocating for the patient in ways that may be tedious but are important in order for the supervisee to become a working member of the patient's team and an active contributor to the treatment plan.

- Supervisees often need supervision regarding management of community resources.

- Community supervision often includes an expanded content of supervision, varying from psychotherapy, to medication management, to social work and case management.

- Countertransference plays a significant role in the community setting.

Expanded Content of Supervision

As in other rotations, supervision requires a focus on the supervisee experience. For the mental health supervisee, this relationship has historically focused on psychotherapy and, additionally for psychiatry residents, medication management. In community mental health, the supervision's scope needs to broaden in order to prepare and support supervisees as they incorporate standards and best practices into their work. Ranz et al. (2012) proposed that the role of the community practitioner should become 1) patient care advocate, 2) team member, 3) information integrator, and 4) resource manager. The content of supervision, therefore, necessarily needs to expand in order to guide supervisees as they develop the skills necessary to master each of these components. This involves emphasizing the importance of information gathering and resource management while understanding that the supervisee may not be accustomed to these roles. Supervisors also need to become familiar with the social, political, demographic, and economic factors that impact the community, and, in turn, the supervisees (Fine and Fine 2011).

Some aspects of supervision may demand more attention. Given the historical maltreatment of patients in the public sector with mental illness, there may be an inherent mistrust that supervisees will need to overcome in order to build a therapeutic alliance. It may be helpful to encourage the supervisee to be attuned to the perspective of the patient, and how his or her unique life experiences and culture may influence their work together.

Countertransference

Countertransference, as in other contexts, is addressed in supervision. Community mental health supervisees may develop strong feelings that can be processed in supervision. They may feel helpless about the plight of their homeless patients, or discomfort in interacting with patients who have been incarcerated or use substances. They may feel frustrated about the choices these individuals make. The supervisor must guide the supervisee to see and understand that some behaviors are not necessarily maladaptive when one considers the context of the patient's life. The supervisor can lay out a concrete picture of the benefits (e.g., survival, safety) of specific behaviors, and the risks (e.g., worsening health, running out of money for food), which in turns aids the patient's understanding as well. The supervisee may then be able to better appreciate the factors that community patients consider when making choices. Discussing competing interests and the patient's core values of freedom and autonomy may also aid in the supervision of a strong countertransference process.

Supervisees may also express frustration about being faced with high no-show rates, carrying out the extensive outreach required for those who are lost to follow-up, having to learn a new formulary, and learning how to incorporate the patient's psychosocial limitations within their system of care. Patient management could involve coordinating with multiple specialties and agencies, completing disability/medical leave paperwork, and even learning new methods of practicing, such as implementing a harm reduction model rather than contingency management for substance use patients, particularly when frequent follow-ups are not an option. Issues with safety, and discomfort with the homeless or incarcerated populations, may also arise. In the public setting, supervisees may also find it challenging to reacquaint themselves with chronic physical illnesses that are not being monitored closely by a primary care physician or specialty physician, in order to differentiate medical from psychiatric complaints. These challenges provide the supervisor with the opportunity to demonstrate the practice of integrated care by creating an active role for the trainee within the multidisciplinary treatment team. The trainee will then have hands-on experience with the coordination of care and services by utilizing the expertise and resources of other team members, including those in external agencies. The supervisor should also familiarize the trainee with the more mundane aspects of community mental health. Trainees will benefit from understanding the details and importance of legal paperwork, including disability forms.

Reframing of Legal Implications

Community mental health systems strive to honor the mission of the community mental health movement of the 1960s, providing the least restrictive services for the mentally ill population. Prevention, deinstitutionalization, and comprehensive care have become the emphases (Fine and Fine 2011). Thus, the threshold for involuntarily committing a community patient might be unsettling for the supervisee. An individual who is chronically homeless, experiencing auditory hallucinations, using substances, but otherwise coming to his or her appointments (albeit sporadically) may not necessarily be considered gravely disabled. This same patient, if seen in the emergency department of an academic institution, may have been immediately placed on a legal hold; the stress of the public insurance system unfortunately leads to a much different triaging system. Supervisees may feel unsettled about the decisions that are requested of them in these situations and may become anxious about their own liability risks at first. Supervision reinforcing the supervisee's multifaceted role, including that of team member, may help the supervisee to utilize available resources, including consulting with other team members and coordinating referrals to appropriate agencies. It is imperative that the supervisee feel validated by his or her assessment of the patient and understand that his or her recommendations for the treatment plan are not inaccurate but instead limited by the walls of the container of the public sector. It may also be helpful to encourage supervisees to study the weaknesses in the systems of care and to pair them with mentors for community-based research or administrative projects that may address some of their frustrations.

Specific Challenges and Strategies

- **The community site doesn't know how to use the trainee.** In some cases, the supervisor may not be co-located with the supervisee at the community site. In other cases, the supervisor may work directly with the supervisee in the field. In either situation, the supervisor should be familiar with the issues and challenges facing the community. Meet with the staff of the community sites in order to develop an on-site curriculum and a clear understanding of the supervisee's role. The trainee's experience will be optimal not only when you understand the community's needs but also when the community site understands the goals of the training program and how this relationship can benefit the community site's overall mission.
- **My supervisee feels less confident working within the community setting.** Working with what may be an entirely new population late in training can bring about changes in confidence levels in the supervisee, and doubts about preparedness for seeing patients independently upon training completion, particularly if supervisees begin to feel as if there are many special populations with which they have not yet been able to work while being supervised closely. Help supervisees identify their weaknesses and/or lack of experience, and work together with supervisees to increase their confidence in those areas. In some instances, you may work with the community site to select specific types of cases that would benefit the trainee's training experience, and ultimately his or her confidence.

- **I can't supervise in a timely manner.** Funding limitations may translate to time-limited experiences for supervisees, because a system already strapped for funds may have difficulty justifying compensation of supervisees. It is not uncommon for supervisees to have supervision at the completion of the clinic day (or week), rather than direct staffing with each patient. Consider brief but more frequent check-ins with the supervisees and provide access to a direct line of communication if possible (i.e., paging, text, or call).
- **My supervisee only saw the patient once!** In working in the academic environment, turnover of providers is frequent. Although this applies to hospital-based care as well, community clinic patients often feel the brunt of it, because the length of time between follow-up visits may not even overlap with the length of time the supervisee is rotating in the clinic. The patients may feel that they are being tossed around to a different doctor each time. Consider optimizing transfer of care in the clinic by facilitating a sign-out process of even the infrequent visitors to the clinic. This could involve protected time for the supervisee to read previous notes on each patient in the morning before seeing them. Also consider reiterating to the patient that the supervisor is consistent throughout and is also involved in his or her care.

Questions for the Supervisee

■ Are there issues around transference and countertransference that interfere with your ability to be a strong advocate for the patient?

■ What do you feel your role is on the team, and what specific learning objectives do you have?

■ Do you know how to obtain the information needed in order to develop and execute a mental health treatment plan independently? If not, how can I help you?

■ Do you know how to help patients access resources that would be beneficial for their mental stability and recovery (health, legal, immigration, disability, financial, or housing benefits)?

Additional Resources

Clarke DM: Supervision in the training of a psychiatrist. Aust N Z J Psychiatry 27(2):306–310, 1993

Community Mental Health Journal (articles on public sector mental health services): https://link.springer.com/journal/10597

Hess AK (ed): Psychotherapy Supervision: Theory, Research, and Practice. New York, Wiley, 1980

LeBlanc AN: Random Family: Love, Drugs, Trouble, and Coming of Age in the Bronx. New York, Simon & Schuster, 2003

Pollack DA, Bigelow DA, Faulkner LR, et al: Psychiatric malpractice and supervision issues in community mental health programs. Hosp Community Psychiatry 41(12):1350–1353, 1990

Shtasel D, Viron M, Freudenreich O: Community psychiatry: what should future psychiatrists learn? Harv Rev Psychiatry 20(6):318–323, 2012

References

Fine P, Fine SW: Psychodynamic psychiatry, psychotherapy, and community psychiatry. J Am Acad Psychoanal Dyn Psychiatry 39(1):93–110, 2011 21434745

LeMelle S, Arbuckle MR, Ranz JM: Integrating systems-based practice, community psychiatry, and recovery into residency training. Acad Psychiatry 37(1):35–37, 2013 23338871

Ranz JM, Weinberg M, Arbuckle MR, et al: A four factor model of systems-based practices in psychiatry. Acad Psychiatry 36(6):473–478, 2012 23154697

Chapter 27   Global Mental Health Supervision

Capacity Building to Achieve Health Equity

Viet T. Nguyen, M.D., M.P.H.

Praqya Rimal, M.A.

Rebecca M. White, M.D.

Bibhav Acharya, M.D.

Global mental health (GMH) is the study and practice of reducing disparities in mental health worldwide, with a focus on low- and middle-income countries, or LMICs (White et al. 2017). As the case for GMH as a field of practice began to develop, growing interest in GMH opportunities among U.S. psychiatric trainees and medical students also began to rise. As a result, the existence of GMH training has become a significant factor when applicants rank training programs (Tsai et al. 2014). As resident demand for GMH training increases, residency program directors and other leadership are tasked with the challenge of appropriate trainee supervision in these contexts. Another common challenge in GMH is the supervision of nonspecialists (e.g., primary care providers [PCPs]) to deliver mental health care. Unfortunately, the topic of GMH supervision is often lacking or insufficient both in the literature and in practice. In this chapter, we explore key strategies and challenges in supervising psychiatric practitioners and non-specialists in GMH.

Key Points

- GMH supervision should be informed by core competencies and values that are aligned with the mission of achieving equity in mental health for all people worldwide, particularly focusing on LMICs and/or on vulnerable populations.

- GMH supervision includes the provision of guidance over the trainee's professional development of working through power differentials across diverse clinical, professional, social, and cultural contexts.

- Some supervision elements that are specific to international work are delivering supervision across different time zones, managing trainee isolation, providing specific direction on ethics of GMH work, developing an interdisciplinary supervisory team, and defining clear expectations among designated supervisors/peers across all sites.

- For clinical and programmatic work in GMH, the supervision of nonspecialist health care professionals in task sharing is vital to the role of GMH psychiatrists and includes competency in models of task sharing and integrated care, such as the collaborative care model.

GMH Competencies

Supervisors and training programs should explore which core components constitute appropriate GMH supervision. Currently, a general consensus in competencies for GMH practitioners is lacking, leaving little direction for appropriate GMH supervision. Competencies should include appropriate use of limited resources to deliver high-quality mental health care, such as appropriate use of World Health Organization (WHO) Essential Medicines (World Health Organization 2017) and other evidence-based therapies for resource limited settings. The supervisor should keep this in mind when supervising cases or providing mentorship and feedback regarding various GMH projects. When the supervisor is discussing competencies, it is important to be mindful of the concept of the "advanced generalist," borrowed from the field of social work (Rondero Hernandez 2013): GMH psychiatrists, in addition to having a minimum requirement of psychiatric training, should possess advanced competencies in a variety of skills, such as clinical supervision skills (especially in the context of task-sharing and supervision of nonspecialists), pedagogy and curriculum development skills, advocacy skills, and cross-cultural skills (including working with interpreters and structural competency in evaluation and treatment), so that they are equipped to work in complex and resource limited environments that are unique to GMH work. Their efforts should also be informed by the work of multidisciplinary experts, such as cultural anthropologists and sociologists (Citrin et al. 2017).

Supervision in GMH is inherently different than traditional psychiatric supervision. GMH supervision requires the provision of guidance over the trainee's professional development in working through power differentials across clinical, professional, social, and cultural contexts. This must be done to actualize equity in mental health for all people worldwide, reduce unintended harm, and promote sustainability. GMH experiences should incorporate specific competencies and values that are in line with the mission and purpose of GMH practice, and should inform how one appropriately supervises trainees in GMH. It is important that competencies be informed by values of justice and equity, in order to address power differentials created by practitioners from high-income countries, or HICs, working in LMICs (Citrin et al. 2017; Kohrt et al. 2016). Prior to a GMH experience being formalized, there should be discussion with the partner sites about bidirectional benefits and expectations from the partnership. Any considerations for appropriateness and oversight of projects should be made explicit with the partner site to address feasibility and need (Datta 2016). One strategy to accomplish this could involve the supervisee conducting a needs assessment at the beginning of the GMH experience to help inform the development of project ideas in partnership with on-site mentors.

Supervisors need to be aware of the ethical concerns and criticisms inherent in GMH practice, which range from lack of competency of cultural challenges in GMH work (Datta 2016) to the preferential allocation of mental health resources above basic necessities such as food and water in LMICs (Citrin 2010; White et al. 2017). Another ethical issue that supervisors should attend to is the concept of "medical voluntourism," which exacerbates inequality and perpetuates the problematic notion that cultural imperialism is maintained through a system that relies on the spread of western conceptualizations of illness, and lacks sustainability (Citrin 2010). There have been numerous examples of unintentional harm that can result from well-intended global health practitioners (Khan et al. 2013). Furthermore, supervision in general global health education is often not sufficient and lacks consistency across training programs of many specialties (Khan et al. 2013), let alone within the emerging subspecialty of GMH. One program (Buzza et al. 2018) has incorporated a multidisciplinary approach to guide curriculum development and the overall mission and purpose of their GMH experiences, including expertise from the humanities and other nonclinical fields, such as sociology, cultural anthropology, and pedagogy.

GMH Supervision Participants

A unique feature of GMH supervision compared with other psychiatric supervision is the diverse team of supervisors involved in supervising the supervisee. Supervision should be provided to practitioners in any stage of medical training who are interested in GMH work, including medical students, psychiatry residents and fellows, and attending psychiatrists. However, it should also incorporate the supervision of nonspecialist providers who will primarily treat mentally ill patients in LMICs, particularly in task-sharing models. This can include primary care physicians and other health care providers from LMICs. These task-sharing models are a key component to scaling up services in low-resource settings.

Given the lack of subspecialists in LMICs, GMH practitioners are most effective as "advanced generalists" and should therefore be supervised by a large and diverse team of mentors and supervisors. An interdisciplinary team with more than one supervisor is essential for multiple reasons: 1) GMH trainees may be in multiple settings, warranting supervisors with national/regional expertise; 2) U.S.-based supervisors may not be readily available, and a large team of supervisors is more likely to provide reliable response for urgent questions from trainees; and 3) the competencies needed for GMH are inherently interdisciplinary, requiring a panel of content experts. Supervisors with dual training (e.g., cultural anthropology and psychiatry) are often a valuable resource to provide interdisciplinary supervision. It is often necessary to incorporate supervisors who may not always have GMH experience but have expertise in a certain competency (e.g., pedagogy).

GMH supervisors within the team might also include clinician-educators with expertise in identified competencies, such as neurology, child psychiatry, consultation-liaison psychiatry, geriatric psychiatry, and HIV psychiatry, even with limited global health experience. In addition, clinicians who have experience with the WHO Essential Medicines and/or WHO mental health Gap Action Programme (mhGAP) intervention guide protocols (WHO's guiding document for nonspecialists delivering mental health services in primary care settings) (World Health Organization 2016) would be important to include in order to bridge gaps in clinical training. Finally, psychiatrists, general physicians, cross-cultural psychiatrists, cultural anthropologists, and other social scientists with relevant experience in partner sites in LMICs should be included in the supervision team (Fricchione et al. 2012). Partner site mentors and supervisors should be explicitly identified and included in supervisory meetings. A lead supervisor or mentor should coordinate the supervisory team if it is large. The lead supervisor should facilitate regular and routine contact with supervisees in person or, if such regular contact is not possible, coordinate indirect communication amongst supervisors and the supervisee. The lead supervisor may often serve as the supervisee's mentor and promote honest self-reflection, support long-term projects, and broach sensitive topics such as power and privilege.

It is essential to clarify the roles of each supervisor prior to departure so that both the supervisor and supervisee are clear about the former's specific area of expertise. The lead supervisor, or another identified supervisor/mentor, should be designated to help the supervisee resolve potential conflicting suggestions from supervisors. The lead supervisor should also check-in regularly with the supervisee to ensure supervision at the partner site is appropriate, as well as regularly check-in with the partner site supervisors.

GMH Supervision Structure

The task of structuring GMH supervision for supervisees requires consideration and should ideally include varied and balanced methods of supervision delivery. Logistical considerations that are specific to structuring GMH supervision, such as where and how often supervision should take place, should be taken into account. Supervision structure will depend on the phase of the GMH experience.

Predeparture

It is important to assess how the trainee will communicate with supervisors prior to their departure. First, an in-person meeting, or at least via phone or e-mail, for predeparture onboarding is critical. It is important to include introductions and communication with the partner site predeparture. If the lead supervisor will be present for a brief period on site, this time should be maximized for in-person supervision, teaching, mentorship, and setting expectations for an ongoing supervision structure.

Prior to the beginning of the rotation, partner site supervisors should provide expectations for the supervisee's role, including expectations about involvement in care delivery. There should be prerotation guidance on ethical concerns of going beyond their scope of practice. Supervisees will need specific strategies for ethical responsiveness when expectations exceed their level of competency (Datta 2016; Marienfeld 2016; Samuel et al. 2014). Supervisors can follow well-recognized frameworks, such as the WEIGHT guidelines for ethical training general global health disciplines (Crump and Sugarman 2010), for standardized protocols in a global setting.

On-Site Experience

During the actual training period in the field, remote supervision can be done synchronously via video conferencing or telephone calls, with time zone differences taken into account. If restricted availability of reliable internet or phone services is an issue, the supervisor can utilize a combination of techniques. Often, supervisors from HICs and home institutions are not physically present at the partner site. If they do visit, they tend to be on site for a brief time compared with the length of the supervisee's rotation. If the lead GMH supervisor will not be on-site, it is imperative that the supervision be structured and routine. It can often be delivered online via videoconference to help meet training goals and reduce trainee isolation.

The frequency of formalized supervision should be made clear at the beginning of the on-site GMH experience and depends on a variety of factors including the structure of the overall training program. For example, an interdisciplinary, clinical, and systems-focused program, such as the UCSF Psychiatry HEAL Fellowship in GMH (Buzza et al. 2018; UCSF 2018), includes biweekly online group supervision, in addition to on-site supervision from site-based supervisors and visiting U.S.-based mentors. In contrast, a program that is primarily research focused, such as the Massachusetts General Hospital Global Psychiatric Clinical Research Training Program (Magidson et al. 2016), will have different demands for supervision that include monthly research seminars to provide supervisees with both peer and supervisor feedback on their research projects.

On-site mentors and supervisors should ensure that ongoing collaboration and bidirectional partnership are maintained during the on-site GMH experience. Meanwhile, the lead supervisor should facilitate online video teleconferencing with various supervisors at a routinely designated interval (e.g., every 2 weeks a few faculty supervisors on a call with supervisees will discuss specific cases/issues on site).

An imperative part of ethical GMH work is ensuring that the supervisee's involvement is sustainable for the partner site. Even if the supervisee is practicing within their scope (e.g., postresidency fellows with a local medical license are legally able to conduct independent patient evaluations), their specific involvement should be dictated by an ethical plan to continue patient care (e.g., if the fellow builds a panel of patients but there is no one to sign off to at the end of the rotation, direct patient care may not be an ethical use of the fellow's time). The supervisor should encourage the supervisee to reflect on the unintended consequences of such scenarios when the supervisee leaves the site, and to think about his or her work through the lens of sustainability and feasibility, especially when he or she is developing programs/projects.

Post On-Site Experience

After returning from the GMH field experience, the lead supervisor will want to gather appropriate data and feedback from on-site supervisors and have the supervisee reflect on his or her experience. Were the supervisee's and training site's goals met during and after the GMH experience? One approach might be to use a combination of 360-degree feedback, competency and ACGME milestone achievements, and self-reflection (Kohrt et al. 2016).

GMH Supervision of Nonspecialists

Task sharing addresses the provision of quality mental health care to patients in LMICs in an attempt to close the existing treatment gap with limited resources (Acharya et al. 2017). Furthermore, formal team-based care with dedicated psychiatrist supervision of nonspecialists has been found to be superior to direct specialist care (co-location or consult/referral models), demonstrating its relevance in HICs and LMICs alike. Because building models of care that utilize task sharing is vital in GMH work, GMH supervisees need to develop clinical supervisory skills in order to appropriately supervise nonspecialists. Such skills include both clinical and administrative/programmatic supervision. In addition, GMH supervisees need competencies in "train the trainer" models to assist in-country specialists to train nonspecialist providers in order to promote sustainability. The role of the GMH psychiatrist as a supervisor, when integrating mental health care into primary care, is detailed in the WHO mhGAP intervention guide (World Health Organization 2016).

The collaborative care model (CoCM) is a task-sharing model that involves a team-based approach with health workers of varying levels of specialization, including a PCP; a behavioral health professional, who is considered the care manager (CM); and a consultant psychiatrist (Acharya et al. 2017). In this model, instead of completely assuming care for the patient, the psychiatrist acts as a consultant or supervisor who gives treatment recommendations for a panel of mentally ill patients comanaged by the PCP and the CM. There must be adequate supervision of primary care staff to ensure that newly trained PCPs and CMs provide high-quality mental health treatment (Acharya and Swar 2016). The GMH psychiatrist's consultation services can range from face-to-face interaction with complex patients to remote case consultation (Zeidler Schreiter et al. 2013). This model leverages the limited time of the psychiatrist to deliver cost-effective mental health care at a population level. Since this is a unique role for the psychiatrist, GMH supervisees would highly benefit from acquiring supervision skills for this context.

When supervising within the CoCM, the GMH supervisor can either have the supervisee present cases in which he or she is supervising the nonspecialist on site, or supervise around the programmatic elements of the CoCM. Common issues that may arise include how to manage cultural and language barriers by adapting standardized training materials and protocols from English, how to use culturally validated scales for the region, how to manage conflict within a team-based model in a culturally appropriate manner, and how to supervise different care providers with varied levels of training and interest in mental health.

Specific Challenges and Strategies

- **My supervisee has restricted availability to reliable internet or phone service.** Backup communication methods must be established (e.g., if live video-conferencing fails, then use mobile phones). Asynchronous communication, such as emails or an online bulletin board, can supplement the structured communication and help address on-demand questions and provide avenues to enhance intrinsically motivated learning. An important strategy is to make sure all apps and technology equipment are in working order prior to departure, so that trouble shooting can be done more easily in person.

- **The supervisee is being asked to go beyond the scope of her training in the field without the appropriate supervision.** Adequate predeparture preparation is imperative to helping the supervisee handle situations in real time without direct supervision of the home supervisor. Prior to departure, clearly communicate expectations to the supervisee and partner site supervisors. You may need to remind the partner site about these expectations as needed. As part of the routine supervision, ask the supervisee about ethical conundrums to promote open dialogue and reflective practice. You might ask, "If you were treating the same patient at your home institution, would you make the same clinical decisions? Why or why not?" Promoting dialogue with the supervisee in a nonjudgmental manner may encourage the supervisee to be more thoughtful about complex ethical challenges in the field. Additionally, ensure that an on-site mentor is available to support the supervisee when such issues arise in real time.

- **My supervisee is getting conflicting messages from the various members of the supervisory team.** It is important that the lead supervisor serve as a mentor to the supervisee. This will help the supervisee problem-solve any potential conflicting messages that he receives in the field. Depending on the nature of the conflict, the supervisor can choose to either intervene or guide the supervisee on how to manage the conflict on his own.

- **The supervisee appears to be suffering from burnout and isolation in her global health and/or research work.** In general, global health work tends to be isolating, as trainees tend to be far away from friends, family members, and the comforts of one's own familiar culture. It is important for the supervisor to structure time for the trainee's own self-reflection and discussion of proactive skills to help identify and combat burnout. This can involve teaching relaxation techniques (e.g., mindfulness meditation) and/or inviting experts on self-reflection and self-care to a supervision session for in-depth guidance. One strategy is to design a program that creates a cohort effect with peers/colleagues to maintain a sense of connection and address supporting the supervisee while minimizing power differentials. For instance, in UCSF's HEAL Initiative Fellowship, a group of interdisciplinary trainees create a 2-year cohort, who interact via in-person trainings, asynchronous monthly journal clubs on an electronic message board, and smaller group "pods" with designated mentors who routinely communicate via video conferencing or phone calls throughout the course of the fellowship (Goldman et al. 2016). Often, the structured interaction between peers in the cohort leads to bonding and informal interaction, which allow for another form of consultation on challenging cases or problems, as well as providing feedback and support. Another strategy is to encourage the GMH supervisee to connect with any affiliated nonpsychiatrist supervisees who may be doing global health work at the same site.

Questions for the Supervisee

■ How may the cultural background of your patient influence their understanding of the presenting problem, expected course of the problem, and expected treatment? Likewise, how does his or her cultural background influence your explanation, assessment, and management of the problem?

■ How can we objectively assess your impact as a supervisee on your training site?

■ Are you finding ways to cope with stress of new cultural environment and isolation from friends/family?

Additional Resources

General Resources for GMH Projects

World Health Organization mental health Gap Action Programme (mhGAP): http://www.who.int/mental_health/mhgap/en/

World Health Organization: WHO mental health Gap Action Programme (mhGAP) Intervention Guide, Version 2.0, for mental, neurological and substance use orders on nonspecialized health settings. Geneva, World Health Organization, 2016. Available at: http://www.who.int/mental_health/mhgap/mhGAP_intervention_guide_02/en/.

WHO Essential Medicines: http://www.who.int/topics/essential_medicines/en/

WHO Project Atlas: Mental Health Atlas: http://www.who.int/mental_health/evidence/mhatlas05/en/

Psychotherapies in Community Settings

World Health Organization, War Trauma Foundation, World Vision International: Psychological First Aid: Guide for Field Workers. Geneva, World Health Organization, 2011. Available at: http://www.who.int/mental_health/publications/guide_field_workers/en/.

WHO Group IPT for Depression: http://www.who.int/mental_health/mhgap/interpersonal_therapy/en/

WHO Problem Management Plus (PM+): http://www.who.int/mental_health/emergencies/problem_management_plus/en/

U.S.-Based GMH Training Experiences and Curricula

Columbia University Global Mental Health Program Resources: http://cugmhp.org/research/redeamericas/#block-2368

UCSF Psychiatry HEAL Initiative Fellowship in Global Mental Health: http://psych.ucsf.edu/ucsf-psychiatry-heal-fellowship-global-mental-health

References

Acharya B, Swar SB: Consultant psychiatrists' role in ensuring high-quality care from nonspecialists. Psychiatr Serv 67(7):816, 2016 27363359

Acharya B, Ekstrand M, Rimal P, et al: Collaborative care for mental health in low- and middle-income countries: a WHO health systems framework assessment of three programs. Psychiatr Serv 68(9):870–872, 2017 28760096

Buzza C, Fiskin A, Breur J, et al: Competencies for global mental health: developing training objectives for a post-graduate fellowship for psychiatrists. Annals of Global Health 84:717–726, 2018

Citrin DM: The anatomy of ephemeral health care: "health camps" and short- term medical voluntourism in remote nepal. Stud Nepali Hist Soc 15(1):27–72, 2010

Citrin D, Mehanni S, Acharya B, et al: Power, potential, and pitfalls in global health academic partnerships: review and reflections on an approach in Nepal. Glob Health Action 10(1):1367161, 2017 28914185

Crump JA, Sugarman J; Working Group on Ethics Guidelines for Global Health Training (WEIGHT): Ethics and best practice guidelines for training experiences in global health. Am J Trop Med Hyg 83(6):1178–1182, 2010 21118918

Datta V: The problem with education in global mental health. Acad Psychiatry 40(4):727–728, 2016 26438236

Fricchione GL, Borba CP, Alem A, et al: Capacity building in global mental health: professional training. Harv Rev Psychiatry 20(1):47–57, 2012 22335182

Goldman RS, Tittle RL, Waters AE, et al: Preparing trainees to practice global health equity: the experience from the first year of the health equity action and leadership (HEAL) initiative. Ann Glob Health 82(3):419, 2016

Khan OA, Guerrant R, Sanders J, et al: Global health education in U.S. medical schools. BMC Med Educ 13(3):3, 2013 23331630

Kohrt BA, Marienfeld CB, Panter-Brick C, et al: Global mental health: five areas for value-driven training innovation. Acad Psychiatry 40(4):650–658, 2016 26983416

Magidson JF, Stevenson A, Ng LC, et al: Massachusetts general hospital global psychiatric clinical research training program: a new fellowship in global mental health. Acad Psychiatry 40(4):695–697, 2016 26108399

Marienfeld C: Considerations of ethics while allowing flexibility for trainees: the model and the rationale for the model of the yale global mental health program (letter). Acad Psychiatry 40(4):731, 2016 26423679

Rondero Hernandez V: Generalist and advanced generalist practice, in Encyclopedia of Social Work. NASW Press and Oxford University Press, 2013. Available at: http://oxfordindex.oup.com/view/10.1093/acrefore/9780199975839.013.160. Accessed August 16, 2018.

Samuel D, Angarita B, Igboeli B, et al: Four international residents' perspectives on working overseas as part of residency training: liberia, myanmar, and saint vincent/grenadines. Ann Glob Health 80(2):143–145, 2014 24976553

Tsai AC, Fricchione GL, Walensky RP, et al: Global health training in US graduate psychiatric education. Acad Psychiatry 38(4):426–432, 2014 24664609

UCSF: UCSF Psychiatry HEAL Fellowship in Global Mental Health. 2018. Available at: http://psych.ucsf.edu/printpdf/1721. Accessed May 21, 2018.

White RG, Orr DMR, Read UM, et al: Situating Global Mental Health: Sociocultural Perspectives, in The Palgrave Handbook of Sociocultural Perspectives on Global Mental Health. Edited by White RG, Orr DMR, Read UM, et al. London, MacMillan, 2017, pp 1–28

World Health Organization: MhGAP intervention guide for mental, neurological, and substance use disorders in non-specialized health settings: Mental Health Gap Action Programme (MhGAP) 2.0. Geneva, World Health Organization, 2016. Available at: http://www.who.int/mental_health/mhgap/mhGAP_intervention_guide_02/en/. Accessed August 16, 2018.

World Health Organization: WHO Model Lists of Essential Medicines. Geneva, World Health Organization, 2017. Available at: http://www.who.int/medicines/publications/essentialmedicines/en/. Accessed August 16, 2018.

Zeidler Schreiter EA, Pandhi N, Fondow MDM, et al: Consulting psychiatry within an integrated primary care model. J Health Care Poor Underserved 24(4):1522–1530, 2013 24185149

Part 5   Nonclinical Supervision Venues

Chapter 28 Administrative Supervision

Joshua Griffiths, M.D.

Joel Yager, M.D.

Psychiatrists need to master administrative skills at various stages of their careers and require suitable supervision along the way. Although much administrative training occurs during residency and fellowship, many psychiatrists first appreciate the need for additional administrative training later on, in early or mid-career, as they assume posts of increasing responsibility at academic medical centers and at hospitals, clinics, and other organizations outside of academia. In this chapter, while emphasizing administrative supervision for residents and fellows, we also address strategies and tactics for administrative supervision for later-career trainees.

Key Points

- Administrative supervision should be formalized, not left to happenstance.

- All trainees having administrative assignments should be formally assigned supervisors.

- Administrative supervisors should discuss with incoming trainees the administrative roles, tasks, expectations, competencies, and challenges specific to each setting and how these experiences fit into bigger systems pictures.

- Administrative skills encompass broad ranges of competencies, useful to increasing numbers of psychiatrists.

- Early- and mid-career learners should access part-time degree or certificate programs and obtain supervision precisely geared to the particular situations and personalities they are likely to encounter in their new or imminent roles.

- Administrative supervision can be structured in several ways, to include apprenticeship, traditional "case-based" supervision, and/or group supervision that might include didactic seminars.

- Challenges focus on helping trainees deal with intractably difficult personnel (including faculty and supervisors), systems of care, and legal/social systems.

- Supervision should include both problem-solving and emotion-focused approaches, addressing both malleable and intransigent individuals, groups, and systems.

Supervision for Residents and Fellows

Administrative supervision for psychiatric residents and fellows ordinarily transpires in the context of their assignments as chief residents, but junior residents can assume administrative responsibilities as well. Many programs sponsor arrays of administrative residency positions; for example, in addition to an education (or administrative, or executive) chief resident, programs often appoint service-based chief residents (who might work in different facilities such as university, county hospital, mental health center, or Veterans Affairs [VA] sites) (Lim et al. 2009; Szuba et al. 1993; Warner et al. 2007). Since administrative assignments also fall to residents who are not specifically designated as "chiefs," to avoid confusion we refer to all these trainees as "administrative residents." Because residents' administrative roles are so diverse, their supervisory needs vary significantly. Here we describe general approaches for supervising administrative residents, focusing solely on issues that transcend specific clinical or programmatic assignments.

We begin with two starting principles: first, all residents having administrative assignments should be formally assigned supervisors, distinct from clinical supervision, to specifically address their administrative work; programs should not negligently throw residents onto services and expect them to figure out what to do on their own. Ordinarily, administrative supervisors are service chiefs to whom the residents are assigned, but third parties can be assigned as well. Supplementing informal access, regularly scheduled supervision should not be left to chance. Group administrative supervision and seminars can supplement service-based teaching. Residents do best when provided with administrative teachers with broad knowledge and hands-on experience from a range of backgrounds, including academic, clinical and, community settings, or with particular expertise such as in planning, budgeting, finance, personnel, and grant management.

Second, administrative supervisors should discuss with incoming residents the administrative roles, tasks, expectations, competencies, and challenges specific to each setting and how these experiences fit into bigger systems pictures. As important, departing administrative residents should orient incoming administrative residents verbally and with written materials to these jobs and their realities. At baseline, residents should be asked about their own goals, expectations, questions, and concerns, and about their longer-term aspirations, so that supervisors can fashion individualized learner-centered teaching.

General Goals and Expectations for Administrative Assignments

Residents taking on administrative assignments are typically tasked in the three domains listed below, regardless of setting. For each domain, subtopics can be developed as specific competencies. Since increasing numbers of psychiatric graduates take positions that require some administrative abilities, these competencies are widely relevant. Competencies can be delineated as traditional knowledge and skill behavioral goals and objectives, for example as specified by "By the end of the rotation, administrative residents should be able to discuss [knowledge]" and/or "By the end of the rotation, administrative residents should be able to demonstrate [skills]" (abbreviated below simply as "Knowledge:...discuss" or "Skill...demonstrate").

Middle Managing

Working effectively as a middle manager of complex teams (communicating in workgroups: receiving instruction, reporting to others, acting as a go-between, mediating, convening, delegating).

Knowledge

Discuss principles of effective one-on-one and small-group communication, including subgroup formation, distortions, theme interference, cognitive biases, and repairing ruptures. These entail the common interpersonal misperceptions and misconceptions that occur in groups, not unlike transference distortions, that produce emotional tensions and behavioral eruptions that detract from work-place efficiencies and effectiveness.

Skill

Demonstrate abilities to competently conduct each of the activities mentioned above.

Planning, Conducting, and Evaluating

Scheduling, assigning, project planning, effecting, quality monitoring, and reporting:

Knowledge

Describe necessary steps to plan, carry out, and evaluate the administrative requirements of the [setting-specific roles].

Skill

Demonstrate competence in planning, conducting, and evaluating the administrative requirements of the [setting-specific roles].

Substituting

Substituting as "junior attending" or "pre-tending," stepping in to accept work for absent juniors:

Skill

Demonstrate competence at being able to fulfill the roles of [setting-specific substitutive roles]. Administrative principles, models, and memes from fields outside academic medicine can helpfully supplement medical setting-specific material. Beyond these generalities, residents face setting-specific (devilish) details that generate commonly encountered administrative challenges that include dealing with difficult personalities (variably superiors, peers subordinates, or all of the above), and work-complexity and total workload burdens, time-pressures, and deadlines. Residents should be tasked with meaningful roles that provide opportunities for mastery. These details determine whether residents experience their administrative assignments as manageable, good learning experiences, competence building, worthwhile, and fun, or, alternatively, as wastes of time and experiences to be endured or avoided.

Supervision for Later-Career Trainees

Beyond residency and fellowship, individuals seeking administrative training and supervision in early or midcareer frequently do so having more refined goals in mind, often in anticipation of taking on a specific new role. Here, career trainees, as we will refer to them, might be expected to assume jobs as supervisors, middle managers, unit directors, program directors, chiefs of service, department chairs, or higher administrative roles in organizations, up to and including those of chief executive officer or president of an organization. At times, career aspirants hope to obtain advanced credentials (e.g., Master of Business Administration, Master of Health Administration, Executive Health Management certificates) not only to learn their trades but also to acquire "street cred"— that is, enhanced credibility with other administrative and financial planners and executives with whom they will be interacting.

Increasingly, psychiatrists in these positions avail themselves of part-time learning programs that might require a few weeks or weekends of live, on-site attendance (if that) followed by distance telelearning, in addition to more usual instruction that may occur through local universities, professional associations, or one's own academic medical center's executive development programs. In all such instances, career trainees need to be selective as to precisely what new competencies they will need in order to be successful in their upcoming or new roles, how they can most efficiently and effectively achieve these credentials and competencies, and whom they might call on for mentoring and supervision.

These curricula are quite diverse and not infrequently entail individualized "case-based" or "problem-based" assignments that focus on the trainee's highly varied specific projects. To the extent that these learners are training for specific roles, in specific locations, involving specific sets of actors, supervisors need to tailor-make their supervision to best address the specific learner-environment niche. Such learner-centered supervision may require several mentors and supervisors, some focusing on technical competencies (e.g., budgeting, planning, personnel, rules and regulations governing the particular role), and some addressing much more nuanced issues such as how to handle unavoidable difficult or quirky personalities entrenched in key organizational positions.

Structuring Supervisory Approaches for Trainees at All Levels

Several models for administrative supervision can be employed, sometimes simultaneously. In "apprenticeship" models, supervisors (ordinarily attending faculty on the service being administered) work alongside their trainees, providing ample opportunities for role modeling. In one approach, mentors teach administration by having trainees sit by their sides for an hour each week as they go through their in-boxes and "to do" lists, discussing each upcoming administrative task in turn. Trainees prefer teachers and supervisors they can quickly access when crises arise, fostering "just in time" learning, which is more useful than "after the fact" learning. Apprenticeships also permit supervisors to help trainees prioritize their "to do" lists and to directly observe and provide direct, immediate, and specific feedback on trainee performance, for example, running team meetings, interacting with various players, developing and disseminating schedules, and planning and conducting various projects.

Traditional regularly scheduled supervision can also be helpful; during this time, trainees should be able to comfortably discuss and openly dialogue about problems they are encountering with individual staff, trainees, and systems, and receive candid opinions and feedback.

Finally, supervising in groups can enhance each trainee's experience. Group supervision can incorporate didactic seminars in which administrative cases, essentially "headaches of the week rounds," are brought for discussion. In one such seminar-group supervision activity, curriculum material included current textbook chapters on administrative psychiatry as well as delightful classics, emphasizing issues of role, authority, responsibility, group dynamics, communication, and personal time management (Brunicardi and Hobson 1996; Caplow 1976; Greenblatt 1991; Schwartz 1982, 1989).

Specific Challenges and Strategies

- **My supervisee is struggling with confronting difficult personnel.** Supervisors can hear out difficulties and learner's frustrations and then try to ascertain the extent to which difficulties are situational or derive from each participant's personality style and/or particulars of the dyadic transaction, and attempt to assist problem-solving accordingly. When working with challenging individuals, supervisors should advocate tact, diplomacy, direct and indirect communications, group pressures, and engaging peers and/or superiors to assist. Here trainees confront their personal limitations and develop communication skills for initiating and conducting difficult conversations and renegotiating job expectations and assignments. Communications-oriented references in the "Additional Resources" list below may help.
- **My supervisee feels overwhelmed by his workload which imposes excessive time burdens.** Supervisors can assist learners in reviewing their calendars, promote efficiencies where possible, set priorities, and effectively address their own unrealistic demands as well as those of superiors and other outside influences regarding the need to alter expectations. Several books by Stephen Covey cited in "Additional Resources" are worth reviewing.
- **My supervisee doesn't have the skill set needed for the work at hand.** These conversations involve creating "safe" spaces in which trainees are invited to honestly and nondefensively reflect on their limitations and where supervisors can realistically appraise trainee's abilities and potentials for mastery. The challenge for supervisors is to find optima—neither selling trainees short on the one hand (premature defeatism) nor setting them up for failure by insisting on unrealistic achievements

on the other (over-optimistic self-delusion). Sometimes supervisors have to encourage trainees to continue who might otherwise give up too soon, Alternatively, supervisors sometimes have to provide frank feedback regarding performance deficiencies to trainees who insist they are doing well when facts say otherwise. In all these instances, which might be taken as personal failures, supervisors should try helping trainees learn through experience to find valuable life lessons and also help minimize the inevitable narcissistic injuries and demoralizations that often ensue.

- **My supervisee has been set up as the "fall guy" by conspiring group dynamics.** Inevitably, rather than accepting responsibility for difficulties or honestly evaluating organizational problems, some leaders at various levels of organizational administration tend to externalize blame. When trainees believe themselves to be unfairly targeted, supervisors should help them analyze situational and interpersonal dynamics, and, where possible, help effect constructive interventions.

- **My supervisee has to manage an undesirable administrative task.** Supervisors frequently help trainees face the drudgery and noncreative repetitiveness accompanying certain inescapable organizational tasks. In some programs, certain administrative assignments characterized as "dumps" require trainees to take on roles and jobs that no one else wants to do. Occasionally, administrative assignments are so undesirable that superiors can rationalize them only by acknowledging the harsh reality that salaries are inextricably tied to certain obligated jobs. Of course, even bad experiences convey life lessons, and, in fact, many trainees realize that taking on undesirable administrative tasks may sometimes be the dues they will have to pay to obtain better recommendations, faculty appointments, or organizational positions later on. But, consistently bad training experiences are never justified. Administrative assignments (and supervisors) that prove intractably malignant should be dropped from the curriculum.

- **My supervisee struggles with handling an intractable administrative task.** Facing intractable noxious difficulties, trainees benefit from realizing what can and cannot be realistically changed. Inventive ingenuity, novel organizational approaches, and energetic persistence can sometimes effect changes that have eluded previous attempts. But some problems remain stuck. Problem-solving approaches might ameliorate some difficulties, or at least better define them for study. One wise mentor advised administrative trainees frustrated by regulations and realities in the VA Medical Center to simply view themselves as anthropologists and sociologists unable to change anything, but learning what they might about human behavior, bureaucracy, and the law. He highly recommended the Serenity Prayer.

Questions for the Supervisee

■ Getting Started

  ■ What have you heard about the job and its expectations?

  ■ What do you hope to get from this experience?

  ■ What goals have you set for yourself?

- ■ What have you been advised to particularly attend to or look out for?

- ■ What apprehensions do you have?

■ Ongoing

- ■ What's come up this week?

- ■ What's causing you the most difficulty right now?

- ■ How are you handling things?

- ■ How are they affecting you?

- ■ How can I help?

Additional Resources

Bernstein AJ: Emotional Vampires at Work: Dealing With Bosses and Co-Workers Who Drain You Dry. New York, McGraw-Hill, 2013

Cover SR: The 7 Habits of Highly Effective People: Powerful Lessons in Personal Change. New York, Simon & Schuster, 1989

Covey SR: Principle-Centered Leadership. New York, Fireside, 1992

Covey SR, Merrill AR, Merrill RR: First Things First. New York, Simon & Schuster, 1994

Stone D, Patton B, Heen S: Difficult Conversations: How to Discuss What Matters Most, 2nd Edition. New York, Penguin, 2010

Ursiny T: The Coward's Guide to Conflict: Empowering Solutions for Those Who'd Rather Run Than Fight. Naperville, IL, Sourcebooks, 2003

References

Brunicardi FC, Hobson FL: Time management: a review for physicians. J Natl Med Assoc 88(9):581–587, 1996 8855650

Caplow T: How to Run any Organization. New York, Holt, Rinehart & Winston, 1976

Greenblatt M: Administrative psychiatry. New Dir Ment Health Serv 49(49):5–17, 1991 2017129

Lim RF, Schwartz E, Servis M, et al: The chief resident in psychiatry: roles and responsibilities. Acad Psychiatry 33(1):56–59, 2009 19349446

Schwartz DA: Administration in psychiatry, in Teaching Psychiatry and Behavioral Science. Edited by Yager J. New York, Grune & Stratton, 1982, pp 455–468

Schwartz DA: A precis of administration. Community Ment Health J 25(3):229–244, 1989 2805637

Szuba MP, Guze BH, Richeimer SH: The postresidency perspective of the psychiatric chief resident. Acad Psychiatry 17(2):113–115, 1993 24443246

Warner CH, Rachal J, Breitbach J, et al: Current perspectives on chief residents in psychiatry. Acad Psychiatry 31(4):270–276, 2007 17626188

Chapter 29   Leadership Supervision

Ella M. Williams, M.D.

Adam M. Brenner, M.D.

Are leaders born or made (Balon 2014)? Leaders most likely result from a combination of innate ability and training. So how are providers taught to become leaders in the clinical setting? And do all clinicians have the potential to become leaders? The goal is to use supervision to develop the clinician into an effective leader. Being an effective clinical leader requires being able to do good clinical work oneself, to effectively respond to adversity, to form trusting relationships, and to negotiate conflicts that arise during change processes. The essential elements of leadership supervision are clarity in these behavioral expectations, clear feedback to the potential leader, and vigorous mentorship around the areas of needed growth.

Key Points

- Good clinical skills are a must.
- Supervisors need to be available to mentor potential candidates.
- Feedback should be professional and sensitive.
- Forming trusting relationships is the foundation of conflict resolution.
- Responding to adversity is crucial.
- Modeling behavior is key for supervisors.

- Change requires a vision.
- Change is always difficult.

Assessing Clinical Skills

The first task in leadership supervising is observing the potential leadership candidate's clinical skills and ensuring that they meet the standard of the institution. This is accomplished by a number of methods. Personal observation is key; however, obtaining information from peers and chart reviews is equally important. We want leaders to make good clinical decisions but also be able to document their decision. As a supervisor of a potential leader, one must be willing to provide feedback in a professional and sensitive manner (Day 2001).

Case Example 1

Dr. E completed his psychiatry residency 2 years ago and is beginning to feel more comfortable as an attending physician in the emergency department. For the first 6 months in this role, he was proactively assigned a mentor to help him with the transition from resident to attending. The mentor directly observed his work, provided feedback, and was available to discuss any difficulties the new attending experienced. During that time, at least two random charts were reviewed by the mentor. The focus of the review was the quality of the H&P [history and physical examination], assessment, and disposition. Dr. E's H&P and assessment were always strong, but initially he had some trouble with disposition. He seemed to be very cautious and reluctant to make definitive decisions. Instead, he often deferred to the attending following him on the next shift to make the final disposition. This was consistent with the direct observation and feedback from peers that he regularly reviewed even routine decisions with more experience attendings. The combination of direct observation, peer feedback, and chart review made clear that his judgment was in fact quite solid and that the difficulty was in his confidence during an important transition in his professional development. He was receptive to this feedback and appreciative of his mentor's encouragement on trusting his decisions.

Through direct observation, the mentor saw him progress from frequently double checking his decisions with more experienced physicians and nurses to generally feeling confident about his judgment, and this growing confidence was reflected in the documentation of the disposition in the chart. Many of the nurses reported that his decisions in caring for patients made them feel more confident in taking care of patients. Now that his clinical work is meeting the expectations of his role, his mentor and he are able to turn their attention to Mr. E's growing in the role of team leader.

Responding to Adversity

The ability to handle adversity is crucial to effective team leadership (Roberts 2009). This is an area where potential leaders may need a great deal of mentoring. Adversity can come in the form of dealing with difficult patients, colleagues, or subordinates. How one deals with these situations can make or break a person's reputation. As the supervisor, the role is to help develop methods for the potential leader to deal with these situations. Practicing different scenarios is helpful. Experience can be the best teacher; so, assigning projects that appear to stretch the potential leader's ability is a good tool

(Day 2001). Providing feedback after dealing with a difficult situation is a must. Many new leaders know intellectually that they will need to grow in their role but may nevertheless expect that this growth will come without mistakes. They may find the perspective of an old adage comforting: "Good judgment comes from experience, experience comes from bad judgment."

The capacity to manage conflicts is a learnable skill, but the foundation is the ability to form trusting relationships with others. As a supervisor, we cannot make someone trustworthy. The potential leader's innate character and integrity cannot be taught (Balon 2014); this is sometimes what divides those who will succeed as leaders from those who will not. We can, however, help the potential leader learn how to show others that he or she is trustworthy, and how to assess the trustworthiness of others. The ability to read and understand others (Day 2001) is vital, and fortunately this is already a strength of most psychiatrists.

It is valuable to instruct new and aspiring leaders in the principles of "win-win" negotiations, since these may not have been covered in previous undergraduate and graduate medical education (Fisher and Ury 1983). Some of the most valuable principles are focusing on interests, not positions; focusing on the problem, not the person; and focusing on optimal and disadvantageous methods of conflict resolution and allowing everyone to save face. Focusing on underlying interests allows the leader to avoid the trap of painting himself or herself into a corner by taking a position before understanding what is really at stake for all parties. This stance allows the leader to focus on the problem and not on the personalities involved.

Similarly, although this may seem obvious, many new leaders (including the authors) benefited from being taught that some strategies are not typically effective when facing heated adversity, such as responding in the heat of the moment or by using text/emails and sacrificing the respect and nuance that are so much easier to convey with tone of voice. The pull to respond to antagonistic emails in kind is so strong that some of us have found that we have had to learn this repeatedly. The illusion of efficiency and efficacy that one feels when firing off a response is short lived. The time saved is a false economy, for in the long run the investment of waiting until one's own temper is calmed and speaking to the sender directly will save a great deal of time.

Finally, all this must always be done while allowing all participants in the conflict to save face and maintain their professional esteem if possible. Taking the moral high ground or leaving a member of the team shamed can take a profound toll on the underlying trust necessary to continue to lead. In the service of this goal, it is often useful to give people the benefit of the doubt when experiencing them as obstructing a change process, and this very often turns out to be more accurate. One of the authors' mentors, Kenneth Altshuler, advised all new leaders to remember that "it is always wiser to assume incompetence than malevolence."

Case Example 2

Dr. A is a junior faculty member leading a team on the inpatient psychiatric unit, which consists of a 16-bed program for dual diagnosis of mental illness and substance abuse. Dr. A has a reputation of being an excellent, efficient clinician. Lately, Dr. A has been feeling that the nurse practitioner on the team, Ms. R, is keeping patients unnecessarily in the hospital to avoid getting new admissions. This has increased Dr. A's own workload, and she is feeling overwhelmed. Dr. A confronted Ms. R in front of staff in an angry accusing manner that embarrassed Ms. R. As a result, tension developed that affected their relationship and had potential implications for optimal patient care.

As Dr. A's supervisors, we met with her to discuss the situation. We provided feedback on how she had handled the situation and alternative methods of dealing with adversity through the principles of collaborative negotiations. She acknowledged that she had made her accusation without proof and should have given herself time to reflect on how she was feeling and asked for assistance. As supervisors, we shared with Dr. A some of our own leadership stumbles so that she did not feel unduly shamed or demoralized. Later, Dr. A apologized to Ms. R for approaching her in front of staff in an angry accusing fashion. This time she waited till emotions were not hot and focused on attempting to understand Ms. R's perspective, where the underlying interest turned out to be previously undiscussed concerns about patient safety. As a result, Dr. A's and Ms. R's relationship did improve and the team was able to return to an atmosphere of mutual respect and optimal function.

Overseeing Change

An important aspect of leadership will include overseeing change processes. The idea of the leader as a visionary who marshals her troops and leads them into battle is one many people have and is often supported by media and popular culture. The reality is far more complicated and also potentially more satisfying. Change does require a vision of the future, but it will not always come from the leader. Sometimes it comes from above, as a mandate of the institution or an accrediting organization, and the leader's task is translational: how to apply this involuntary change to her own team or department in a way that is ultimately generative and retains the integrity of their core values. Sometimes the new vision comes from below, and it is the leader's subordinates who come to her with an idea that has developed in the trenches.

Regardless of the source, change is always difficult because, while everyone is excited about doing things better, relatively few feel comfortable with the other side of that coin—that they had not previously been doing things as well as they could have been. When the issues involve patient care and our deepest values and identities as caring clinicians, it can be especially hard to acknowledge blind spots or deficits. How can supervision of leaders help in these challenges?

It is important that leaders have their own opportunity to discuss with mentors, or in peer mentoring groups, the resistance to change that they experience, both from within and from their colleagues and subordinates. Having supportive and safe opportunities to share their frustrations makes it easier to then help their team do the same. It is also valuable to frequently remind new leaders that change is a process, not an event; it will take time, and it will be messy. And finally, mentors of leaders often can help by encouraging the new leader to loosen their grip on the reins. The most natural thing when stressed and anxious about a process is to tighten control. However, the more that the stakeholders are empowered and given freedom to solve problems themselves, the more likely it is that the plan will have buy-in and address the actual interests of those on the ground.

Referring to the previous example, an unspoken part of the conflict between Dr. A and Ms. R is that Dr. A is aware that the hospital administration is putting pressure on the department to increase the turnover of patients on the team, because the unit has been consistently over budget. After repairing her relationship with Ms. R, Dr. A realizes that she has been putting off addressing this issue because she was anxious about how the other staff would react, and because she did not see how they would actually be able to achieve this. Dr. A now responds by sharing this situation with the rest of the team and asking them for volunteers to form a working group with her. She is careful to reach out to members of each discipline so that the working group will be representative of the team, and is very gratified to find that in brainstorming together the group is able to generate ideas about increasing efficiency that Dr. A never before considered.

Educating New Leaders

As supervisors of new leaders, much of this is teaching done through modeling (Roberts 2009). Throughout the process of leadership development, mentors must listen, be patient, be honest (Day 2001), and demonstrate appropriate conflict management in their own interactions. Potential leaders are encouraged to take advantage of leadership course work at their institution (Johnson and Stern 2013) or elsewhere, and to read books on management and leadership. Although some residency training programs may include seminars on these topics, this is not universal, and many junior faculty do not enter their new roles understanding that, as with psychiatric assessment or psychotherapy, leadership comprises a set of learnable skills with a rich and evidence-based literature to draw upon. Similarly, new leaders are encouraged to engage in testing to learn more about their leadership style and personality. Assessment tools such as What's My Communication Style (Russo 2008), Emotional Intelligence Test (Bradberry and Greaves 2009) and Exploring Your Personal Strengths (Buckingham and Clifton 2001) are quite helpful and readily available. Having emotional intelligence is a key to separating "good" from "great" leaders (Johnson and Stern 2013).

Specific Challenges and Strategies

- **My supervisee feels I micromanage him.** Whether it's asking your supervisee to send you a document to review before it goes public or another matter, the supervisee may feel that such requests create undo pressure. In situations where emotions may run high, you might first thank the supervisee for expressing concerns that relate to the supervisee's perceived micromanagement by the supervisor instead of becoming grumpy. Open communication is always key between a supervisor and supervisee. When a supervisee is assigned a new task, it is important to initially monitor to ensure all *i*'s are dotted and *t*'s are crossed. This is especially important if the person ultimately responsible for the task is the supervisor. This monitoring would only be temporary, allowing the supervisee to ask and the supervisor to answer any questions up front instead of trying to put out fires after they arise. Once the task becomes routine and both are comfortable, then the supervisee can complete the task independently.
- **My supervisee is frustrated by perceived additional duties placed on her.** The addition of new duties to one's clinical workload can be overwhelming, especially if they appear to impinge on personal time. Additional duties can be mandates from higher-level hospital management or learning tools to enhance clinical skills.

In either case, they are not optional. You will have to work with the supervisee to find a win-win approach to the additional task. Strategies will need to be developed to help her improve her efficiency in her clinical work to reduce her stress. It is also important to provide a good understanding of the value of the task. You might also brainstorm with the supervisee about other ways to make an otherwise adversarial experience become more palatable, such as finding systems approaches that might alleviate undue burden and/or working to support her need for possible increased protected time for the added task.

Questions for the Supervisee

- What are your overall goals at this institution?

- What kind of mentoring do you find most useful?

- What have you learned about conflict management in the past?

- What have you learned about leading change?

Additional Resources

Bradberry T, Greaves J: Emotional Intelligence 2.0. San Diego, CA, TalentSmart Publishing, 2009
Buckingham M, Clifton D: Now, Discover Your Strengths. New York, Free Press, 2001
Russo E: What's My Communication Style? Self-Assessment, 3rd Edition. West Chester, PA, HRDQ, 2008

References

Balon R: Leadership versus management. Acad Psychiatry 38:720–722, 2014
Bradberry T, Greaves J: Emotional Intelligence 2.0. San Diego, CA, TalentSmart Publishing, 2009
Buckingham M, Clifton D: Now, Discover Your Strengths. New York, Free Press, 2001
Day DV: Leadership development: a review in context. Leadersh Q 11(4):581–613, 2001
Fisher R, Ury W: Getting to Yes: Negotiating Agreement without Giving In. New York, Penguin Books, 1983
Johnson JM, Stern TA: Preparing psychiatrists for leadership roles in healthcare. Acad Psychiatry 37(5):297–300, 2013 24026366
Roberts LW: Leadership in academic psychiatry: the vision, the "givens," and the nature of leaders. Acad Psychiatry 33(2):85–88, 2009 19398615
Russo E: What's My Communication Style? Self-Assessment, 3rd Edition. West Chester, PA, HRDQ, 2008

Chapter 30 Supervising Scholarship

Francesco N. Dandekar, M.D.
Belinda S. Bandstra, M.D., M.A.

The supervision of scholarship is an important part of psychiatry, given the quickly changing and vastly expanding nature of the field. Properly understood as encompassing discovery, integration, application, and teaching (Boyer 1990), scholarship is an integral part of the learning and practice of psychiatry. It is also a multifaceted topic not only because of the breadth of types of scholarship but also because of the breadth of types of supervision.

Key Points

- Create a clear mutual understanding of the goals of the supervisory relationship around scholarship, whether it be broad mentorship or direct management of a scholarly project.

- Thoughtfully negotiate supervisory styles and be aware of how supervisory needs may shift over time.

Negotiating Supervisory Roles in the Context of Scholarship

There are multiple roles that a supervisor may play in the development of a supervisee's scholarship, and a supervisee may be looking for different types of guidance from a supervisor.

- **Mentor**—supervisors may help their supervisees understand types of scholarship and explore their own proclivities within scholarship.
- **Liaison**—supervisors may connect supervisees with others who share similar scholarly interests or approaches to scholarship.
- **Collaborator**—supervisors and supervisees may have common scholarly interests and pursue them jointly.
- **Primary investigator**—a supervisee may participate in the supervisor's project.

Thus, it is important for a supervisor and supervisee to negotiate the goals of their supervisory relationship up front and recognize potential conflicts of interest.

Negotiating Supervisory Styles in the Context of Scholarship

Beyond clearly defining roles in the supervision of scholarship, it is also important to recognize that there are a wide range of styles of supervision, perhaps even more so in scholarship than in clinical work given the breadth of the field. In particular, supervision may range from extremely structured to allowing the supervisee a high degree of autonomy. This too must be negotiated between the supervisor and the supervisee.

Hersey and Blanchard (1969) advanced a model of Situational Leadership that defines four styles of leadership: directing, coaching, supporting, and delegating (or empowering). Directing is providing clear, concise directions with less focus on giving nurturing support, and is thought to be useful for highly committed supervisees with low competence in the field. Coaching is both highly directive and highly supportive, providing supervisees with clear directions but also moving them toward being masters of their own work. Supporting does not involve a lot of direction, but rather it provides a lot of nurturance and is more helpful for seasoned supervisees who may have variable commitment or lower morale. Finally, delegating or empowering is lower in both direction and support and is designed for supervisees who are able and willing to work independently and autonomously. Supervisors typically have their "preferred" style or styles and should understand what those are; they should also strive to become adept at all four styles so as to be able to adjust to supervisees' needs.

Of note, supervisees enter into supervisory relationships with variable skill sets and prior experiences. It is helpful to discuss this with supervisees in detail so as to gain a more informed understanding of each supervisee's individual strengths as well as areas in which he or she may need more guidance and/or oversight. From this foundation, supervisors can foster a supervisee's aptitudes as well as keep in mind areas in which supervisees are likely to need more assistance and guidance.

It follows that these areas may evolve over time, because a supervisee may need more direct supervisory involvement in certain contexts or for certain projects or undertakings. While it is certainly a supervisee's responsibility to communicate needs to the supervisor, it can behoove the supervisory relationship for a supervisor to periodically check-in with the supervisee to ascertain if more or less support is desired. Specific issues to be discussed include frequency and content of check-in meetings, as well as ways in which the supervisee will report his or her progress (e.g., formal document, informal email, in-person meeting; see "Additional Resources" below). Whiteside and colleagues (2007) advocate for an explicit set of formal documentation, including signed informed consent, descriptive syllabus of expectations and responsibilities, and delegation of some supervisory responsibilities to senior supervisees. Each supervisor can assess what level of formality works best for him or her and for each individual supervisee.

The role of a supervisor in a context of scholarship is complicated by the reality that the supervisor potentially stands to benefit from the work of his or her supervisee. For example, a supervisor may expect or desire a supervisee to take a lead role in a specific research project the supervisor needs assistance with, while the supervisee simply desires to learn about the possible options in a given field of research. Or, a supervisee may want to gather information about a given field and potentially work with another supervisor but may feel embarrassed about sharing this with his or her current supervisor. As Löfström and Pyhältö (2012) describe, the supervisory relationship can be fraught with ethical dilemmas. It is vital that supervisors facilitate transparent and thorough communication with their supervisees. In doing so, potential conflicts can be avoided and both parties have the information and means to shape the supervisory relationship or, in some cases, to decide if a better fit could be found elsewhere.

Specific Challenges and Strategies

- **My supervisee has difficulty articulating scholarly goals.** The supervisor should inquire as to the specific goals a supervisee has regarding his or her scholarly pursuit, as these will likely influence the nature and tenor of the supervisory relationship. There are numerous intentions a supervisee can bring to a supervisory relationship, such as a clear aim to pursue a research project or become involved in a specific clinical experience. However, whereas some supervisees will be very clear about their goals, others may still be gathering information about possible scholarly interests they have. It can be somewhat challenging for a supervisor to meet needs that are not yet well formed, yet the principle of open communication remains relevant: an ongoing dialogue with a supervisee can be instrumental in developing and shaping future scholarly work.

- **I'd like my supervisee to take interest in *my* project.** Ideally, the supervisor's primary goal would be to support his or her supervisee's educational goals and interests. Some supervisors will be content with simply serving as a resource for their supervisee, sharing knowledge and experience without desiring anything in return. Some supervisors will expect a supervisee to help with their own scholarly projects. This unintentional conflict of interest may also arise if a supervisee is working on a project of particular interest or value to his or her supervisor. Supervisors should be aware of the potential personal gain that can arise from a supervisee's interest and involvement and make good-faith decisions in the supervisee's best interests. Of course, mutual benefit in these types of mentorship relationships is not uncommon; however, supervisors must be diligent about frequently assessing the goals and desires of their supervisees so as to not let the inherent power dynamic affect the fidelity of the supervisory relationship. Regardless of the expectation, it behooves supervisors to be upfront, both with themselves and with their supervisees; this helps avoid misunderstandings and establishes a stable foundation for the supervisory relationship.

Questions for the Supervisee

- What type(s) of scholarship most appeal to you?

- What role are you hoping scholarship will take in your professional life and career?

- What are you looking for in this supervisory relationship?

- What do you hope our relationship will look like?

- What would you like to gain from this relationship (and what would I like to gain from this relationship)?

- How do you best learn and grow?

Additional Resources

Eberly Center for Teaching Excellence and Educational Innovation, Carnegie Mellon University: https://www.cmu.edu/teaching/designteach/teach/instructionalstrategies/independentstudentprojects/index.html
Mentoring styles tool: https://www.icre.pitt.edu/mentoring/docs/Tool_Mentoring_Styles.pdf

---

References

Boyer EL: Scholarship Reconsidered: Priorities of the Professoriate. Princeton, NJ, Carnegie Foundation for the Advancement of Teaching, 1990
Hersey P, Blanchard KH: Life cycle theory of leadership. Train Dev J 23:26–34, 1969
Löfström E, Pyhältö K: The supervisory relationship as an arena for ethical problem solving. Education Research International 2012:1–12, 2012
Whiteside U, Pantelone D, Eland J, et al: Initial suggestions for supervising and mentoring undergraduate research assistants at large research universities. Int J Teach Learn High Educ 19:325–330, 2007

Chapter 31 Quality Improvement

Supervising Trainees to Lead Change

Melissa R. Arbuckle, M.D., Ph.D.

According to the Accreditation Council for Graduate Medical Education (ACGME) (2017), all residents are expected to "systematically analyze practice using quality improvement methods, and implement changes with the goal of practice improvement" (p. 10). The ACGME clarifies that "experiential learning is essential to developing the ability to identify and institute sustainable systems-based changes to improve patient care" (Accreditation Council for Graduate Medical Education 2017, p. 18). Highlighting the importance of training in quality improvement (QI) to psychiatry, the ACGME and the American Board of Psychiatry and Neurology (ABPN) have set specific milestones in psychiatry for resident participation in "formal practice-based quality improvement" (Accreditation Council for Graduate Medical Education and American Board of Psychiatry and Neurology 2015). However, QI is often focused on systems of care, making training in QI critical for a diverse set of learners, including psychologists, social workers, and nurses in addition to medical students and physicians.

Teaching QI is more effective when trainees are actively involved in developing their own QI project (Philibert 2008). Following adult learning principles, this allows students to consolidate their learning through the immediate application of core concepts (Knowles 1979). Success of any QI project depends, in part, on the ability of the faculty supervisor to guide trainees through the QI process from setting appropriate goals, to identifying methods for tracking and measuring outcomes, to selecting and implementing changes. Although some trainees may have a specific project in mind and seek out individual supervision, QI is particularly well suited to group supervision. Within a group, trainees may take on individual projects or work together toward a common goal. Regardless, there are several relevant key principles when supervising QI in groups or with individuals.

Key Points

- Set a frame and a timeline.
- Select feasible projects and achievable aims.
- Identify measures for tracking.
- Engage stakeholders and select opportunities for change.
- Follow-up regularly.

Setting a Frame and a Timeline

As with any supervision, it is critical to set a frame. What is the overall timeline for the project? Is the project a year-long effort, or is it limited to a 2-month clinical rotation? Supervisors also need to establish how frequently they will meet and how long each session will be. It is also important to ask trainees about any prior experience with QI, particularly what worked well and what did not work well, to consolidate and build on prior learning.

Selecting Feasible Projects and Achievable Aims

The first order of business is to help learners choose a project and set measurable aims. Trainees, often on the frontlines of clinical care, are well versed in the clinical microsystems in which they work and can provide greater insight into gaps in clinical care (Philibert 2008). Designing and developing their own QI initiatives gives trainees an opportunity to identify clinical challenges that are particularly relevant and meaningful for them. Treatment guidelines, consensus standards of care, and quality indicators can all guide trainees toward potential gaps in care and inform project aims (Haan et al. 2008). Specific aims might also be drawn from the Institute of Medicine recommendations for improvement in health care (Institute of Medicine Committee on Quality of Health Care in America 2001). Choosing goals early and allowing trainees to meet during protected time provides a structure that promotes and enhances the opportunity for successful projects.

Creating a positive QI experience is contingent on helping the learners to select a feasible project given the time and resources of the group. Supervisors should allow learners to brainstorm, while helping them to think critically about the feasibility of their ideas. Attempting a project that is too large in scope or focusing on too many projects may lead to failure. Determining if a project is feasible requires an accurate assessment of potential barriers (e.g., the time commitment required, the resources available, the level of support from faculty and administrators).

Identifying Measures for Tracking

In setting goals, supervisors should ask, "What is the baseline data or current performance measure?" If trainees do not know the baseline data, or if they do not know how to obtain baseline data, then they will not be able to measure progress or determine project outcomes. Supervisors should encourage trainees to consider who will collect the data, when the data will be collected (and how often), and how the data will be collected. The feasibility of the project could hinge on the plan for data collection. Although the availability of data from an electronic medical record (EMR) makes tracking QI outcomes more feasible, the lack of EMR data is not an absolute barrier. For certain projects, trainees may be able to self-report or extract their own clinical data (Houston et al. 2009). With the expanding availability of simple, free survey systems (e.g., Google Docs), it could be fairly easy for teams to develop and implement alternative electronic reporting systems. Regardless, developing novel measurement systems does add another layer of complexity that may limit project success.

Engaging Stakeholders and Selecting Opportunities for Change

As with any QI project, the next step is to help learners identify potential interventions to facilitate system change. Trainees should brainstorm possible barriers and facilitators and propose a variety of potential interventions. Identifying the root cause of the problem is essential for planning and focusing interventions. It is important to understand why the system does not already meet expected goals. In developing potential interventions, trainees should review whether the current lack of alignment with project goals is due to clinical uncertainty (based on a lack of consensus or evidence regarding the most effective treatments), a lack of awareness or education, or a breakdown in the systems or processes of care (Oldham et al. 2008).

This review of barriers and facilitators is followed by a plan to implement changes, to measure outcomes, and to monitor the impact of interventions. It is important for students to review the state of the current system, the cost of implementing a change, and who the stakeholders are. Including key stakeholders early in the planning is critical (Houston et al. 2009; Patow et al. 2009) because the success of proposed interventions and QI projects often requires the support of faculty and administrators and access to clinical data.

Following Up Regularly

Each subsequent session should be structured around the Plan-Do-Study-Act model (Institute of Healthcare Improvement 2007). Meeting regularly validates QI as a training priority, reminds every one of the goals at hand, and builds momentum. Follow-up sessions should begin with a brief review of the latest plan, followed by a review of the data, and a discussion of the value and impact of the most recent changes. The team then collectively identifies additional changes that might improve outcomes. During this process, the specific tasks to implement are listed along with an identified team member who will take responsibility for the task and a deadline for when the task should be completed. The supervisor should encourage prompt follow-up on the plan. This may mean checking in and sending out reminders to participants regarding their assigned duties between sessions. It is important that deadlines be reasonable but that they also allow for enough time to see potential impact of the intervention prior to the next meeting.

Specific Challenges and Strategies

- **My supervisee is unclear if Institutional Review Board (IRB) approval is necessary.** Supervisors should help trainees determine whether their proposed project could be considered research and requires IRB approval. Those projects that are intended to drive local changes and improve internal systems are generally consistent with QI and do not represent research; however, those aiming to discover new knowledge and disseminate and publish results may require IRB approval. Although QI is generally not considered research, it is still useful to present the proposed project to the IRB for confirmation, particularly any study requiring access to medical records and protected health information. Proposed changes that require IRB approval may be worth pursuing by the group; however, they should not be the only QI initiative planned, because IRB approval alone could take months and delay or supplant the opportunity for students to implement a proposed QI project.
- **My supervisee can't get buy-in from others impacted by the project.** A major challenge with trainee-led initiatives is the lack of authority in the settings where they work. Trainees often have limited ability to implement "bottom up" changes, particularly if the project is not seen as a priority among faculty and other key stakeholders (Philibert 2008). Trainees should be encouraged to engage faculty members early to ensure that they are pursuing goals that are supported by clinical leadership and synergistic with other efforts. In some cases, the supervisor may serve as a valuable liaison with other faculty in terms of helping to better integrate the perspective of faculty members and enhance buy in. Supervisors may also need to advocate for access to data reports (from the EMR) and information technology support, if it is a critical component of the project.
- **My supervisee seems less engaged and committed to the project.** QI projects can be labor intensive, and improvements take time (Houston et al. 2009). A lack of positive results can be demoralizing and lead to disengagement in the process. Keeping the group (or individual) engaged and motivated requires that follow-up review sessions be led with a positive, collaborative tone. Encouraging trainees to share stories of success can motivate and inspire others and enable everyone in the group to learn multiple alternative strategies for how the proposed changes could work for them. Focusing on the clinical impact and the clinical relevance of the work can also be motivating. However, it is also possible that the proposed plan does not translate into an improvement in patient care. In some cases, the appropriate "action" may be to discontinue the project and focus efforts on another goal.

Questions for the Supervisee

■ What is the overall timeline for the project?

■ What is the aim of the project?

■ What will we measure to track outcomes?

■ Who are the important stakeholders?

■ What are feasible changes you could make?

Additional Resources

Fixsen DL, Naoom SF, Blase KA, et al: Implementation Research: A Synthesis of the Literature. Tampa, FL, University of South Florida, Louis de la Parte Florida Mental Health Institute, National Implementation Research Network, 2005

Massoud R, Askov K, Reinke J, et al: A modern paradigm for improving healthcare quality. 2001. Available at: https://www.usaidassist.org/sites/assist/files/modern paradigm_2001_0.pdf. Accessed August 16, 2018.

National Implementation Research Network: http://nirn.fpg.unc.edu/

References

Accreditation Council for Graduate Medical Education: Accreditation Council for Graduate Medical Education common program requirements. July 1, 2017. Available at: http://www.acgme.org/Portals/0/PFAssets/ProgramRequirements/CPRs_2017-07-01.pdf. Accessed August 16, 2018.

Accreditation Council for Graduate Medical Education, American Board of Psychiatry and Neurology: The Psychiatry Milestone Project. 2015. Available at: https://www.acgme.org/acgmeweb/Portals/0/PDFs/Milestones/PsychiatryMilestones.pdf. Accessed August 16, 2018.

Haan CK, Edwards FH, Poole B, et al: A model to begin to use clinical outcomes in medical education. Acad Med 83(6):574–580, 2008 18520464

Houston TK, Wall TC, Willet LL, et al: Can residents accurately abstract their own charts? Acad Med 84(3):391–395, 2009 19240454

Institute of Healthcare Improvement: How to improve. 2007. Available at: http://www.ihi.org/resources/Pages/HowtoImprove/default.aspx. Accessed August 16, 2018.

Institute of Medicine Committee on Quality of Health Care in America: Crossing the Quality Chasm: A New Health System for the 21st Century. Vol 21. Washington, DC, National Academy Press, 2001

Knowles M: The Adult Learner: A Neglected Species. Houston, TX, Gulf Publishing Company, 1979

Oldham JM, Golden WE, Rosof BM: Quality improvement in psychiatry: why measures matter. J Psychiatr Pract 14(May)(Suppl 2):8–17, 2008 18677195

Patow CA, Karpovich K, Riesenberg LA, et al: Residents' engagement in quality improvement: a systematic review of the literature. Acad Med 84(12):1757–1764, 2009 19940586

Philibert I: Involving residents in quality improvement: contrasting "top-down" and "bottom-up" approaches. ACGME Bulletin September 2008, p 25 Available at: https://www.acgme.org/Portals/0/PFAssets/bulletin/ACG11_BulletinSep08_F.PDF. Accessed August 16, 2018.

Part 6   Special Issues in Supervision

Chapter 32 How to Select an Individual Psychotherapy Supervisor

A Practical Guide

Joshua J. Hubregsen, M.D.

Adam M. Brenner, M.D.

It is important to have good supervision in psychotherapy training. Good supervision has a significant impact on therapeutic success. Compared with the importance of having effective supervision, the amount of literature about how to ensure that your supervision will be meaningful is surprisingly scant. For the supervisee, this chapter serves as a practical approach to how to select an appropriate supervisor. Of course, sometimes in training programs, choice of a supervisor is not possible, but the ideas presented in this chapter may be helpful to those supervisees in assessing how well the supervision is meeting their needs. For the supervisor, this chapter may provide some insights on what supervisees perceive to be useful.

Key Points

- The process of selecting a supervisor includes identifying one's needs, identifying options, and meeting with at least one prospective supervisor.

- Supervisees should understand the basics of what constitutes high-quality supervision to assist in selecting a good supervisor.

- Supervisees should focus their efforts on selecting a supervisor who will form an alliance with them around goals and will be affirmative and supportive of their growth.

- Meeting with a prospective supervisor can help to frame the goals and expectations of long-term supervision and is an opportunity to confirm the supervisee's choice of supervisor.

What to Know Before Selecting a Supervisor

Before you select a supervisor, it is important to clarify your supervision needs. Try to think of your needs in two ways: you will want to fulfill any logistic requirements, and you will want to be well trained. The first set of needs are your specific content needs, such as the type of psychotherapy training required. The second set of needs involves selection of a good supervisor—one with whom you can build a strong supervisory alliance. This alliance will enable you to work on shared goals that make sense to you, and it should promote the feeling that your supervisor is generally affirmative and supportive of you in your training. Literature suggests that trainee satisfaction is of utmost importance in supervision (Allen et al. 1986; Carifio and Hess 1987; Fernando and Hulse-Killacky 2005; Ladany et al. 1999). Your satisfaction with training should directly relate to this idea of building a strong supervisory alliance.

Some of your training content needs, such as the kind of psychotherapy experience required (e.g., psychodynamic, cognitive behavioral), will be prescribed. If this is the case, your first selection criterion will be to find a supervisor expert in that specific modality. Alternatively, you may not be under any requirement regarding the school of therapy but may feel that the evidence base suggests that your patient's presentation is best managed through a specific approach. In addition, your program may have other longitudinal requirements related to the training of your supervisor or related to specific patient populations. Be sure to first understand these basic program rules to help you plan which supervisors will be available to you.

Beyond these required needs, you will want to have a wide variety of supervisory experiences in your training to provide exposure to different styles, foci, and goals (Borders 1994). As you think of how to broaden exposure with a variety of supervisors, consider aspects such as the supervision setting, supervisor gender, and supervisor areas of expertise. Such content expertise can include not only types of psychopathology (e.g., trauma, psychosis, anxiety, personality disorders) but also issues such as stages of life, spiritual life, cultural diversity, or LGBT identities, among many others. Supervisors will also have different styles related to the degree of countertransference exploration, the focus on specific psychotherapy tasks and techniques, and the control and direction of the supervisory encounter. In regard to the last mentioned, at one end of the spectrum

TABLE 32–1. **Diversifying the supervisory experience**

Factor	Options
Type of therapy	Psychodynamic, cognitive-behavioral therapy, dialectical behavior therapy, interpersonal psychotherapy, EMDR (eye movement desensitization and reprocessing), prolonged exposure therapy, among others
Supervisor gender	Male, female, gender-nonconforming
Supervision setting	Private, academic, public
Supervisor practice location	Inpatient, outpatient clinic, private practice
Supervisor strengths	Expertise with type of psychotherapy, specific types of patients, cultural or life stage issues, and so forth
Diagnostic challenges	Trauma, psychosis, anxiety, mood, personality, and so forth
Supervisor style	Facilitative versus directive

are supervisors who uses their content expertise to determine the focus and provide instruction to the supervisee. In the other end of the spectrum are supervisors who position themselves more as consultants who encourage the supervisee to set the agenda and emphasize assisting the supervisee in clarifying his or her thinking and finding his or her own voice as a therapist (Shanfield and Gil 1985). Supervision factors are summarized in Table 32–1.

The next thing that you will want to know is what makes a good supervisor. Knowing the basics of what constitutes good supervision will help you select a supervisor with whom you can build a strong alliance. In surveying graduate student experiences, Allen et al. (1986) found that "the best discriminators of quality were perceived expertise and trustworthiness of the supervisor, duration of training, and an emphasis on personal growth issues over the teaching of technical skills" (p. 91). Carifio and Hess (1987) concluded that the ideal supervisor is appropriately empathetic, respectful, genuine, concrete, supportive, noncritical, and self-disclosing, while setting clear and explicit goals, giving appropriate feedback, and avoiding conflating supervision with psychotherapy. Shanfield et al. (1993) found additionally that highly rated supervisors were those best able to track trainee's affectively charged concerns. Table 32–2 summarizes elements of effective and ineffective supervision.

Knowing what to expect from good supervision, you should select supervisors who will help you to set goals for your learning and who will be affirmative and supportive of your growth. In assessing whether you have selected wisely, you should expect the following positive outcomes from an effective supervision: increased confidence, a sense of a supportive "safety net" as you practice, and a growing capacity for independent work.

How to Select a Supervisor

It is never too early to start the selection process, since all supervisors have limited availability. If you are part of a training program, be aware that each program may approach supervision differently. In general, start by gathering a list of available supervisors.

TABLE 32–2.   **Assessing quality supervision**

Effective supervisor	Ineffective supervisor
Is empathic, genuine, respectful, supportive	Is authoritarian
Prepares for and is involved in session, enjoys supervisory role	Lacks time to prepare, or frequently cancels sessions
Understands his or her own strengths and weaknesses (open)	Has limited self-awareness; is not accepting of feedback (closed)
Adheres to ethical guidelines	Exhibits sexist behaviors or violates boundaries
Communicates goals and expectations clearly	Sets vague expectations or changes expectations
Adapts to supervisee's learning needs, style, and personal character (flexible)	Uses prescribed supervisory style (rigid)
Avoids providing psychotherapy during session	Conflates supervision with psychotherapy

Slowly narrow the list by comparing with your previously identified needs, remembering that you will want a variety of good supervisors. Many supervisors may be geographically close or have availability that matches your schedule, but avoid the temptation to select someone purely for the sake of convenience. Review your list and select several candidates. Take time to speak with your peers and colleagues to learn about supervisor styles, experience, reputation, and adaptability. A trusted faculty member or mentor may also have specific suggestions about good supervisors. Taking time to speak with others should provide you with important perspective. Use all this information to narrow your selection to just a few choices.

After deciding on a supervisor with whom you feel you would work well, arrange a meeting and ask questions provided at the end of the chapter to help you decide if this will be a good match for your supervision needs. It is perfectly reasonable to decide at this point that your ideas on paper do not match the reality of the supervisory encounter. Ultimately your experiences in supervision will be enriched by having taken preparatory steps and allowing yourself, whenever possible, to pay attention to your own sense of whether the supervisor is a "good fit" for your own temperament and needs.

Specific Challenges and Strategies

- **I'm not affiliated with a training program, and I don't know who can supervise me.** Try reaching out to your local professional society or network, or to national psychotherapy-specific organizations such as the American Psychoanalytic Association or the Academy of Cognitive Therapy. They may be able to suggest local options specific to your training needs.
- **I live in an area without supervisors readily available.** Remote videoconferencing may be a viable alternative (Gammon et al. 1998). In a rapidly changing landscape, various online services and organizations offer remote supervision (Rousmaniere et al. 2014). The prospective supervisee will need to be careful in assessing qualifica-

tions and quality of such offerings as well as the privacy and security of the technology utilized.

- **My supervisor has been assigned to me by my program.** Request to have a say in who your supervisor will be. In many cases, supervisors have been selected by the program to make the decision easier for you. If you still don't have a choice, try to learn about the supervisor and be clear about what your own goals of supervision will be.

Questions for a Potential Supervisor

- What do you enjoy about supervising?

- How do you like to structure our supervision time?

- How would you describe your supervision style?

- What do you expect of me as a trainee?

- Could we set some goals for supervision?

- Do you have enough time to supervise me?

Additional Resources

The following associations have websites that may be helpful for identifying clinicians in a geographic area who have expertise in specific psychotherapies:

American Psychoanalytic Association: apsa.org
National Association of Cognitive-Behavioral Therapists: nacbt.org

References

Allen GJ, Szollos SJ, Williams BE: Doctoral students' comparative evaluations of best and worst psychotherapy supervision. Prof Psychol 17(2):91–99, 1986
Borders LD: The good supervisor. ERIC Digest, ED372350. April 1994. Available at: https://www.ericdigests.org/1995-1/good.htm. Accessed August 16, 2018.
Carifio MS, Hess AK: Who is the ideal supervisor? Prof Psychol 18:244–250, 1987
Fernando DM, Hulse-Killacky D: The relationship of supervisory styles to satisfaction with supervision and the perceived self-efficacy of master's-level counseling students. Couns Educ Superv 44:293–304, 2005
Gammon D, Sørlie T, Bergvik S, et al: Psychotherapy supervision conducted by videoconferencing: a qualitative study of users' experiences. J Telemed Telecare 4(1)(Suppl 1):33–35, 1998 9640727
Ladany N, Lehrman-Waterman D, Molinaro M, et al: Psychotherapy supervisor ethical practices: adherence to guidelines, the supervisory working alliance, and supervisee satisfaction. Couns Psychol 27(3):443–475, 1999
Rousmaniere T, Abbass A, Frederickson J, et al: Videoconference for psychotherapy training and supervision: two case examples. Am J Psychother 68(2):231–250, 2014 25122987
Shanfield SB, Gil D: Styles of psychotherapy supervision. J Psychiatr Educ 9:225–232, 1985
Shanfield SB, Matthews KL, Hetherly V: What do excellent psychotherapy supervisors do? Am J Psychiatry 150(7):1081–1084, 1993 8317580

Chapter 33 The Supervisee

Making the Most of Supervision

Amanda M. Franciscus, M.D.

The supervision-supervisee dyad introduces a new framework for learning, one that is often not experienced in a trainee's previous didactic-focused study. The supervisee can share in the responsibility of making the most out of supervision by learning the fundamentals of supervision and strategies for preparing and engaging in supervision sessions (Berger and Buchholz 1993; Bernard and Goodyear 2013; Crocker and Sudak 2017; Johnson 2017). This chapter focuses on techniques for the supervisee in clinical settings, but the techniques can be adapted for application in a variety of settings.

Key Points

- Develop an understanding of supervision, including the role of the supervisor and the supervisee, to promote a positive and effective supervision experience.

- Begin the supervision relationship by attending to the relationship, reviewing a supervision agreement, and creating supervision goals.

- Prepare for each supervision session to enhance the experience for both supervisee and supervisor.

- Learn to elicit feedback from the supervisor to enrich learning in supervision.

- Be prepared to deal openly with anxieties and conflicts that arise in the relationship.

Strategies Before Supervision Starts

Learn About the Supervisor

Gathering information about the supervisor prior to supervision can lead to a better understanding of what to expect and guide learning goals. The supervisee can review the supervisor's clinical biography online or from a program's list of supervisors and ask prior trainees about a supervisor (Berger and Graff 1995; Pearson and Students 2004). Consider the following in gathering supervisor information: focus of work, background and training, and experience level in domains of clinical environments, patient populations, theoretical stances, and past research. Consider asking past trainees: "Can you describe the supervisor's style?" "How did you present your work?" "How did the supervisor provide feedback?" "What were the supervisor's knowledge, skills, and attitudes about diversity (or other relevant topics)?" "How were conflicts, if any, resolved with your supervisor?" (Berger and Graff 1995; Pearson and Students 2004).

Complete a Self-Assessment

Consider completing a self-assessment before starting supervision. Many programs have milestones or competencies to reach by the end of training that can be used as a self-assessment. Through careful self-assessment, supervisees' insight into their motivations, strengths, and areas for improvement can lead to the development of learning goals, help them prepare for feedback sessions, and compare and contrast assessments completed by supervisors and program directors (Jardine et al. 2017).

Strategies for the First Supervisory Session

Establish a Supervisory Alliance

Once supervision begins, consider the alliance with the supervisor, review the supervision contract (if used), and discuss learning goals. Establishing an alliance with the supervisor is extremely important to maximize the supervisee's experience. Supervision uses the relationship between supervisor and supervisee to model, teach, and mentor. Partnering with the supervisor to create a clear understanding of the supervision and evaluative processes, as well as methods for conflict resolution, will help maintain the relationship. One way to accomplish this is to use a supervision agreement: a formal contract to establish a working relationship (Table 33–1). If a supervisor does not use one, you might suggest reviewing a contract together. Whenever possible, a written agreement is recommended over a verbal agreement (Sutter et al. 2002).

Develop Learning Goals

At the start of supervision, develop specific learning goals based on identified strengths, areas for improvement, training gaps, unique training and characteristics of the supervisor, and the current clinical environment and population (Johnson 2017). Write these goals down and discuss them with your supervisor, asking the supervisor what additional areas he or she see are opportunities for growth (Johnson 2017).

TABLE 33–1. **Components of supervision contract**

Practical and procedural aspects	Duration of supervision-supervisee relationship
	Frequency and duration of supervision sessions
	Context of the supervision (e.g., for patient care, for scholarly project)
	Emergency procedures and contact numbers
	Cancellation policy
	Fees (if relevant)
	Confidentiality (and its limitations)
Supervisor's qualifications	Supervisor's education, training, clinical interests, areas of expertise, and qualifications as a supervisor
	Supervisor's goals for supervision
Supervisee's qualifications	Supervisee's education, training, clinical interests, and areas of expertise
	Supervisee's strengths and areas of growth
	Supervisee's goals for supervision
Review of responsibilities	For the supervisor
	For the supervisee
	Example: For patient care: case load requirement, documentation format, presentation frequency, who returns phone calls, who does refills, etc.
	Example: For scholarly concentration projects: who sets up meetings, who keeps project deadlines and deliverable on track, etc.
Expectations	Session framework
	What to bring to supervision (e.g., video, transcripts, articles)
Feedback/evaluations	Frequency of feedback
	Frequency of evaluation
	Review of evaluation forms
	How competencies will be assessed
	How any professional concerns will be reported and managed
	Conditions where confidentiality is limited
Conflicts and concerns	Procedures for addressing disagreements (if conflict is not resolved in session, outline for next step)

Source. Adapted from Berger and Buchholz 1993; Crocker and Sudak 2017; Johnson 2017; Pearson and Students 2004.

Strategies for Supervision Sessions Following the First Session

In supervision, a supervisee should anticipate doing the work. This often takes the form of a supervisee bringing in questions, topics, concerns or materials from a patient case, scholarly work, or administrative issue, while the supervisor facilitates learning by layering considerations, professional knowledge or organizational standards (Milne 2007).

Come Prepared

Making the most of the supervision session takes preparation before each session, active participation throughout the session, and the openness to discuss experiences, failures, and feedback. Prior to a supervision session, reflect on material to guide the upcoming supervision session. For example, to prepare for supervision related to a scholarly project, reflect on questions such as "What has been challenging in meeting the next project deliverable?" If the supervision is for therapy or medication management, reflect on questions such as "What patient am I often thinking about (or seldom think of)?" or "What challenges have I encountered in recent session (Pearson and Students 2004)?" Based on this reflection, develop questions to ask the supervisor during the upcoming supervision. Be specific and avoid vague statements like "What should I do with X?" Take the time to carefully consider possible approaches to challenges without simply asking the supervisor. Be proactive in trying to problem solve around a difficult issue by thoughtfully analyzing the issue and applying knowledge or researching a response instead of relying passively on the supervisor for answers. Prepare needed material to bring to session that correlates with the supervision question, such as handouts, manuscripts, relevant readings, or therapy videos. It is advisable to limit the material provided to the supervisor to ensure sufficient time to have specific questions answered. For example, case presentations might be limited to 2 minutes or therapy video transcripts to 10 minutes. Work with the supervisor to determine how the supervision time can be best used. Remember to also read and review previously discussed topics assigned during the last supervision session. If needed, come to session with questions to clarify what was read and assigned.

Set an Agenda

To actively participate in a supervision session, arrive promptly and work with the supervisor to set an agenda for the supervision time. The start of an agenda should address immediate needs, which might include patient safety (suicidal patients) or ethical dilemmas, and include an update on prior supervision's suggestions or assignments (Pearson and Students 2004). As part of the agenda setting, request time for specific questions or prepared material. As a supervisee, do not expect to have all the answers; be open about gaps in knowledge or challenging material, and consider your supervisor's feedback thoughtfully (Crocker and Sudak 2017; Rodenhauser et al. 1989). One common error of supervisees is the tendency to focus exclusively on material or topics that are "going well." Instead, by bringing up mistakes and problems, you can give an accurate representation of the situation and more effectively learn how to respond to challenges and learning edges (Crocker and Sudak 2017).

Seek and Integrate Feedback

Lastly, feedback is one of the core fundamentals of supervision. Ideally, feedback should be done throughout the supervision process and within each supervision session. If you are not getting sufficient feedback, ask for it early and often. It is helpful to ask directly after completing a task, whether this is an interview, presentation, or new technique. Supervisees can enhance their learning by applying the feedback as soon as possible. Consider asking the supervisor for help in developing an action plan or a goal, informed by the feedback, to target a change within a specific timeline: "How can we monitor my performance based on the feedback I received?" Translate learning and feedback during supervision into study objectives and next steps outside supervision. For example, in clinical supervision, make note of techniques you want to implement during your next patient encounter. Or to further guide self-learning, collaboratively discuss relevant resources or readings to be completed before the next supervision session. Consider making a specific plan for these assignments: "I would like to set a goal for myself to review one of these resources by next week." Review goals and progress with your supervisor at regular intervals.

Ways to Use Supervision Techniques to Your Advantage

As discussed throughout this book, there are many supervision techniques that promote and enhance learning. Two techniques a supervisee can prompt are modeling and role-playing. A supervisee could say the following, "I had difficulty explaining the risk and benefits of treatment X today. Can I hear how you would explain it?" By observing the supervisor model an intervention, the supervisee learns how to approach an issue. Similarly, the supervisee might ask, "As chief of the service, a junior said '*X*' to me, and I did not know how to respond. Can I role-play with you? Then maybe we could switch and I can hear how you would respond?" Role-playing allows the supervisee not only to observe the supervisor model an intervention but also to rehearse a skill (see Chapter 7, "Role-Play" and Chapter 8, "Modeling, Rehearsal, and Feedback: A Simple Approach to Teaching Complex Skills").

Other techniques used in clinical supervision include staying alert to the phenomenon of the parallel process and addressing transference/countertransference. Parallel process occurs when the supervisee unconsciously presents himself or herself to the supervisor as the patient presented himself or herself to the supervisee (Berger and Buchholz 1993). Consider the following, "As I am presenting this case, I feel *X*; I wonder if this is how the patient feels?" Regarding transference/countertransference, the supervisee could attend to, reflect on, and potentially discuss countertransference toward a patient or even transference the supervisee has toward to the supervisor (see Chapter 37, "The Supervision of Countertransference").

Strategies to Manage Conflict

Conflict in collaboration occurs in all relationships (Bernard and Goodyear 2013), including with patients and with supervisors. Literature highlights themes that may arise between a supervisee and supervisor, including feelings of rivalry, issues of authority, pressure to have similar view points, and personality conflicts (Berger and Buchholz 1993). In the case of conflict with a supervisor, a supervisee should bring up concerns as early as possible, using direct feedback (Crocker and Sudak 2017). If issues are not resolved within the supervision relationship, the supervisee should consider seeking support from the program director, a chief resident, or other members of the training team (see Chapter 36, "Ruptures in the Supervisory Relationship").

Reflecting on Experiences of Supervision

At the completion of supervision, the supervisee should reflect on the process. Consider keeping a log of your reflections including helpful and unhelpful strategies, skills/attitudes obtained, conflict resolution techniques, and the impact supervision had on continued learning or career trajectories (Johnson 2017). This can be used for final feedback to the supervisor and guide your expectations and goals for future supervision.

Specific Challenges and Strategies

- **My supervisor is very supportive, but I wish I could get more constructive feedback about how to improve.** Start asking! One way is to ask for specifics. For example, supervisors might say, "Great job on the interview." Follow up with: "Which particular part of the interview did you think was done well?" or "On X part, I felt it went Y. What was your perception of it?" Another way is to ask for balanced feedback. If the supervisor is delivering all glowing or all constructive feedback, probe for the opposite: "What could I have improved on during that interview?" "Was there anything I did well?"
- **I'm nervous about sharing some of my difficulties and areas of growth with my supervisor.** Practice self-compassion! It's a learning process—a supervisee is not expected to know how to do this. Supervisee anxiety is a common occurrence; areas include evaluation anxiety, performance anxiety, anxiety when trying new techniques/clinical duties, and anxiety with interpersonal dynamics in the supervision (Liddle 1986; Pearson and Students 2004). Normalizing and accepting anxiety is a part of supervision. It's recommended that supervisees discuss anxieties with the supervisor to develop ways to cope, explore sources of the anxiety (e.g., patient projection, feelings of vulnerability, burnout), and problem-solve.
- **The supervision feels unstructured, and I often leave feeling unsure about what I learned or how to move forward.** First, have you prepared for the supervision experience by creating learning objectives? Stop anytime and create or regroup on these goals. Second, are you preparing for each session? Do you come in with a "supervision question" based on reflection, research, or something read? Third, have you proposed an agenda for the session? Last, have you made clear end-of-session objectives? Discuss all four strategies and brainstorm with your supervisor; if it still feels unstructured, provide this feedback to the supervisor and try to develop an alternative approach to supervisory sessions.

Questions for the Supervisee

■ What are your learning goals for this year?

■ How can you use supervision to help you move toward these goals?

■ What challenges have you experienced in the past during supervision, and how can you strategize around these for this new experience?

Additional Resources

Goal-Setting Tools

Accreditation Council for Graduate Medical Education and American Board of Psychiatry and Neurology: The Psychiatry Milestone Project, July 2015. Available at: http://www.acgme.org/Portals/0/PDFs/Milestones/PsychiatryMilestones.pdf.

Johnson EA: Working Together in Clinical Supervision. New York, Momentum Press, 2017

Strategies to Enhance Reflection and Skill Development

Rousmaniere T, Goodyear RK, Miller SD, et al: The Cycle of Excellence: Using Deliberate Practice to Improve Supervision and Training. Chichester, UK, Wiley, 2017

Psychology Tools, Supervision (Clinical/Professional Supervision): Psychology Tools Cognitive Behavioral Therapy (CBT) Worksheets for Clinical Supervision. Available at: https://psychologytools.com/download-supervision-materials.html.

References

Berger SS, Buchholz ES: On becoming a supervisee: Preparation for learning in a supervisory relationship. Psychother Theor Res Pract Train 30:86–92, 1993

Berger N, Graff L: Making good use of supervision, in Basics of Clinical Practice: A Guidebook for Trainees in the Helping Profession. Edited by Martin DG, Moore AD. Prospect Heights, IL, Waveland Press, 1995, pp 408–432

Bernard JM, Goodyear RK: Fundamentals of Clinical Supervision. Pearson College Division. Boston, MA, Pearson Education/Allyn & Bacon, 2013

Crocker EM, Sudak DM: Making the most of psychotherapy supervision: a guide for psychiatry residents. Acad Psychiatry 41(1):35–39, 2017 27909977

Jardine D, Deslauriers J, Kamran SC, et al: Milestone Guidebook for Residents and Fellows. Accreditation Council for Graduate Medical Education, June 2017. Available at: https://www.acgme.org/Portals/0/PDFs/Milestones/MilestonesGuidebookforResidentsFellows.pdf. Accessed August 16, 2018.

Johnson EA: Working Together in Clinical Supervision. New York, Momentum Press, 2017, pp 19, 33–55

Liddle B: Resistance in supervision: a response to perceived threat. Couns Educ Superv 26:117–127, 1986

Milne D: An empirical definition of clinical supervision. Br J Clin Psychol 46(Pt 4):437–447, 2007 17535535

Pearson QM, Students C: Getting the most out of clinical supervision: strategies for mental health. J Ment Health Couns 26(4):361–373, 2004

Rodenhauser P, Rudisill JR, Painter AF: Attributes conducive to learning in psychotherapy supervision. Am J Psychother 43(3):368–377, 1989 2683811

Sutter E, McPherson RH, Geeseman R: Contracting for supervision. Prof Psychol Res Pr 33:495–498, 2002

Chapter 34 Psychotherapy Supervision by a Psychologist

Benefits and Potential Challenges

Kristine H. Luce, Ph.D.

Kathleen M. Corcoran, Ph.D.

Psychologists have extensive theoretical and clinical training in both psychotherapy and psychotherapy supervision that is derived from established psychological principles. Foundational training generally begins while pursuing the undergraduate degree and continues beyond licensure. Given their dedicated training and expertise, psychologist clinicians are particularly well qualified to teach and supervise the practice of psychotherapy, and their expertise can be helpful in psychiatry residency training. Because there are many differences between psychologists and psychiatrists in educational background, clinical training, and professional guidelines and standards, it is helpful to understand and address potential challenges at the outset of supervision.

Key Points

- There are important differences in the training of psychiatrists and psychologists that are helpful to understand.

- Supervision is a core competency for licensure as a psychologist.

- Psychologists are expected to provide competency-based clinical supervision and maintain best practice standards as they evolve.

- There are challenges that can arise given the differences between the disciplines that are helpful to plan for and address at the outset of the supervision experience.

Educational Differences Between Disciplines

The educational background of psychologists tends to be quite different from that of psychiatrists. Prior to medical school, students who plan to apply to medical school generally take rigorous undergraduate courses in biological science, physics, and chemistry. After 4 years of medical school education, students apply for specialized residency training, for example, psychiatry. Given this educational trajectory, psychiatry residents may have limited opportunity to learn foundational psychological principles before they begin providing psychotherapy to clients. Furthermore, little or no specialized training is provided with regard to teaching or supervising psychotherapy.

In contrast, most psychologists earn bachelor degrees in psychology before they apply for doctoral studies. A 2016 survey by the National Science Foundation indicated that of psychologists surveyed who earned doctorate degrees in clinical and counseling psychology ($n=1,540$) and who reported their first bachelor's degree on the survey ($n=1,269$), 77.8% earned bachelor degrees in psychology (National Science Foundation 2016). The American Psychological Association (2017) defines psychology as the "study of the mind and behavior" and asserts that the "discipline embraces all aspects of human behavior" in "every conceivable setting." The *APA Principles for Quality Undergraduate Education in Psychology* (American Psychological Association 2011) recommend that, in addition to a comprehensive introductory course that introduces the entire field, and subfields, of psychology and serves as a prerequisite upon which future courses and concepts are built and sequenced, undergraduate psychology programs teach psychology as a scientific discipline that includes basic research design and statistics. Consistent with these and the 2007 *APA Guidelines for the Undergraduate Psychology Major* (American Psychological Association 2007), Stoloff and colleagues (2010) reviewed the curriculum for 374 B.S. or B.A. psychology degree programs and found that a course on research methods was offered by all programs. Thus, the majority of licensed psychologists not only begin learning the foundational principles of psychotherapy at the beginning of their undergraduate psychology education, but also start learning about scientific inquiry and how to evaluate the effectiveness of various psychotherapies, teaching methods, and supervision models.

Psychologists who practice psychotherapy generally earn either a Ph.D. (Doctor of Philosophy) or a Psy.D. (Doctor of Psychology) in clinical or counseling psychology. To prepare students for the independent practice of psychotherapy, doctoral programs are required to teach graduate coursework about the history and theories of various psychotherapies and coordinate clinical practicum training opportunities during which doctoral students will complete at least 2,000 supervised face-to-face therapy contact hours during graduate school. Face-to-face therapy contact hours generally include a variety of psychotherapy tasks and modalities, including psychological assessment and individual, group, and family therapy modalities and often include various theoretical orientations, although only one orientation is typically taught during a particular therapy training experience. Prior to being granted the doctoral degree, students are required to complete a full-time clinical internship during which they accrue an additional 2,000 supervised face-to-face therapy contact hours. Although specific psychologist licensure requirements vary by state, postdoctoral psychology therapists are required to obtain additional supervised face-to-face therapy contact hours to register for and take the Examination for Professional Practice in Psychology, which, in addition to other state requirements, is used in most U.S. states and Canadian provinces to license psychologists.

Training Differences Specific to Psychotherapy Supervision

To obtain accreditation from the APA, doctoral programs are required to teach courses that equip doctoral students to achieve competence in measuring, evaluating, and implementing effective strategies for supervision (American Psychological Association 2006). Thus, not only are psychologists required to obtain competency in the provision of psychotherapy, they are expected to learn to competently teach psychotherapy to other mental health providers and to evaluate the effectiveness of their teaching and supervision. Furthermore, the Association of State and Provincial Psychology Boards (ASPPB) (2017) recommends that state licensing boards and colleges include supervision as a competency that is expected of psychologists at the point of licensure; therefore, questions about supervision models and best practices are asked on the Examination for Professional Practice in Psychology. After licensure, psychologists are expected to provide competency-based clinical supervision and to maintain best practice standards as they evolve. Consistent with this expectation, some states, including Arkansas, California, and Washington, require that primary supervisors complete continuing education coursework about psychotherapy supervision as part of licensure renewal.

As a way of promoting the provision of competency-based clinical supervision, elements of best practices were identified and the following supervision guidelines were adopted and published: the APA Guidelines for Clinical Supervision in Health Service Psychology (American Psychological Association 2014) and the ASPPB Supervision Guidelines for Education and Training Leading to Licensure as a Health Service Provider (Association of State and Provincial Psychology Boards 2015). The supervision guidelines are intended to provide a framework for competence-based psychotherapy supervision and to articulate a standard of excellence by which supervision practices can be evaluated. Not only are psychotherapy supervisors expected to obtain education and training in the best practices for competent psychotherapy supervision, they are expected to maintain their expertise by incorporating any revisions to best practice standards as may be indicated by new research evidence.

Procedural Differences Between Disciplines
Supervision of Trainees

It is recommended that psychotherapy supervisors approach supervision relationships with empathy, responsiveness, and openness that invites residents to ask questions and disclose when they are unfamiliar with a psychological principle that may be taken for granted by a psychologist supervisor. As with walking, advanced clinicians often do not recall when they first learned the fundamentals. Furthermore, it is advisable to approach supervision with a beginner's stance and directly ask residents if they are familiar with foundational principles rather than assume previous acquisition of learning. A more formal needs assessment is recommended, but this may restrict evaluation to particular therapeutic techniques. Distributing handouts and assigning brief readings about essential foundational principles constitute an efficient and beneficial strategy to help residents acquire foundational knowledge upon which psychotherapy competency builds.

Length and Timing of Psychotherapy Rotations

Psychology trainees typically have 6- or 12-month rotations in a single placement (e.g., within a psychology department student clinic, a hospital, a Veterans Administration mental health clinic, or a community mental health center), whereas psychiatry residents may have multiple co-occurring psychotherapy rotations using different therapy models and the rotations may range from 3–12 months. Residents' psychotherapy rotations are typically only one of many other overlapping rotations, such as medication management clinics, and they have responsibilities across all rotations that sometimes make it difficult for them to focus as comprehensively on their psychotherapy training.

Supervisor Duties

In psychotherapy supervision, the clinical supervisor is responsible for directing the treatment and is ultimately responsible for the quality of care (Alban and Frankel 2007). Furthermore, the duty of care rests on the psychotherapy supervisor such that the supervisor may be legally and ethically liable for acts or omissions of their supervisees (Saccuzzo 1997). As indicated in the ASPPB supervision guidelines (Association of State and Provincial Psychology Boards 2015), written supervision contracts between the supervisor and supervisee are recommended. Explicit clarification of expected duties and responsibilities of supervisees, especially in cases when known discrepancies in professional expectations are likely to occur, reduces miscommunication and enhance the supervisory relationship.

Working Within Different Educational Systems

Beginning the Supervision Experience

As indicated previously, it is recommended that psychotherapy supervisors approach the supervision relationship with empathy, responsiveness, and openness. It is beneficial to model and encourage a beginner's stance to create an environment that values and facilitates mutual growth and learning. While maintaining this relational frame, the supervisor will find it useful to discuss the following in the first meeting: 1) relevant educational background and clinical experience (e.g., therapy model, supervision model) of both the supervisor and supervisee (e.g., psychotherapy didactics, previous or concurrent psychotherapy rotations); 2) goals of both the supervisor and supervisee for supervision; 3) procedural differences between disciplines and supervisor expectations (e.g., consultation with other clinicians about therapy cases); 4) structure and process of supervision (e.g., audio, video, process notes); and 5) assignments (e.g., transcription of sessions, written case formulation, readings). A written supervision contract is recommended to clarify roles, responsibilities, and supervision goals. Parallel to the process of psychotherapy, supervision goals and expectations should be reviewed regularly to evaluate progress and to consider revisions based on changing training goals.

Aligning Clinical Training With Didactics

Residency didactic curriculum may not match psychotherapy supervision. Psychiatry residents have multiple overlapping didactic courses and clinical demands that may not always proceed in sequential order, and the didactic or theoretical psychotherapy curriculum may not match the resident's current psychotherapy rotation (e.g., exposure strategies are taught in the fall, but the exposure-based therapy rotation occurs in spring). In supervision, it is helpful, first, to review the syllabi of psychotherapy courses and ask residents to review their notes and highlight concepts that require further instruction. Then, it is beneficial to structure supervision in two parts, theoretical and applied. It is suggested that the theoretical portion include a review of or introduction to case conceptualization, discussion of the session-by-session and overall structure of the psychotherapy model, review of or instruction about foundational psychological principles of the psychotherapy model, and specific psychotherapy techniques. It is recommended that the applied portion include review of residents' conceptualization of cases, review of and feedback on therapy audio/video recordings, experiential exercises (e.g., role-plays) and collaborative treatment planning.

Specific Challenges and Strategies

- **My supervisee is mixing different psychotherapy approaches and is confused about how to focus on one approach.** It is confusing for trainees to learn two therapies simultaneously and unreasonable to expect competency without immersion in one model at a time. If possible, the supervisor should encourage the residency program to limit this practice.
- **The duration of my supervisee's rotation is only 4 months, and the case that was assigned is quite complex clinically.** Although it is difficult to coordinate and predict case complexity, it is advisable to request involvement in the identification of short-term training cases for residents who have brief psychotherapy rotations. This strategy better serves patients and enhances the consolidation of learning for residents.
- **My supervisee is overwhelmed trying to provide cognitive-behavioral therapy–based therapy without sufficient didactic training in the residency program.** If possible, it is ideal to request involvement in psychotherapy course development and consider teaching a foundational course to increase the likelihood that supervisees have equivalent foundational knowledge in the psychotherapies that will be taught.
- **My supervisee is not interested in learning psychotherapy.** This is not unique to psychiatry, as many psychologists choose to specialize in research, teaching, or

consulting. To best serve the patients of trainees who are not as invested in learning psychotherapy, it may be important to focus efforts on evaluating and strengthening the therapeutic relationship. We know from psychotherapy research that a strong therapeutic relationship alone will benefit the patient and will reinforce essential psychological literacy. It may be beneficial to help residents determine how psychotherapy training may align with their broader training goals. For example, one goal could be learning to strengthen and maintain the therapeutic relationship knowing that these skills will be beneficial in medication management settings. Another example is learning specific treatment interventions such as behavioral activation for depression or the basics of exposure for anxiety, which can be used in many psychiatric settings, including inpatient wards, outpatient medication management settings, or community mental health.

- **When I reviewed my supervisee's videotape, I observed a technique that contradicted what we had agreed on in our last supervision meeting.** In the author's experience, it is a common and encouraged practice for psychiatry residents to "consult" with multiple supervisors, classmates, and workshop educators about cases. Because the primary psychotherapy supervisor is directly legally liable for patient care, supervisors may request that supervisees refrain from this practice or establish clear expectations and agreements about how additional information and opinion will be incorporated in supervision and treatment planning. It may also be beneficial to discuss the supervision process and supervision relationship to determine if there is agreement between the supervisor and supervisee about the case formulation and treatment plan and invite feedback about supervision. Ultimately, however, if there is lack of consensus, the psychotherapy supervisor is responsible for treatment decisions.

- **My supervisee acts more independent than most trainees. My supervisee and I discussed the content of a letter addressed to a patient. During the next supervision meeting, I asked to review and sign the letter, but my supervisee had already mailed it to the patient.** It is common practice that psychiatry residents independently author and sign correspondence to patients; in contrast, psychology supervisees include their supervisor as a cosigner until they are independently licensed in the professional practice of psychology. This is generally resolved by openly discussing this difference between the disciplines and explicitly clarifying expectations.

Questions for the Supervisee

- What kind of training (e.g., didactic, clinical) have you had in psychotherapy?

- Are you interested in learning psychotherapy? If so, tell me about your hopes for this training experience. If not, can we think together of ways this training experience might enhance your other professional goals?

- Tell me about previous supervision experiences? What worked best to enhance your learning? Was there anything that inhibited your learning?

- Is there anything that would be helpful for you to know about my training and background before we begin our work together?

Additional Resources

Sudak DM, Trent Codd R, Ludgate JW, et al: Teaching and supervising cognitive behavior therapy. Hoboken NJ, John Wiley and Sons, 2015

Wright JH, Brown GK, Thase ME, et al: Learning Cognitive-Behavior Therapy: An Illustrated Guide. Arlington, VA, American Psychiatric Association, 2017

References

Alban A, Frankel AS: Supervision vs. consultation: what you need to know. June 3, 2007. Available at: https://www.clinicallawyer.com/2007/07/supervision-vs-consultation-what-you-need-to-know/. Accessed on August 16, 2018.

American Psychological Association: Guidelines and Principles for Accreditation of Programs in Professional Psychology. Washington, DC, American Psychological Association, 2006. Available at: http://www.apa.org/ed/accreditation/about/policies/guiding-principles.pdf. Accessed on August 16, 2018.

American Psychological Association: APA Guidelines for the Undergraduate Psychology Major. Washington, DC, American Psychological Association, 2007

American Psychological Association: APA Guidelines for the Undergraduate Psychology Major. Washington, DC, American Psychological Association, 2011. Available at: http://www.apa.org/education/undergrad/principles-undergrad.pdf. Accessed on August 16, 2018.

American Psychological Association: Guidelines for Clinical Supervision in Health Service Psychology. Washington, DC, American Psychological Association, 2014. Available at: https://www.apa.org/about/policy/guidelines-supervision.pdf. Accessed on August 16, 2018.

American Psychological Association: About APA. Frequently asked questions about the American Psychological Association. 2017. Available at: http://www.apa.org/support/about-apa.aspx. Accessed on August 16, 2018.

Association of State and Provincial Psychology Boards: Supervision guidelines for education and training leading to licensure as a health service provider. 2015. Available at: http://c.ymcdn.com/sites/www.asppb.net/resource/resmgr/Guidelines/Final_Supervision_Guidelines.pdf. Accessed on August 16, 2018.

Association of State and Provincial Psychology Boards: 2017 ASPPB competencies expected of psychologist at the point of licensure. 2017. Available at: http://c.ymcdn.com/sites/www.asppb.net/resource/resmgr/guidelines/2017_ASPPB_Competencies_Expe.pdf. Accessed on August 16, 2018.

National Science Foundation, National Center for Science and Engineering Statistics: Survey of Earned Doctorates (Custom Tabulation, January 2018). Alexandria, VA, National Science Foundation, 2016

Saccuzzo D: Liability for failure to supervise adequately mental health assistants, unlicensed practitioners and students. California Western Law Review 34(1), Article 10, 1997. Available at: http://scholarlycommons.law.cwsl.edu/cwlr/vol34/iss1/10. Accessed on August 16, 2018.

Stoloff M, McCarthy M, Keller L, et al: The undergraduate psychology major: An examination of structure and sequence. Teach Psychol 37:4–15, 2010

Chapter 35 Cultural Issues Within the Supervisory Relationship

Belinda S. Bandstra, M.D., M.A.

Ripal Shah, M.D., M.P.H.

Megan Tan, M.D., M.S.

The value of diversity and creating a physician workforce that more closely resembles the people and populations served is finding increasing traction in academic medical centers and training contexts (Roberts et al. 2014). Efforts to increase the number of underrepresented minorities and first-generation professionals in training contexts, coupled with individuals moving to different regions for specialty training and the presence of international supervisees, have led to an increasing number of circumstances in which supervisor and supervisee are not from the same cultural background.[1] Whether supervisors and supervisees feel that cultural differences between them are important

---

[1]For the purposes of this chapter, we will utilize the definition of culture put forth by the Cultural Formulation section of DSM-5 (American Psychiatric Association 2013): "*Culture* refers to systems of knowledge, concepts, rules, and practices that are learned and transmitted across generations. Cultures include language, religion and spirituality, family structures, life-cycle stages, ceremonial rituals, and customs, as well as moral and legal systems. Cultures are open, dynamic systems that undergo continuous change over time; in the contemporary world, most individuals and groups are exposed to multiple cultures, which they use to fashion their own identities and make sense of experience" (p. 749).

to address is, itself, a question that may be affected by cultural factors. One study suggested that among supervisors and supervisees who identified as black/African American, 53% found conversations about race to be very beneficial, compared with only 25% of those who identified as white/Caucasian (White-Davis et al. 2016). Nonetheless, there are a number of additional reasons, which extend across cultures, for why the discussion of culture is important in the supervisory relationship.

Given the power difference between the supervisor and the supervisee, it is incumbent on the supervisor to open the dialogue about culture, just as it is the supervisor's position to clarify expectations and roles, anticipate potential barriers, and otherwise guide the supervisee through the process of entering supervision. Garrett et al. (2001) note that even supervisors who are members of a minority group act symbolically in a majority position in the supervisory relationship; in contrast, even a supervisee who is a member of a majority group is in a minority position by status, and thus it is important for the supervisor to set the intentionality of the dyad in addressing these issues. Considering issues of culture is an important supervisory practice whether or not a supervisee is perceived to be from a different culture.

Key Points

- Supervisors must recognize that how they view the process, relationship, and content of supervision may be different from how their supervisees view them, and that these views may be heavily mediated by the supervisors' and supervisees' respective cultures.

- Given the power differential between supervisor and supervisee, it is the supervisor's responsibility to make space for the conversation about culture.

- It is important to be aware of issues of culture in all supervisory relationships, not only when a supervisee is "obviously" from a different culture.

- Because talking about culture carries a high degree of affective potency, humility and the development of mutual trust are imperative for these conversations.

Culture Impacts Our Assumptions About the Process of Supervision

Adult learning theory principles such as self-directed learning, drawing on one's own life experiences, learning in the context of assuming new roles, and learning in a problem-centered, immediately applicable way (Knowles 1984) are accepted as the ideal in many supervisory settings. However, educators and educational theorists have criticized adult learning theory as arising from a particular cultural context and debated its merits across cultures (Merriam 2001; Pratt 1991). Supervisees from certain cultural contexts may be more accustomed to different modalities of learning, and brokering shared goals and approaches is essential to the effective transmission of knowledge and skills. How supervisees express their need for help, and how quickly they feel they can express this need, may be culturally informed. What they know about where to turn for resources, information, and support may vary as well.

Culture Impacts Our Assumptions About the Supervisory Relationship

Supervisors should be aware of certain value dimensions (Hofstede 1997) that may impact the relationship that they have with supervisees across different cultures.

Power Distance

Power distance is the extent to which people accept an unequal distribution of power and status. For example, a supervisor coming from a low power-distance culture may view a supervisee as "an equal" and expect supervisees to be comfortable questioning, disagreeing, or otherwise making their supervisory needs known. However, a supervisee coming from a high power-distance culture may need more explicit permission to participate openly in the conversation. Conversely, a supervisee coming from a low power-distance culture may enter a supervisory relationship expecting to make many of his own decisions, while a supervisor from a higher power-distance culture may expect the supervisee to defer more to expertise.

The meaning of feedback is also impacted by power distance. A supervisor from a low power-distance culture may be intending to provide feedback in a supportive, formative way, but this may be interpreted by a supervisee from a high-power distance culture as a more conclusive or impactful judgment than was intended. Conversely, a supervisor from a high power-distance culture may be surprised to find that feedback intended to effect change was received by a supervisee from a low power-distance culture as "merely a suggestion."

Uncertainty Avoidance

Uncertainty avoidance is the extent of discomfort with ambiguous situations. A supervisor coming from a low uncertainty-avoidance culture may feel quite comfortable leaving expectations or guidelines vague, whereas a supervisee coming from a high uncertainty-avoidance culture may become frustrated to not have more formalized policies and procedures. Conversely, a supervisor from a high uncertainty-avoidance culture may present clear expectations, which a supervisee from a low uncertainty avoidance culture may interpret as disapproval or lack of trust.

Culture Impacts Our Assumptions About the Content of Supervision

Beyond views of the supervisory process and relationship, supervisors' and supervisees' respective cultures may also broadly influence perceptions of the world and interpretations of experiences, and therefore their selection of goals of treatment and ways of working toward goals (Garrett et al. 2001). (See Chapter 41, "Supervising Cross-Cultural Topics in a Clinical Setting" for a fuller discussion of supervising clinical issues pertaining to culture.)

Specific Challenges and Strategies

- **My supervisee identifies as belonging to a minority culture, but I identify as belonging to a majority culture.** Some supervisors from majority cultures may feel uncomfortable bringing up issues of culture, or suspect that they lack the information needed to engage in a productive conversation. It may be helpful for majority-culture supervisors to recognize that everyone has a culture, not just minorities, and to reflect on their own cultural contexts. The questions below may be a helpful starting point. Additional complexities may arise in supervision when the supervisee and patient come from similar cultural backgrounds. Making space for the supervisee to express reflections on the cultural components of the case, and to give the supervisor feedback on cultural understanding, is highly important and, given the affective potency of culture, requires a high degree of mutual trust.

- **My supervisee identifies as belonging to a majority culture, but I identify as belonging to a minority culture.** Although it is not always the case that minority-culture supervisors are more adept at or interested in talking about culture, supervisors who do wish to address these issues may benefit from being aware of the personal meaning of addressing culture and their motivations in teaching. Supervisors may also face the challenge of convincing their supervisees of the importance of cultural issues. Employing the DSM-5 Cultural Formulation, sharing narratives with clinical and nonclinical content, and supporting supervisees in reflecting on their own cultural contexts are strategies for bringing the conversation to the table. Specific challenges for this dyad may arise when the supervisor and the patient come from similar cultural backgrounds, and the supervisee comes from a different background. Again, a high degree of mutual trust is valuable for giving and receiving feedback on cultural dynamics that may arise.

Questions for the Supervisor and the Supervisee

- How might cultural factors be impacting the way that you and I work together in supervision?

- What are my cultural assumptions about the way we learn in supervision? What are yours?

- What are my cultural assumptions about what our supervisory relationship should be like? What are yours?

- To what extent do I emphasize cultural issues in the provider-patient relationship, and to what extent do you?

Additional Resources

American Psychiatric Association: Cultural formulation, in Diagnostic and Statistical Manual of Mental Disorders, 5th Edition. Arlington, VA, American Psychiatric Association, 2013, pp 749–759

Institute of Medicine Committee on Institutional and Policy-Level Strategies for Increasing the Diversity of the U.S. Healthcare Workforce: In the Nation's Compelling Interest: Ensuring Diversity in the Health-Care Workforce. Edited by Smedley BD, Butler AS, Bristow LR. Washington, DC, U.S. National Academies Press, 2004

Lewis-Fernandez R, Aggarwal N, Hinton L, et al: DSM-5® Handbook on the Cultural Formulation Interview. Washington, DC, American Psychiatric Association Publishing, 2016

Shweder RA: Thinking Through Cultures: Expeditions in Cultural Psychology. Cambridge, MA, Harvard University Press, 1991

References

American Psychiatric Association: Cultural formulation, in Diagnostic and Statistical Manual of Mental Disorders, 5th Edition. Arlington, VA, American Psychiatric Association, 2013, pp 749–759

Garrett MT, Borders LD, Crutchfield LB, et al: Multicultural SuperVISION: a paradigm of cultural responsiveness for supervisors. J Multicult Couns Devel 29:147–158, 2001

Hofstede GH: Cultures and Organizations: Software of the Mind, 2nd Edition. New York, McGraw-Hill, 1997

Knowles MS: Andragogy in Action: Applying Modern Principles of Adult Learning. San Francisco, CA, Jossey-Bass, 1984

Merriam SB: Andragogy and self-directed learning: pillars of adult learning theory, in The New Update on Adult Learning Theory: New Directions for Adult and Continuing Education. Edited by Merriam SB. San Francisco, CA, Jossey-Bass, 2001, pp 3–13

Pratt DD: Conceptions of self within China and the United States: contrasting foundations for adult development. Int J Intercult Relat 15(3):285–310, 1991

Roberts LW, Maldonado Y, Coverdale JH, et al: The critical need to diversify the clinical and academic workforce. Acad Psychiatry 38(4):394–397, 2014 24989990

White-Davis T, Stein E, Karasz A: The elephant in the room: Dialogues about race within cross-cultural supervisory relationships. Int J Psychiatry Med 51(4):347–356, 2016 27497455

Chapter 36   Ruptures in the Supervisory Alliance

C. Edward Watkins Jr., Ph.D.

Ruptures, potentially affecting the entirety of the supervisory relationship, have most often been identified as being particularly problematic with regard to the supervisory working alliance. The working alliance has long been recognized as consisting of three fundamental components: 1) the supervisor-supervisee bond, 2) the shared goals that guide the supervision process, and 3) the shared tasks by which those goals are pursued. The alliance—that crucial relational mediator that has the potential to make or break the supervision experience—has been referred to as the "heart and soul of supervision" (Watkins 2014). Ruptures pose a particular threat to the supervisory alliance because they have the power to interrupt, disrupt, or even derail the viability of the alliance altogether (Watkins et al. 2015, 2016). The unrepaired rupture may well be a primary, if not the preeminent, reason that supervision relationships fail.

Although both supervisor and supervisee can introduce ruptures into the supervisory situation, this chapter will focus on supervisor ruptures. Any supervision relationship is, by definition, hierarchical, evaluative, and power disproportionate in nature: The supervisor is in a power position, tasked with evaluating the performance of the supervisee (e.g., via assigning a grade or providing a performance evaluation). Because of that power dynamic, supervisees may understandably be hesitant to point out supervisor ruptures or relational issues that do occur. Because ruptures can be so relationally destructive, it behooves supervisors to be ever mindful that 1) there is real possibility of alliance ruptures and alliance rupture impact, 2) they may indeed (often unwittingly) create such ruptures themselves, and 3) their best course of action then is to take reparative measures. Whatever the supervisory perspective, repairing ruptures is of primary concern (cf. Watkins 2016; Watkins and Scaturo 2013).

Key Points

- Ruptures can be hazardous to the health of the supervisor-supervisee relationship; they possess fester capacity.

- Supervisees may respond to supervisor rupture by means of either confrontation or withdrawal.

- Supervisee withdrawal—because of the power differential in the supervision relationship—may be the behavioral response most apt to occur.

- Supervisors respond differentially to rupture events, dependent upon whether supervisee confrontation or withdrawal is made manifest.

- The supervisor ideally initiates or is open to a supervisee-initiated rupture discussion and actively processes any such rupture events as fully as possible with the supervisee.

- Ruptures are ideally repaired with dispatch so that the supervisory relationship can be restored to good working order.

- Supervisor humility is a crucial variable in making rupture repair increasingly likely.

Supervision Alliance Ruptures and Repair

Ruptures

Current understanding about supervision ruptures largely involves reasoned extrapolations from the therapeutic alliance rupture literature to supervision. A *supervision alliance rupture* refers to some sort of relational strain or conflict between supervisor and supervisee that has a negative impact on the nature of their working interaction. Ruptures can fester (i.e., if left unaddressed, they only worsen in impact). They corrode and erode the supervisory alliance. Research about conflict and negative experiences in supervision suggests that rupturing interactions may be far more prevalent than we would like to think, with, for example, about 100% of supervisees having experienced inadequate supervision and 50% having experienced harmful supervision (Ellis et al. 2014).

Ruptures can potentially result from a wide range of interpersonal possibilities: supervisor mistakes or errors, neglect, excessive task orientation, empathic failures, or multicultural insensitivities. Four major sources of rupture are 1) mismatched expectations and miscommunications, 2) developmentally normative conflicts, 3) problems of interpersonal dynamics, and 4) cultural differences (Bernard and Goodyear 2019). Role conflict due to mismatched supervisor-supervisee expectations may well be the most common reason for rupture (Friedlander 2015). Some specific examples, seemingly ready-made to induce rupture, include supervisors making insensitive, disrespectful remarks with regard to difference and diversity variables; supervisors regularly being late for or cancelling supervision sessions; or supervisors (when not on call or in emergency situations) routinely taking personal phone calls or texting during supervision sessions. Some quite different examples, in which good-intentioned supervisor behaviors may actually result in ruptures, include when supervisors, in excitedly sharing possible intervention after intervention, end up overwhelming instead of helping their supervisees; or when supervisors, in an effort to leave ample space for and provoke independent thought and judgment in supervision, leave their supervisees feeling unanchored and poorly contained.

Supervisees may be most likely to react to supervisor ruptures in one of two ways: confrontation or withdrawal. Confrontation ruptures involve the supervisee directly expressing dissatisfaction to the supervisor about some aspect of supervision. For example, "Our supervision time together is very important to me. You are very helpful. But when you (supervisor) spend time on your phone, taking personal calls and texts, it bothers me because I believe that I am missing out on your helpful feedback." Because confrontations are, by definition, direct, they accordingly allow supervisors the opportunity to directly engage supervisees about the rupture event and ideally work toward repair and resolution. But as indicated earlier, the power differential in supervision can make confronting supervisors a much more difficult proposition for supervisees. Withdrawal ruptures involve the supervisee disengaging or pulling back from supervision in some way. For example, the supervisee may ask fewer questions of the supervisor, be less responsive, or be less involved overall. Withdrawal ruptures can be more difficult to identify, not being immediately evident, and can take a period of time to detect.

Repair

A *rupture repair* refers to the effort made to acknowledge, address, and resolve the conflict that has given rise to the supervision rupture. By means of such effort, the supervisor hopes to restore the supervisory alliance to good working order. Two fundamental action steps seem preeminently pivotal in making rupture repair more likely: The supervisor 1) willingly initiates a rupture discussion with the supervisee or is open to a supervisee-initiated rupture discussion; and 2) actively processes any rupture events as fully as possible with the supervisee (Watkins et al. 2015, 2016). The repaired rupture may indeed be a critical, if not the critical, reason that troubled supervision relationships are often successfully rescued from failure.

Specific Challenges and Strategies

- **I'm not sure that a supervision rupture has even happened.** With withdrawal ruptures typically not being immediately evident, the challenge for supervisors understandably becomes being able to see and draw possible meaning from that which is interactionally more invisible than visible. Supervisor withdrawal rupture response includes at least six components: 1) being willing to engage in self-reflection and openness to examining one's own supervisory work; 2) maintaining a sensitivity to interactional changes, possible signs of conflict, in supervision (e.g., recognizing supervisee diminished responsiveness); 3) considering the possibility of rupture, identifying a possible rupture event, and internally reflecting on how best to proceed; 4) bringing up the possibility of rupture, or something perhaps being wrong, in supervision for joint consideration; 5) jointly processing and discussing the rupture event or events (where present) with the supervisee; and 6) working to achieve a rupture resolution that is satisfactory to the supervisee and restores the good standing of the supervision alliance. The acronym, O/D—WID—R and R—Observe/Detect—Wonder, Inquire, Discuss—Repair and Resolve, might be useful to hold in mind when thinking about withdrawal rupture detection and repair. With Observe/Detect, supervisors ask "What do I see happening (or not happening) in our relationship?" With Wonder, Inquire, Discuss, supervisors, respectively, ask themselves what might have been the cause of any observed/detected changes; ask the supervisee if that which was possibly detected might be so; and invite supervisees to discuss those detected changes—in hopes of making Repair and Resolve increasingly likely. In essence, the supervisor forever strives to maintain sensitivity to the very possibility of withdrawal behavior, monitor the supervision relationship closely, and check in periodically with the supervisee to gauge her/his perspective about the supervision process.

- **It's so hard not to feel defensive when confronted by a supervisee.** Perhaps the greatest challenge in effectively responding to a confrontation rupture is maintaining a supervisory stance of openness and nondefensiveness. Supervisor confrontation rupture response includes at least six components: 1) being willing to engage in self-reflection and openness to examining one's own supervisory work; 2) maintaining a sensitivity to interactional changes, signs of conflict, identified by the supervisee (e.g., listening to supervisee's expression of dissatisfaction); 3) recognizing the reality of rupture (as expressed by the supervisee), understanding the rupture event or events involved, and internally reflecting upon how best to proceed; 4) openly expressing recognition of and willingness/desire to jointly consider the rupture event; 5) jointly processing and discussing the rupture event or events with the supervisee; and 6) working to achieve a rupture resolution that is satisfactory to the supervisee and restores the good standing of the supervision alliance. The acronym L–ID–R and R, for Listen—Inquire, Discuss—Repair and Resolve, might be useful to hold in mind when thinking about confrontation rupture detection and repair. With Listen, supervisors strive to hear clearly and completely the concerns of the supervisee. With Inquire, Discuss, supervisors 1) ask questions to gain further clarity and fuller understanding and 2) invite supervisees to engage in discussion about those very concerns, in hopes of making Repair and Resolve increasingly likely. In essence, the supervisor forever strives to hold fast to a supervisory attitude in which 1) the supervisor is a learner, not a finished product, 2) supervision is accordingly viewed as a lifelong learning endeavor, 3) supervisees are considered valuable sources of feedback about the supervision experience, and 4) supervisee feedback, viewed as highly facilitative of the supervisor's lifelong learning, is thereby desired (Watkins et al. 2018).

- **It's hard to stay humble.** Whether dealing with confrontation or withdrawal ruptures, the supervisor can understandably feel challenged and unsure about what exactly to do, and may protectively respond defensively. It can indeed be very difficult to stay humble. But maintaining proper perspective, a stance of humility in the face of adversity, looms large in making supervision work. And humility, a foundational virtue in clinical supervision, is arguably the specific prerequisite for making any rupture repair efforts possible (Watkins et al. 2018). Supervisor humility involves four basic features: openness, other orientation, accurate self-assessment, and recognizing one's own imperfections. In responding to either supervisee confrontational or withdrawal behavior, the supervisor ideally responds from a humble place that privileges and prioritizes the supervision relationship and strives to safeguard its integrity (Hook et al. 2016; Watkins and Hook 2016; Watkins et al. 2018). Research suggests that wise supervisors are foremost humble, are open to and desire supervisee feedback, and make use of such feedback to better themselves and the supervisory relationship (Nelson et al. 2008). Apology, grounded in humility, is one intervention that can have reparative, relationship-restoring effects (Watkins et al. 2015). Consisting of up to 10 elements (e.g., naming the offense, taking responsibility), apology can be either simple (involving fewer elements) or complete (involving more such elements) (see Watkins et al. 2015). Any supervisor-offered apology ideally matches the severity of the involved offense.

- **My supervisee will not respond to my rupture repair efforts.** Rupture repair efforts are at their best when preeminently invitational, where supervisees feel invited to freely and safely engage—with immunity and impunity—in a discussion about the rupturing event and its potential repair. But in some cases, rupture repair efforts may not work. The critical questions then become: Why is the supervisee not in any way responsive to supervisor attempts to repair the relationship? What can be done in such situations? For example, it may be that a rupturing event—when occurring within the context of a marked supervisor-supervisee personality mismatch—can further exacerbate relational tensions and make any sort of repair increasingly improbable. Or it may be that harmful supervisor actions (e.g., sexual advances made toward supervisee, verbal abuse; Ellis 2017; Ellis et al. 2014) have rendered repair beyond the pale of possibility. In such situations, to best ensure protection of and provide safeguard for both the patient and supervisee, transferring the supervisee to another supervisor is often the most viable, even necessary, course of action.

Questions for the Supervisor

- When the supervisee perceives me to have engaged in relationship-rupturing behavior and is accordingly confrontive, how do I wish to respond?

- How can I prepare or ready myself to appropriately respond to my supervisee's confrontation?

- When I perceive my supervisee to be withdrawing in the supervisory relationship, perhaps because of a rupture event, how do I, as the supervisor, wish to respond?

- How can I prepare or ready myself to appropriately respond when possible rupture-induced supervisee withdrawal occurs?

- When my supervisee engages in rupture-inducing behavior, what responsibility do I have in initiating and instigating reparative measures?

Additional Resources

Kirchhoff J, Wagner U, Strack M: Apologies: Words of magic? The role of verbal components, anger reduction, and offence severity. Peace and Conflict Journal of Peace Psychology 18(2):109–130, 2012

Watkins CE Jr, Reyna SH, Ramos MJ, et al: The ruptured supervisory alliance and its repair: on supervisor apology as a reparative intervention. The Clinical Supervisor 34(1):98–104, 2015

Watkins CE Jr, Hook JN, Ramaeker J, et al: Repairing the ruptured supervisory alliance: humility as a foundational virtue in clinical supervision. The Clinical Supervisor 35(1):22–41, 2016

References

Bernard JM, Goodyear RK: Fundamentals of Clinical Supervision, 6th Edition. Upper Saddle River, NJ, Pearson, 2019

Ellis MV: Narratives of harmful supervision: synthesis and recommendations. The Clinical Supervisor 36(1):20–87, 2017

Ellis MV, Berger L, Hanus AE, et al: Inadequate and harmful clinical supervision: testing a revised framework and assessing occurrence. The Counseling Psychologist 42:434–472, 2014

Friedlander ML: Use of relational strategies to repair alliance ruptures: How responsive supervisors train responsive psychotherapists. Psychotherapy (Chic) 52(2):174–179, 2015 25111380

Hook JN, Watkins CE Jr, Davis DE, et al: Cultural humility in psychotherapy supervision. Am J Psychother 70(2):149–166, 2016 27329404

Nelson ML, Barnes KL, Evans AL, et al: Working with conflict in clinical supervision: wise supervisors' perspectives. Journal of Counseling Psychology 55(2):172–184, 2008

Watkins CE Jr: The supervisory alliance: a half century of theory, practice, and research in critical perspective. Am J Psychother 68(1):19–55, 2014 24818456

Watkins CE Jr: A unifying vision of psychotherapy supervision: part II—pan-theoretical markers and modules for supervision practice and supervisor education. Journal of Unified Psychotherapy and Clinical Science 4(1):36–47, 2016

Watkins CE Jr, Hook JN: On a culturally humble psychoanalytic supervision perspective: creating the cultural third. Psychoanal Psychol 33:487–517, 2016

Watkins CE Jr, Scaturo DJ: Toward an integrative, learning-based model of psychotherapy supervision: supervisory alliance, educational interventions, and supervisee learning/relearning. J Psychother Integration 23:75–95, 2013

Watkins CE Jr, Reyna SH, Ramos MJ, et al: The ruptured supervisory alliance and its repair: on supervisor apology as a reparative intervention. The Clinical Supervisor 34(1):98–104, 2015

Watkins CE Jr, Hook JN, Ramaeker J, et al: Repairing the ruptured supervisory alliance: humility as a foundational virtue in clinical supervision. The Clinical Supervisor 35(1):22–41, 2016

Watkins CE Jr, Hook JN, Mosher D, et al: Humility in clinical supervision: fundamental, foundational, and transformational. The Clinical Supervisor August 2, 2018 [Epub ahead of print]

Chapter 37 The Supervision of Countertransference

Carlos C. Greaves, M.D.

The concepts of transference and countertransference denote a psychodynamic approach to psychotherapy in their more formal connotations. Yet, regardless of the therapeutic approach applied by the practitioner, aspects of these two phenomena are always present when two human beings gather to study, treat, or try to understand psychological realities and their disturbances.

Transference refers to the conscious and unconscious projections, displacements, and ascriptions with which, on the basis of prior conditionings, the patient distorts the reality of the therapist. *Countertransference* refers to the conscious and unconscious responses, reactions, assumptions, and intentions toward patients with which therapists either accurately understand or distort them, or avoid or overemphasize their psychological expressions. Another aspect of countertransference is the coloring and emphasis given to any particular clinical interpretation, resulting from prior life experiences, conditionings, world views, values, and philosophy of life, that therapists hold for themselves.

A science of the subjective is oxymoronic: to attempt to objectify subjectivity will render it no longer such, yet understanding, clarification, and implications are very much worthwhile, even necessary, for effective dynamic psychotherapy (Hayes and Gelso 2001).

Given that some degree of entanglement between the patient and therapist's inner worlds takes place, the development of an intersubjective realm is unavoidable. Awareness and understanding of this intersubjective realm are critical in order to avoid undue influence, paternalism, dependency or interdependency, the fostering of erotic energies, or the imposition of values and ethical views. Transference and countertransference are the conduits through which intersubjectivity manifests. The therapist-supervisee is in a very powerful and influential position as an authority in psychological matters, to which the patient readily submits, tending to be receptive to all sorts of positions, especially if these positions are emphatically presented as the proper approach to living. If this is tied with a therapist-supervisee in need for power or under the effects of hubris, a truly dangerous situation for both could unfold. Characterological idiosyncrasies need to be attended to and thoroughly explored (Betan et al. 2005).

In the individual supervision of countertransference, a somewhat parallel process to that between patient and therapist occurs, inasmuch as the supervisee and the supervisor are developing an intersubjective realm as the supervision progresses. Thus, it behooves them both to be aware of this phenomena to the point they can objectify and understand it, and, hence, be a model of what is actually happening between the supervisee and the patient. For this to be successful, aspects of the inner worlds of both, especially that of the supervisee, need to be available.

Key Points

- The construct and formulation of any case are directly dependent on the unique psyche of the examiner/therapist.

- The supervisor can use various strategies to help the supervisee develop self-awareness and clarify their subjectivity.

- Several ethical issues that arise in the context of the relationship between therapist-patient and supervisor-supervisee are relevant to any relationship defined by a power gradient between two people.

Strategies to Explore Countertransference

The supervisor needs to be aware that this supervision experience requires a higher level of commitment than most others, one characterized by greater emotional investment, focus on the unique needs of the supervisee, tact and kindness given the supervisee's vulnerability, and the willingness to be open with personal psychological material. The modeling involved by the supervisor may have a deeper impact on the supervisee than otherwise. The supervisor should explain his or her conceptual frame regarding countertransference in order to facilitate the supervisee's understanding of what is to take place in supervision, with an emphasis on openness and trust. The supervisee must be assured that the material revealed in the sessions will remain confidential and not be part of any evaluative process. Likewise, whatever private aspect of the supervisor's world is revealed, the supervisee would agree, should be kept confidential.

The following strategies enhance the supervision of countertransference:

Share Life History

The supervisory experience would be best accomplished when both supervisee and supervisor share some of their life history from the outset; a bond of trust and reciprocity will thus be established, the first step toward an intersubjective connection between the two.

Use Questions to Explore the Subjective Impact of a Patient on the Supervisee

As cases are presented, a series of questions can be useful to emphasize the inward focus of the supervision. Examples include: "What was your first impression of this person?" "What is your understanding of that impression?" "Does it relate to previous encounters you've had? In what way?" "How has that impression shifted, now that you better know your patient; what accounts for the shift?" "Do you look forward or not to seeing this individual and why?" "Are you indifferent?" "Do you dread it?" "Does the patient remind you of any particular person in your past or current life?" and/or "What are your feelings for such a person, either now on in the past?" (Linn-Walton and Pardasani 2014).

The key to supervision of countertransference is an ongoing focus on the subjective impact the patient is generating on the supervisee, the plausible reasons for this, and the ways in which these reasons are tied to past experiences, personal encounters, interpersonal difficulties, compatible characters/ personalities, preferences, family myths, values, religious beliefs, political affiliations, and world views.

Link Subjectivity to Case Conceptualization

Particularly helpful clarifications involve the supervisor helping the supervisee see the connection between not only his or her own subjectivity (as projected onto the patient) and interpretation of the patient's emotions and behavior, but also the supervisee's conceptualization of the case, formulation, and approach to the therapy: What is it that is emphasized? What is avoided? Which technique(s) is used and why? What is deemed to be relevant and what is not, for what reasons?

Help Clarify Intent Toward Patient

Helping the supervisee connect his or her own subjectivity to interpretations of the patient's emotions and behaviors, case conceptualization, formulation, and approach to therapy is particularly important. Questions might include: "Do you wish this patient well? Why?" "Have you developed a prognostic vision for your patient?" "What do you see as their potentials?" "What do you see as realistic?" "Are you underestimating their possibilities?" "Do you see any link between what you aspire for your patient and your own aspirations?" "Are you avoiding in your patient what you avoid in your own life?" "Are your patient's substitute objects for intimacy in your life?" and/or "Are there ways in which you encourage your patient to fulfill unfulfilled aspects of your own life?"

Consider Other Approaches to Enhance Supervisees' Self-Awareness

In addition to personal psychotherapy, the supervisee might also be encouraged to engage in personal journaling, individual supervision, group supervision, consultation with colleagues, and meditation and mindfulness exercises. Self-awareness can also be enhanced by contact with art, literature (both fiction and nonfiction), transcultural travel, experiences with nature and with appropriate readings in psychology, sociology, philosophy, and anthropology.

The supervisor might also encourage the supervisee to candidly ask others (colleagues, teachers, friends, acquaintances) for feedback. This can gradually enlarge the body of self- knowledge and understanding required for effective, nonbiased, freedom-enhancing psychotherapy.

Attend to Supervisory Boundaries

The supervision of countertransference borders on psychotherapy. It is up to the supervisor to be aware of this and to attempt to keep the boundaries between the two clearly defined. An important difference exists. In the psychotherapy of patients, the goal for the insights into the nature of the patient's subjectivity, behaviors, and interpersonal dynamics is the growth and better adjustment of the patient. However, in supervision, the goal for insights is professional development, directed at the interface between supervisee and the patient. The supervisee's personal growth is a welcome side effect, not the direct aim of the supervision. Should a particularly difficult emotional insight reflecting intrapsychic struggles in the supervisee occur, the supervisor might recommend individual psychotherapy—a recommendation, ideally universal to all supervisees in the field of psychotherapy.

Group Supervision Strategies

Another approach to developing the supervisee's self-awareness through understanding his or her countertransference is the use of group supervision. There are certain advantages to training future psychotherapists in a group context, not necessarily as a substitute for individual supervision, but as a complementary approach. As supervisees react intellectually and emotionally to a given case history in their own idiosyncratic fashion, they are encouraged to share these reactions in a group setting. Through this modality, they are able to realize, compare, and analyze, in a direct experiential way, how the realities of such a case are distorted by their individual consciousness. The consequence of such awareness is a degree of humbleness vis à vis their own theories and approach to their patients, the willingness to revise them, to keep them malleable and update them regularly, and to enter into consultation with colleagues and with the professional literature.

Participants in group supervision of countertransference would ideally be in their last year of training, by which time they have had ongoing contact with one another, participated in process groups, had more clinical experience, done group presentations, and been casually socializing with one another for some time. They are also presumably more mature and have a greater understanding of the value of subjective awareness. Therefore, this type of group experience can be successful because the group participants have already developed a significant amount of trust with one another and may be willing to share some intimate aspects of themselves. Cohesiveness in the group may increase significantly during the development of the experience.

The contents of group sessions should remain confidential, and the supervisor-facilitator would not be involved in any evaluative role within the training program and, ideally, would have had a modicum degree of familiarity with the group participants beforehand. Thus, an adjunct voluntary faculty member who has taught a course or two and/or has led some group experiences for the class would more likely be trusted for this group supervision experience than would an academic faculty member. The supervisor-facilitator needs to be an experienced clinician.

During a group supervision session, a supervisee presents a case, shows a video interview, or performs a face-to-face live interview while others observe. Ideal cases for group presentation would be those that are difficult, disturbing, or complex. The facilitator would then lead a discussion of the various responses in the group and of the subjective reasons for such. The supervisor might model by offering his or her own reactions and discuss the intrapsychic reasons for those reactions. The supervisor can then encourage the participants to do so as well. See the appendix to this chapter for an example of a group countertransference supervision approach.

Specific Challenges and Strategies

- **My supervisee is not psychologically minded and is unwilling to engage in an in-depth exploration of interpersonal issues/dynamics.** This is a serious problem that puts into question the appropriateness of this individual's work in the field of psychotherapy, regardless of whether his or her focus is psychodynamic or in the more instrumental techniques. Offer a solid rationale for the need to understand interpersonal dynamics regardless of the nature of any two human's interaction, particularly in the healing professions. If resistance continues, recommend a change of profession.
- **My supervisee has an emotional impasse toward a specific patient.** Through gentle inquiry, help the supervisee explore the nature of the difficulty. Through a deeper understanding, strategies can collaboratively be devised to resolve the issue. If several approaches fail in a seemingly intractable problem, encourage the supervisee to disqualify himself or herself from continuing therapy with this person, followed by a strong suggestion, if appropriate, to engage in individual psychotherapy.
- **My supervisee misses supervision sessions without notice, is apathetic or rigid, is unwilling to accept suggestions or criticisms, is defensive, or is rude or disrespectful.** Gently focus on these issues within the supervision and help the supervisee work through them. If these issues are left unaddressed, the supervision will become a superficial, useless exercise, at best. At worst, the therapy represents a danger for those patients under this individual's care. You would be wise to see these behaviors and resistances from a parallel-process perspective and assume they might be happening in the supervisee's office as well.
- **There is an impasse in the supervisory relationship itself.** You, as the supervisor in the power position, need to be careful and gentle in pointing out your perspective on the difficulty, while receptively encouraging the supervisee to do so as well, mindful that these represent unique opportunities to model conflict resolution, openness, kindness, acceptance, and freedom from judgments. On the other hand, were the situation to persist after adequate discussion and analysis, you ought to recommend a different supervisor for the supervisee, making sure of reassuring him or her of the confidentiality of your interactions.
- **Romantic feelings arise in the relationship.** Whether one sided or reciprocal, these situations are, by far, problematic if not downright destructive, unless one or both parties are willing to develop proper boundaries, discipline, sublimating de-

fenses, postponement, or acts of renunciation for the impending affair. Professionalism must be the guiding principle. If such an affair develops, the system is likely to become aware of it, with serious consequences for both faculty and supervisees. Reputations will be at stake, trust eroded, the department criticized, and positions threatened. The maxim that "sex is never part of therapy" would be put into question, given the close parallelisms between the supervisory relationship and the doctor-patient one. The impact on the character of the supervisee, especially, could have longlasting consequences. It is best to dissolve the supervisory relationship or wait 2 years post training before judging that the affair is now unrelated to the power dynamic between the two.

Questions for the Supervisor

■ Do I like this supervisee? Why do I feel this way about him or her?

■ Does he or she remind me of someone I trained with? A friend? A family member?

■ Am I competitive with, threatened by, controlling of, attracted to, repelled by, or uninterested in this supervisee?

■ Do I want him or her to be, think, and/or do therapy like I do?

■ How can I foster the supervisee's unique strengths, temperament, and knowledge into the development of an effective compassionate and ethical therapist?

■ What psychiatric literature or experiences can I suggest that would further my supervisee's growth and openness to the great variety of human conditions that he or she will encounter professionally?

Additional Resources

Alexandris A, Vaslamatis G: Countertransference: Theory, Technique, Teaching. New York, Routledge, 2018
Gelso CJ, Hayes JA: Countertransference and the Therapist's Inner Experience: Perils and Possibilities. Mahwah, NJ, Lawrence Erlbaum, 2007

References

Betan E, Heim AK, Zittel Conklin C, et al: Countertransference phenomena and personality pathology in clinical practice: an empirical investigation. Am J Psychiatry 162(5):890–898, 2005 15863790
Hayes JA, Gelso CJ: Clinical implications of research on countertransference: science informing practice. J Clin Psychol 57(8):1041–1051, 2001 11449387
Linn-Walton R, Pardasani M: Dislikable clients on countertransference: a clinician's perspective. Clin Supervisor 33(1):100–121, 2014 25798024

Appendix A Group Countertransference Supervision Model

This model represents one example of a group supervision focused on countertransference used successfully by this author for several years within a psychiatric residency training program with PGY-IV residents. It is an intense experience for participants and facilitator alike. The intensity increases proportional to the length of the seminar, as each session builds on the previous one, deepening the openness, trust, and emotional tenor of the experience.

Goals

The overall goal of this model is to intensively train the participants in subjective and intersubjective awareness. This seminar aims at the concomitant awareness of subjective phenomena in the context of an objective function. These two opposite conscious attitudes are in need of greater integration for the practice of effective psychotherapy: "to become better aware of what is happening with me as I fully focus on what my patient is saying and doing."

Preparation

The format is a weekly, 1.5-hour seminar. There should be twice the number of sessions as there are members of the seminar. The facilitator should distribute a schedule of days and assigned roles to account for vacations and expected absences. There are two parts of the exercise, and ideally every participant will experience each of the four roles in each part. Regular attendance is key, and the facilitator should ask for a weekly commitment.

A confidentiality agreement at the start is essential. A preparatory session prior to the start of the seminar is of great help to clarify the process, explain the roles, and invite the participants to muster trust, openness, and candid feedback to one another.

Roles

The facilitator identifies four members each session to assume four roles, which rotate weekly:

- **Presenter:** This person presents his or her own clinical case (current or past). This case should be difficult, disturbing, or complex.
- **Observer:** This person spends the session writing down, in a purely objective, phenomenological fashion, what he or she sees happening in the room with no opinions or reactions of a personal nature.
- **Recorder:** This person spends the session writing in a free association manner the thoughts, impressions, emotions, and so forth, that arise for the Recorder throughout the session. The Recorder becomes the following week's Reader (see below). This person must be able to attend the following week's session.
- **Reader:** This person, who was last week's Recorder, reads slowly to the group whatever he or she wrote in the previous session so that reactions in the group can be experienced more thoroughly. No editing of the writing should happen.

The role of Recorder/Reader, the carrier of the subjective function, is in contrast to the role of the Observer, the carrier of the objective function.

Part I: Preparation

Part I prepares the group for Part II, where the group will go deeper as safety and trust become well established.

For the first session, only, the Recorder will be the supervisor-facilitator, while the group talks about any particular topic of their choice. In the next session, thus, he or she will be the Reader. This offers both a model of what is expected and a way for the supervisor-facilitator to become more of a group participant. The session starts with the Reader reading last week's written account; meanwhile, today's Recorder begins recording and the Observer begins observing. After the reading is over, the participants are encouraged to ask clarifying questions and to share their reaction to the reading. The supervisor then shares thoughts about the reading, focusing on those relevant traits revealed which are pertinent to the participant's therapeutic work in general. These supervisor comments should be made in the form of suggestions (e.g., aspects to keep track of or elements to be aware of while performing therapy). Tact, kindness, and gentleness are of the essence; these comments, at best, should be used as examples that all supervisees can relate to and would want to be aware of. The supervisor should avoid judgments but rather point out the uniqueness of each mind and how best to utilize that idiosyncrasy for therapeutic goals. This part lasts an average of 20–30 minutes.

Following the reading from last session, the Presenter presents a case lasting no more than 20 minutes. The emphasis should be on the subjective experience of the Presenter-therapist about the patient and the patient's issues. A general discussion follows that includes reactions to the case, reactions to the presenter, and formulations according to each participant's take on the presentation. The facilitator then offers his or her formulation and rationale for it. The discussion section generally takes an average of 40 minutes.

Lastly, the Observer reads what has been observed without processing the data. This takes about 5–10 minutes. It is imperative that the Recorder attends the following week's session for their Reader role. Other roles do not require such strictness in sequencing.

Part II: Operation

The roles and rotation remain the same, yet the tasks are somewhat different:

*   **Presenter:** The Presenter correlates his or her subjective sense of the patient presented, as well as his or her formulation, to the Presenter's life's upbringing events, peer experiences, past conditionings and so forth.
*   **Observer:** The Observer focuses objectivity more on group process and dynamics than on the individuals behaviors, (e.g., changes in general mood, shifts in group affect, such as boredom, excitement, humor, participation, or quietness).
*   **Recorder:** The Recorder is asked to associate as many impressions experienced at the present moment to aspects of his or her developmental history and past experiences.
*   **Reader:** During the week between writing and reading, the Reader is welcome to add clarifying notes that help clarify the Reader's impressions as informed by his or her past, convictions, values, and so forth.

Chapter 38 Boundaries

Management of Supervisory Roles and Behaviors

Randolph S. Charlton, M.D.

Boundaries in all forms of mental health supervision involve experiences in which the structure of supervision (the frame), the behavior of the supervisor (professional role and responsibility) and the subjective, emotional experience of the participants (the relationship) intersect with the educational and professional needs and development of the supervisee. Boundary issues can be understood to exist in the physical, psychological, emotional, and social space within which supervision takes place (Jain and Roberts 2009). Supervision of issues surrounding boundary experiences involves unique challenges and requires particular skills on the part of a supervisor. In this chapter, I address the basic nature of boundaries in psychotherapy, comparing and contrasting the core concepts to the management of boundaries in the supervisory experience.

Key Points

- A secure supervisory alliance and frame are necessary for managing boundaries.

- Supervision involves a spectrum of role behaviors and modes of listening which influence the management of boundaries.

- Boundary issues around teaching, self-disclosure, therapy, and sexuality in the course of supervision require special attention.

- Boundary crossings are inevitable and at times deliberate interventions. Attention to the meaning and management of boundary crossings and boundary violations is a central, ongoing aspect of supervision.

- Boundary violations are, by definition, harmful to a patient or supervisee and require immediate and deliberate intervention.

The Supervisory Alliance and Frame

The alliance between supervisor and supervisee, much like that between therapist and patient, begins with consciously shared goals, general agreement on how to proceed to reach those goals, and the creation of an empathic relationship of safety, trust, and concern. The supervisee wants to become a more competent practitioner, trusts that the supervisor has the skills and desire to help, and agrees that presenting and discussing case material is an effective way to accomplish the goal.

Revealing what we actually do, say, and feel, especially around boundary issues, leaves supervisees and supervisors alike vulnerable to permutations of anxiety, guilt, embarrassment, and shame. These feelings and the attendant desire to avoid them are part of the experience of supervision. Fear of a negative evaluation and a desire to avoid narcissistic injury lead supervisees to withhold and even lie to their supervisors when a sense of trust is lacking (Heru et al. 2004). Creation and maintenance of a relationship of trust, safety, empathy, and honest communication is the starting point for successful supervision.

The frame of supervision delineates the pragmatic and relational boundaries within which the experience and meaning of supervision are played out. Reviewing the elements of the frame with a supervisee sets the ground rules for his or her work with patients and tacitly for supervision itself. The way in which a supervisor structures and frames the supervisory experience, especially around boundary issues, is a key learning tool for the supervisee. Learning the meaning and importance of boundaries involves three basic components:

- Didactic understanding of the core components of boundaries between the practitioner and the patient. This includes knowing the areas in which boundaries exist, the possible conflicts and problems within each area, and appropriate and useful ways to manage and work with boundary crossings and violations.
- Repeated experiences working with boundaries in the practitioner's professional setting.
- Experience in supervision and therapy of what it is like to be on the "other side" of boundary issues.

Instead of assuming a supervisee already knows and understands the elements related to boundaries in his or her work, a supervisor should go over how structural elements will be handled in supervision. When the supervisor becomes aware of a boundary conflict, a need for a boundary crossing, or an impending boundary violation, it should be addressed directly, with empathy and understanding. Knowing what a client "feels" when boundary issues arise is an essential aspect of all mental health work.

Teaching a supervisee how to structure his or her work with clear boundaries related to location, confidentiality, not acting on information provided by a patient for personal gain, acceptance of gifts, setting times and dates, beginning and ending sessions, clothing, and language is essential. The three remaining boundary conditions of the frame—physical touching (and, more importantly, the feelings of affection, love, and desire that promote touching), professional role and responsibility, and self-disclosure—are complex and involve particularly vulnerable and often powerful emotions on the part of supervisee and supervisor. Boundary crossings and violations exist in relation to all of these areas, and while in many situations problems begin as simple practical matters, they have the potential to become emotionally charged, conflicted, and potentially destructive (Gabbard 2009).

Boundary Issues and Supervisory Roles and Behaviors

Experiences that touch and cross interpersonal and intrapsychic boundaries occur each time a provider and patient, or supervisor and supervisee, relate and react to each other. Empathy, projection, identification, introjection, and projective identification all involve boundary crossings that are integral and potentially useful aspects of both supervision and therapy (Gutheil and Gabbard 1998). Because every supervisee is different and each supervision is unique, the specifics involved in managing the boundaries of supervision are not hard and fast rules of conduct, but general principles mediated through the context and meaning of a particular experience.

In a general sense, the function of a supervisor has been variously categorized as that of "teacher, expert, therapist, supportive colleague, self object, and container" (Frawley-O'Dea and Sarnat 2001). Supervision involves a spectrum of role behaviors and interventions that involve boundary crossings. It is particularly important to understand the relationship between role, activity, and boundary vulnerability in the areas outlined below.

Teaching Is the Core of Supervision

Critiquing a supervisee's performance is a responsibility of supervision and involves potential boundary problems related to neutrality, confidentiality, and dual relationships. When a supervisor believes that the supervisee is not managing a therapeutic situation adequately or appropriately, it becomes necessary to criticize, correct, or even admonish. This introduces the potential for narcissistic injury on the part of a supervisee. When a supervisor reports to a training or promotion committee, the frame around confidentiality is crossed, albeit with permission, and issues of power differential, fear of negative consequences, and loss of trust can occur. Finally, when a supervisor is also a supervisee's didactic instructor, problems of a dual relationship occur. Constant attention to the supervisory alliance in relation to the conflicts inherent in the teaching role of supervision is an ongoing responsibility of the conscientious supervisor.

Self-Disclosure by the Supervisor Is Commonplace

Self-disclosure by the supervisor is common, but it is a highly debated tool in supervision. Opinions vary from restricting disclosure to clinical matters directly related to casework (Meissner 2002) to visualizing the complementary flow of personal experience and clinically insightful self-disclosure between supervisee and supervisor as a unique and effective teaching tool (Weinstein et al. 2009). Examples from a supervisor's clinical experience are often pertinent and excellent teaching tools. Learning through imitation and identification is a valuable aspect of supervision. However, if the content of disclosure strays too far from relevant clinical matters, there is the potential for a break in the professional role necessary to maintain a secure supervisory alliance. There is a difference between the legitimate supervisory role of a supportive colleague and the slippery slope of using the supervisee as a friend. A supervisor's needs for narcissistic validation, positive regard, and even love can arise in supervision, but they need to be used as information that the supervisor is experiencing internal pressures to violate the primary responsibility of supervision. The appropriate response is to examine the feelings and impulses as a countertransference reaction and deal with the attendant conflicts. If it becomes difficult or impossible to manage these narcissistic needs, a supervisor should seek supervisory consultation or psychotherapy.

Therapy in Supervision Is Sometimes Unavoidable

The incorporation of therapy in supervision is a delicate and controversial topic. Clearly, supervision is not therapy, but every supervisor sees ways in which a supervisee's unconscious conflicts and defenses affect work with patients. Intellectual information, while helpful, is sometimes not powerful enough to address clinical missteps and problems with boundary issues in a supervisee's work. Walking the line between supervision and therapy can be difficult. The supervisory alliance differs from a psychotherapy therapeutic alliance in that the "contract" of supervision limits the supervisor to helping a supervisee with issues related to professional competence and identity and not treating the spectrum of the supervisee's underlying emotional conflicts. The fact that supervisees are vulnerable to anxiety over narcissistic insult and injury is well known (Heru et al. 2004). Watkins (2016) presents a cogent and useful model of supervision directed toward the maintenance of a supervisee's self-cohesion, self-esteem, and management of self-doubt in supervision. He points out that a supervisor's listening should move across a spectrum from an empathic immersion in the supervisee's experience to an objective understanding of the experience of what it is like to work with the supervisee. Included in this is an evaluation of how the supervisee is experienced by his or her patient. When limitations or problems in the supervisee's technique, relationship to the client, and/or handling of boundaries appear, utilizing an empathic understanding of the supervisee's internal experience takes into account a supervisee's narcissistic vulnerability while helping to resolve difficulties and conflicts in the supervisee's professional self.

Sexual Attraction and Fantasy Topics Are Fraught With Anxiety for Both Supervisee and Supervisor

When supervisors in an academic psychiatry program were asked if they would ask about a supervisee having sexual fantasies about a patient, they responded: 19% never, 55% occasionally, 23% usually, and 3% always. The residents responded even more negatively. Both supervisors and residents predominately selected never or occasionally when asked about discussing sexual feelings between resident and supervisor (Heru et al. 2004). Clearly, feelings of sexual desire are problematic, and it is important to realize that it is often the fear of sexual desire that makes even talking about sex unsafe. The danger of losing appropriate boundaries around physical touching and emotional engagement that goes beyond a professional relationship is at times significant enough to make supervisees and supervisors avoid the topic of sex entirely. Learning how to work with sexuality in therapy and supervision is a necessary prerequisite for a competent supervisor.

Boundary Crossings and Violations in Supervision

Thomas Gutheil and Glen Gabbard were pioneers in the exploration of boundary crossings and violations, explicating the dimensions of the therapeutic frame as it defines relevant physical and psychological boundaries and writing about the specific problem of sexual boundary violations (Gutheil and Gabbard 1993). They defined a *boundary crossing* as a therapeutic experience or action that varies from the "usual behavior" of therapy that may be helpful to the patient and most importantly does no harm. A *boundary violation* involves clear harm to the patient, ranging from poor and ineffective treatment to lasting trauma. Boundary violations can occur along the entire spectrum of therapeutic and supervisory interactions. They involve harmful transgressions of the supervisory alliance on the part of the supervisor and indicate significant problems in the supervisor's ability to manage his or her own emotions, impulses and needs.

Narcissistic vulnerability and narcissistic injury are common underlying causes of difficulty with boundary issues. It is well known that even competent, experienced therapists and supervisors in the throes of stressful or traumatic life events, illness, divorce, family, or financial problems are more likely to have difficulty with boundaries, both personally and professionally (Coen 2007). Supervisors with acute or chronic issues of self-cohesion and self-esteem are more likely to use a supervisee's admiration or affection to shore up their wounded self-image and attendant depressed and lonely feelings. Boundary violations spring from a supervisor's conscious and unconscious needs and desires, and a narcissistically wounded supervisor is more vulnerable to misinterpret experiences of transferential love (or hate) as "real" and more likely to fall into a pattern of repeated boundary crossings which can end in boundary violations.

In a survey of senior psychiatry residents in Australia, almost 5% indicated that they had been sexually involved with a supervisor/teacher (Ryan 1988). In a nationwide survey of members of the American Psychological Association's psychotherapy division, 10% acknowledged sexual contact with a faculty member when they were students, and 13% acknowledged sexual contact with a student while functioning as a teacher/supervisor (Pope et al. 1979) In a separate representative sample of members of the American Psychological Association, 19% reported unwanted sexual advances in a supervisory relationship, 51% reported knowing of peers who have been involved in a sexual relationship with a supervisor, and 9% reported having been involved sexually with a supervisor (Brown 1993).

Every supervisor needs to be aware of his or her emotional state and if there is an awareness of incipient or significant narcissistic vulnerability to address the situation.

Consultation, collaboration with colleagues, and therapy should always be options for those of us who teach and supervise.

Specific Challenges and Strategies

- **What do I do if there is a significant disruption in the supervisory alliance?** Address (or readdress) the supervisory alliance and how you have dealt with the frame of supervision. Do you understand the supervisee's expectations, feelings about being in supervision, and his concerns about you as a supervisor? Examine how your personality, teaching style, and theoretical orientation are affecting the supervision. Figure out a way to talk about the problems from an empathic (what's the supervisee's experience) and an "other" perspective (what are the problems you're experiencing with the supervisee).

- **A supervisee wants to change to another supervisor, and I'm hurt and angry. How do I handle it?** If you are surprised by the announcement, something has been seriously missing in the supervision. Either the supervisee is an expert at concealing his experience (a real possibility) or you have not been able to perceive clearly what is going, or not going, on. There is work to do with feelings of hurt and anger, yours and likely the supervisee's. If you cannot get to a manageable place on your own, find a consultant and talk it through. Direct dialog about the motives and feelings behind the supervisee's desire to stop working with you is necessary. The experience will revitalize the supervision, perhaps change the way you've been working, or end up in a mutual decision to stop.

- **I find myself daydreaming about a supervisee. How do I deal with my feelings of attraction?** Ask yourself what is going on in your personal life and how might your needs be leaking into your work? If you're experiencing difficulty in your primary relationship, pay attention and address the problems. Look carefully at how your feelings are influencing your interactions with the supervisee. Are you more solicitous? Less open and available? Subtly seductive? Consider immediate consultation and/or personal therapy.

Questions for the Supervisor

■ What is most gratifying about being a supervisor? Most discouraging?

■ Who was the most difficult individual I've ever supervised? Why?

■ How would I feel about asking a supervisee about his or her sexual fantasies about a patient?

■ What boundary of supervision have I deliberately crossed recently?

■ What boundaries of supervision do I unconsciously (and recurrently) cross?

■ What have I said or done as a supervisor that I would have difficulty telling or keep secret from a colleague?

Additional Resources

Celenza A: Sexual Boundary Violations: Therapeutic, Supervisory, and Academic Contexts. Northvale, NJ, Jason Aronson, 2007

Sarnat J: Supervision Essentials for Psychodynamic Psychotherapies. Washington, DC, American Psychological Association, 2016

Watkins CE: Listening, learning, and development, in psychoanalytic supervision: a self psychology perspective. Psychoanal Psychol 33(3):437–471, 2016

References

Brown M: Sexual intimacies in the supervisory relationship. Unpublished doctoral dissertation. School of Education, Boston College, 1993

Coen SJ: Narcissistic temptations to cross boundaries and how to manage them. J Am Psychoanal Assoc 55(4):1169–1190, 2007 18246758

Frawley-O'Dea MG, Sarnat JE: The Supervisory Relationship: A Contempory Psychodynamic Approach. New York, Guilford, 2001

Gabbard GO: Professional boundaries in psychotherapy, in Textbook of Psychotherapeutic Treatments. Edited by Gabbard GO. Washington, DC, American Psychiatric Publishing, 2009, p 896

Gutheil TG, Gabbard GO: The concept of boundaries in clinical practice: theoretical and risk-management dimensions. Am J Psychiatry 150(2):188–196, 1993 8422069

Gutheil TG, Gabbard GO: Misuses and misunderstandings of boundary theory in clinical and regulatory settings. Am J Psychiatry 155(3):409–414, 1998 9501754

Heru AM, Strong DR, Price M, et al: Boundaries in psychotherapy supervision. Am J Psychother 58(1):76–89, 2004 15106401

Jain S, Roberts LW: Ethics in psychotherapy: a focus on professional boundaries and confidentiality practices. Psychiatr Clin North Am 32(2):299–314, 2009 19486815

Meissner WW: The problem of self-disclosure in psychoanalysis. J Am Psychoanal Assoc 50(3):827–867, 2002 12434873

Pope KS, Levenson H, Schover LR: Sexual intimacy in psychology training: results and implications of a national survey. Am Psychol 34(8):682–689, 1979 496089

Ryan CJ : Sex, lies and training programs: the ethics of consensual relationships between psychiatrists and trainee psychiatrist. Aust NZ J Psychiatry 32:387–391, 1998

Watkins CE: Listening, learning, and development in psychoanalytic supervision: a self psychology perspective. Psychoanalytic Psychology 33(3):437–471, 2016

Weinstein LS, Winer JA, Ornstein E: Supervision and self-disclosure: modes of supervisory interaction. J Am Psychoanal Assoc 57(6):1379–1400, 2009 20068245

Chapter 39 Unprofessional Behavior

Identification and Remediation in Supervision

Ann C. Schwartz, M.D.

Definitions of the term *professionalism* vary in the literature, and professional organizations have worked both to define professionalism and to develop standards for the assessment and teaching of professionalism (ABIM Foundation et al. 2002; American Board of Internal Medicine 1995). Professionalism is a complex competency including a set of core beliefs and values that guide the work of providers who are treating patients (Lucey and Souba 2010). Attributes associated with professionalism include altruism, accountability, excellence, duty, honor, integrity, and respect for others (Schwartz et al. 2009). Problems in professionalism are often serious and can be challenging to remediate. Identifying and addressing professionalism concerns early is crucial in the development of supervisees (Schwartz et al. 2009), because difficulties in this domain in training predict more serious problems over the education and training life cycle and may extend beyond the training years (Murden et al. 2004; Papadakis et al. 2004). Supervisees with professionalism problems require substantial administrative and supervisory resources (Kaslow et al. 2007) and negatively impact others in the training environment. Therefore, procedures and strategies must be available to identity, supervise, and remediate supervisees with unprofessional behaviors.

Key Points

- Early identification and intervention of professionalism concerns are crucial in the development and supervision of supervisees.

- A low threshold for reporting professional lapses should be expected and promoted by supervisors across all training sites.

- Supervisor and supervisee awareness and training regarding professionalism should be optimized.

- A formal structure for dealing with lapses and/or unprofessional behavior should be developed.

- Remediation or learning plans should be individualized and targeted based on the nature and severity of the professionalism problems and developed in collaboration with the supervisee, with the areas of weakness/deficiency clearly identified.

- Ongoing assessment of performance and behavior, a defined timeline, and defined next steps are critical components in developing a remediation plan.

- Careful and thorough documentation at each step of the remediation process is critical.

- Supervisors should be familiar with and adhere to institutional policy and procedures.

Overall Approach

While professionalism has become a central theme in medical education, little is known about the best practices in supervising those who have lapses in this domain. The overall approach in the supervision of unprofessional behavior includes identifying professionalism problems, assessing and investigating concerns, having feedback conversations, and designing interventions to address subsequent lapses (e.g., remediation plans) (Papadakis et al. 2012). The specific concern or issues that need to be improved must be correctly identified so that any future remediation or learning plans can target those issues (Katz et al. 2010). The overall approach will vary depending on the behavior and severity of the professionalism lapse and the theorized cause of the unprofessional behavior (Schwartz et al. 2009).

Once professionalism problems have been assessed and identified, the next step is to further investigate the concerns to further characterize the behavior and determine whether it is a single unprofessional incident or repetitive (Roberts and Williams 2011). The severity and impact of the difficulties should be assessed and classified as mild, moderate, or severe, as the interventions may differ depending on level of unprofessional behavior. Mild problems in professionalism could include supervisees who are late to supervision, refer to patients in a disrespectful manner, or who do not wear appropriate clinical attire. Mild problems may be reclassified as moderate if the behaviors escalate in frequency or severity, or the supervisees are unresponsive to feedback given (e.g., supervisees are routinely late or miss supervision following feedback on these behaviors).

Examples of moderate professionalism problems include inadequate documentation of clinical encounters or failure to seek supervision when appropriate. Severe violations of professionalism may include illegal (e.g., stealing property) or unethical (e.g., having sex with a patient) behaviors and may require immediate action, including remediation, probation, or termination (Hickson et al. 2007; Katz et al. 2010).

Once unprofessional behaviors have been identified, the lapses should be reviewed and discussed immediately and directly with the supervisee. In relatively mild cases of unprofessional behavior, the interventions may begin on a basic level, with the supervisor simply commenting on attitudes and behaviors of concern and monitoring. The aim of the discussion is for the supervisor to share the concerns regarding professionalism, using specific and concrete examples. A collaborative approach that acknowledges the possibility of disagreements about the claims regarding professional lapses may facilitate these potentially difficult conversations. Following the feedback, the supervisee should be given the opportunity to respond and share their perspective about the concerns raised and encouraged to reflect on their own behavior and why it may have occurred (Hickson et al. 2007; Lucey and Souba 2010). The supervisor should engage in ongoing monitoring and feedback and discuss the potential consequences if the problematic attitudes and behaviors persist (Buchanan et al. 2012; Hauer et al. 2009). These informal discussions should be documented in writing (and their informal, unofficial status noted) and placed in the supervisee's file should the issue recur in the future (Papadakis et al. 2012).

When informal conversations and feedback are not sufficiently effective in ameliorating the mild or moderate problems of professionalism and the problematic attitudes and behaviors persist or escalate, additional interventions are warranted. Training programs generally use a combination of strategies to remediate professionalism lapses (Ziring et al. 2015). The elements in successful remediation include expectation setting, identifying and investigating deficiencies, developing an individualized learning plan, monitoring, effecting resolution, and developing a remediation document (Katz et al. 2010).

A remediation or individualized learning plan should be individually tailored, considering the nature and severity of the professionalism problems and taking into account supervisees' learning styles and institutional resources (Carrese et al. 2015; Hauer et al. 2009). Remediation plans should mention the core competency (e.g., professionalism) being addressed and a detailed description of the event/behaviors that led to the remediation. Plans should include the problem, described in concrete, nonjudgmental terms with examples, the goals including examples, and how to get there (e.g., supervision, readings). Remediation or individualized learning plans must clearly delineate attainable expectations related to professionalism, methods and frequencies of assessments, timeline, and consequences of failing to meet expectations (e.g., second remediation, probation, termination) (Buchanan et al. 2012; Hauer et al. 2009). The process and the desired outcomes should be concrete and measurable (Katz et al. 2010) (Figure 39–1).

Remediation and individualized learning plans should enumerate the intervention(s) that will be used to remediate the unprofessional behavior(s). Problems with professionalism may be better addressed through a behavioral approach that involves identifying the problematic behaviors, offering rationales for the dysfunctional nature of those behaviors, and practicing new behaviors, such as courtesy, respect, and reliability. Examples of prescribed learning activities include more intensive supervision and/or

Date of Remediation Plan Meeting:
Names of All Persons Present at the Meeting:
Name of Supervisee:
Supervisor/Advisor: **Date for Follow-up Meeting(s):**

Item	Description	Plan
Characterization of the lapse(s) or problem(s)	Use competencies to characterize issue(s)	
Date(s) the problem(s) was brought to the supervisee's attention and by whom		
Expectations for acceptable performance	Describe in terms of specific competency or competencies	
Supervisee's responsibilities/actions	Activity or activities for supervisee, why it is important, what behaviors define success	
Supervisor's responsibilities/actions	Expectations of the supervisor in the remediation process	
Timeframe for acceptable performance		
Assessment methods	Examples include supervisor feedback, observed interviews, reflective writing assignments, etc.	
Requirements: Monitoring	Who, frequency, expectations for follow-up meetings	
Consequences for unsuccessful remediation	Additional disciplinary measures that may include probation, nonrenewal of contract, termination	

I, _____, have reviewed the above remediation plan with my supervisor(s) and director of training. My signature below indicates that I fully understand the above and agree to participate in the plan as outlined above. My comments, if any, are below:

_____   _____
Supervisee name/signature   Date   Training Director name/signature   Date
Supervisee's comment:

FIGURE 39–1. Sample remediation plan.

the assignment of a mentor, practice with standardized patients, reading assignments or additional coursework, experiential activities, reflective writing, repeating a clinical rotation, and encouraging personal therapy (Hauer et al. 2009; Ziring et al. 2015). Coaching and observation with immediate feedback and monitoring are likely to be more effective strategies for addressing any lapses in professionalism than are technical solutions that involve enforcement of the rules and reminders (Lucey and Souba 2010).

The remediation plan should be developed in collaboration with the supervisee. Supervisors should emphasize that the goal of the plan is not to punish, but rather to enhance growth and improve professionalism-related attitudes and behaviors to meet competency standards. The remediation plan should be in writing, signed by the involved parties, and placed in the supervisee's file. Supervisee progress should be monitored and documented throughout the remediation process to ensure that acceptable levels of performance have been achieved (Hauer et al. 2009; Wu et al. 2010). The methods utilized in monitoring should be objective, measurable, realistic, and feasible.

Advisory panels such as clinical competency committees (CCC) within residency programs or progress and promotions committees (PPC) in training programs may be used to guide the decision-making process regarding remediation and can minimize the perception of bias and allow for more objective and defensible decisions. The committee can be helpful in developing advisory, supportive, and insight-giving strategies.

At the conclusion of the remediation period, it must be determined whether the remediation was successful. Remediation ends when the supervisee successfully incorporates new behavior and information that put his or her professionalism above the minimal standards, or when the supervisee fails to successfully achieve the terms of remediation (Katz et al. 2010). If the supervisee is not meeting the goals of remediation, further disciplinary action will be necessary. In these cases, excellent documentation, adherence to due process, and fair and equitable treatment are essential (Katz et al. 2010). If the professionalism lapses are severe (e.g., missing shifts, dishonesty), the supervisee may be less amendable to remediation and more punitive approaches may be necessary. Early involvement of administration (e.g., Graduate Medical Education in medical education) and legal counsel is recommended, and institutional policies and procedures should be considered throughout the remediation process (Hauer et al. 2009).

Specific Challenges and Strategies

- **I am often unclear about what qualifies as a professionalism issue or am reluctant to address one.** There is a lack of validated tools to assess professionalism, and there are no strict criteria for defining what performance cutoffs require formal remediation. Professionalism can be difficult to define, and individuals may disagree about what behaviors are appropriate in different situations (Katz et al. 2010; Schwartz et al. 2009). Supervisors may often be uncomfortable providing feedback on and addressing professionalism issues or think that others are addressing the issues. For these these challenges to be addressed, faculty members should be provided with training to enhance their skills in providing feedback and addressing professionalism lapses. A cultural shift within the institution may be needed to develop an environment where faculty play an integral role in identifying and addressing professionalism lapses and are encouraged to report offenses (Ziring et al. 2015).

- **What do I do about the hidden curriculum?** The hidden curriculum in educational settings exposes supervisees to instances of unprofessional behavior and learners then inadvertently emulate their role models (Hickson et al. 2007). For example, faculty members may speak of patients in a derogatory manner, teaching students and residents that such behavior is acceptable. Supervisees, supervisors, clinicians, and physicians in all training and practice settings at times display unprofessional behaviors; therefore, we must work to create a culture in which reflection, acknowledgment of mistakes, and recommitment to the highest standards of professionalism are goals to which all aspire throughout their careers (Adams et al. 2008).

- **My supervisee lacks insight into the problematic behaviors.** Without resident buy-in, problematic attitudes and behaviors may continue, and remediation is unlikely to be successful. In instances where the trainee lacks insight, gathering clear and consistent supporting data from multiple observers can be helpful. Confrontation by a group of faculty can help reinforce that the problems are a consistent perception rather than just one person's perception (Katz et al. 2010). Involvement of trainees in the remediation or individualized learning plan may help with compliance, and trainees are more likely to be receptive to remediation if they feel they are being supported rather than threatened or punished (Katz et al. 2010).

- **There is not enough supporting documentation.** Limited supporting documentation could lead to difficulties in pursuing disciplinary action including warnings, probation, or termination. To address this challenge, supervisors should be expected to provide honest and direct feedback, and their final written evaluation should reflect the supervisees' performance and include any professionalism concerns (Katz et al. 2010). Documentation is essential throughout the entire remediation/probation period and can minimize any potential legal questions in the future. All lapses in professionalism should be clearly documented, and meetings and important discussions with the trainee should be summarized in writing.

- **The remediation plan is unsuccessful.** An unsuccessful remediation plan may be related to issues in the creation or implementation of the plans. In these cases, the supervisor should assist in ensuring that the problem has been correctly identified. Adjustment problems related to supervisees personal lives, substance use, personality disorders, and mental illness may affect resident performance and initially manifest as unprofessional behaviors and yet may be difficult to identify in supervisees (Katz et al. 2010). The remediation plan would differ based on the theorized cause of the behavior, and supervisees should be assisted in receiving the appropriate treatment rather than being punished (Schwartz et al. 2009). Remediation is resource-intensive and may involve faculty mentorship and increased supervision, and programs may have limited time and resources to develop and implement optimally individualized plans (Katz et al. 2010). Ultimately, some deficiencies may not be amenable to successful remediation, and despite everyone's best efforts, remediation plans and promotion are not always successful (Roberts and Williams 2011).

Questions for the Supervisor

■ Have I correctly identified the problem with the supervisee?

■ Have I reviewed the professional lapses and discussed immediately and directly with the supervisee?

■ Have I heard both sides of the story?

■ Have I been monitoring the supervisee's behavior since the last feedback session?

■ Does the action plan developed for the supervisee allow me to observe measurable behaviors?

■ Have I thoroughly documented each step of the remediation process?

Additional Resources

Katz ED, Dahms R, Sadosty AT, et al: Guiding principles for resident remediation: recommendations of the CORD remediation task force. Acad Emerg Med 17(suppl 2):S95–S103, 2010

Schwartz AC, Kotwicki RJ, McDonald WM: Developing a modern standard to define and assess professionalism in trainees. Acad Psychiatry 33(6):442–450, 2009

Ziring D, Danoff D, Grosseman S, et al: How do medical schools identify and remediate professionalism lapses in medical students? A study of U.S. and Canadian Medical Schools. Acad Med 90(7):913–920, 2015

References

ABIM Foundation, American Board of Internal Medicine, ACP-ASIM Foundation, et al: Medical professionalism in the new millennium: a charter for physicians. Ann Intern Med 136:243–246, 2002 11827500

Adams KE, Emmons S, Romm J: How resident unprofessional behavior is identified and managed: a program director survey. Am J Obstet Gynecol 198(6):692.e1–692.e4, discussion 692.e4–692.e5, 2008 18538156

American Board of Internal Medicine: Project Professionalism. Philadelphia, PA, American Board of Internal Medicine, 1995

Buchanan AO, Stallworth J, Christy C, et al: Professionalism in practice: strategies for assessment, remediation, and promotion. Pediatrics 129(3):407–409, 2012 22371458

Carrese JA, Malek J, Watson K, et al: The essential role of medical ethics education in achieving professionalism: the Romanell Report. Acad Med 90(6):744–752, 2015 25881647

Hauer KE, Ciccone A, Henzel TR, et al: Remediation of the deficiencies of physicians across the continuum from medical school to practice: a thematic review of the literature. Acad Med 84(12):1822–1832, 2009 19940595

Hickson GB, Pichert JW, Webb LE, et al: A complementary approach to promoting professionalism: identifying, measuring, and addressing unprofessional behaviors. Acad Med 82(11):1040–1048, 2007 17971689

Kaslow NJ, Rubin NJ, Forrest L, et al: Recognizing, assessing, and intervening with problems of professional competence. Prof Psychol Res Pr 38:479–492, 2007

Katz ED, Dahms R, Sadosty AT, et al; CORD-EM Remediation Task Force: Guiding principles for resident remediation: recommendations of the CORD remediation task force. Acad Emerg Med 17(Suppl 2):S95–S103, 2010 21199091

Lucey C, Souba W: Perspective: the problem with the problem of professionalism. Acad Med 85(6):1018–1024, 2010 20505405

Murden RA, Way DP, Hudson A, et al: Professionalism deficiencies in a first-quarter doctor-patient relationship course predict poor clinical performance in medical school. Acad Med 79(10)(Suppl):S46–S48, 2004 15383387

Papadakis MA, Hodgson CS, Teherani A, et al: Unprofessional behavior in medical school is associated with subsequent disciplinary action by a state medical board. Acad Med 79(3):244–249, 2004 14985199

Papadakis MA, Paauw DS, Hafferty FW, et al; Alpha Omega Alpha Honor Medical Society Think Tank: Perspective: the education community must develop best practices informed by evidence-based research to remediate lapses of professionalism. Acad Med 87(12):1694–1698, 2012 23095921

Roberts NK, Williams RG: The hidden costs of failing to fail residents. J Grad Med Educ 3(2):127–129, 2011 22655131

Schwartz AC, Kotwicki RJ, McDonald WM: Developing a modern standard to define and assess professionalism in trainees. Acad Psychiatry 33(6):442–450, 2009 19933884

Wu JS, Siewert B, Boiselle PM: Resident evaluation and remediation: a comprehensive approach. J Grad Med Educ 2(2):242–245, 2010 21975628

Ziring D, Danoff D, Grosseman S, et al: How do medical schools identify and remediate professionalism lapses in medical students? A study of U.S. and Canadian medical schools. Acad Med 90(7):913–920, 2015 25922920

Chapter 40 Termination

Supervising a "Good Goodbye"

Cheryl Yund Goodrich, Ph.D.

Teaching supervisees how to end mental health care with a patient seems to always come last in training if addressed at all. Even referring to these endings as "termination" has an unfortunate legalistic tone, perhaps chosen in an attempt to avoid painful, emotional experiences of limitation and loss. It is important to teach that preparation for endings is an integral part of a treatment from its start and that a 'good goodbye' is a developmental achievement.

Key Points

- Teach termination planning as part of the patient evaluation phase and emphasize that treatment is an arc with a beginning, middle, and end.

- Demonstrate goal setting in order to describe the "goal posts" of termination.

- Use attachment styles as a guide to understand how patients and therapists end relationships including treatment relationships.

- Identify signs of a pretermination phase.

- Model and describe alliance building and rupture/repair skills to prevent premature terminations.

- Give examples of how to cope with abrupt, unready and dismissive patient responses to ending.

Begin With the End in Mind

A central training antidote for the neglect of termination skills is planning for a good ending during the evaluation phase of meeting with a patient. Supervisors can describe an arc of treatment and how beginning, middle, and end are, at best, integrated. A psychotherapy or medication management termination should not be simply a stopping point; it can embody the achievements of a successful treatment. Supervisors can help their supervisees, and in turn the supervisees' patients, approach the ending as a "good goodbye" (Novick and Novick 2006). A supervisor can model, perhaps in role-play with their supervisee, how to integrate planning for termination during the evaluation phase. It can be helpful to have supervisees reflect on what signs would suggest a patient was nearing the goalposts, such as when the patient intervenes with himself or herself the way the therapist does or checks out his or her assumptions with others. During the assessment phase, it is also helpful to encourage supervisees to hone in on their patients' attachment styles. For example, the supervisee might ask the patient how important relationships have ended in the past, to help determine how the patient may react to the termination of the therapeutic relationship.

Invite Discussion of Supervisee's Reactions to Termination

Avoidance of the emotional pain of accepting one's limits and the loss of the therapeutic relationship is an important challenge not only for the patient but also the provider. The supervisor should make it routine practice to talk with the supervisee about the real threat of avoidance—in terms of planning for both the calendar end and the emotional end of treatment—for their patient *and themselves*. The supervisor and supervisee can discuss *their own* attachment styles or tendencies—secure, or insecure, preoccupied or avoidant—and how these tendencies may affect their approach to termination. Supervisees with more preoccupied attachment styles may react to impending terminations by doubting their competence or feeling abandoned. Supervisees with more avoidant styles tend to minimize the importance of termination and delay planning for it. Supervisors need to be adept at recognizing and managing their own natural and specific reactions to endings, and be able to model that kind of attention to the supervisee.

Develop Supervisee's Termination Skills
Identify and Repair Ruptures

Key termination skills are the abilities to identify and address ruptures in the treatment relationship and to repair the relationship in order to assist the patient to stay for an optimal dose of treatment and prevent premature termination (see Chapter 36, "Ruptures in the Supervisory Alliance"). One in five patients drop out of therapy prematurely (Swift and Greenberg 2012). The supervisor can help the supervisee identify impending ruptures by pointing out, for example, a patient's chronic lateness or puzzlingly long silences and encourage the supervisee to be alert for signs of possible ruptures. Furthermore, the supervisor can help the supervisee understand that treatment, including medication management, occurs within a relationship and that the health of this relationship is primarily the responsibility of the provider. The supervisor can teach alliance building skills, such as encouraging the supervisee to ask for feedback from the patient throughout treatment and to attend to subtle shifts of emotion in the room. Should a rupture occur in the relationship, it can be helpful to role play with the supervisee how to manage repairing the rupture.

Identify and Work Within the Pretermination Phase

The concept of "pretermination" can be a game changer in learning and conducting effective psychotherapies (Novick and Novick 2006). Pretermination is described as an identifiable phase during which patients are effectively taking responsibility for their own well-being but have not yet become explicitly aware of their capacity for independence from the provider. In psychological terms, this is evident when the patient actively balances attention to self and other, internal and external, cognition and affect; in sum, the capacity to mentalize. During this phase, supervisors can ask supervisees to identify signs of pretermination in their cases and help supervisees recognize the hallmarks of pretermination, including patients' increased capacity for self-care and self-regulation, and when patients assume more responsibility for progressive joint work with the provider. Signs of a pretermination phase give the supervisee a guidepost for beginning a termination phase.

Prepare for a Successful Termination Experience

Accepting the limitations of what can be achieved in a psychotherapy is difficult, especially when a supervisee may only see a patient for less than a year. But time-limited therapies offer opportunities to supervisees to explicitly face frustrations and disappointments about the limits that time and resources impose. Supervisors can actively model awareness of their own characteristic style of dealing with limitation and loss. For example, the supervisor might say, "I went into this work with pretty heroic ambitions to help people change. But with time, I've learned to respect the complexity and subtly of a person's life and I've come to believe that they will carry on as best they can given all that's come before and what they are yet to confront. Now I feel satisfied to see I've helped them become more reflective. I've taught them to 'fish' and I need to trust they'll continue to refine their own way of 'fishing.'" This practice can embody for the supervisee how to deal with the all-too-human impulse to cling to omnipotent beliefs in perfection, including the idea of becoming a fully rational and controlled person. It is ongoing psychological work to face the ordinary conflicts, pain, and losses of real life.

When there is joint agreement about planning an end to the treatment, the depth of the relationship is a gauge of how far in advance to set the end date. It can be useful to teach supervisees to be concrete about termination and get out their calendars with their patients to count the weeks or months remaining in the treatment and mark the date of the planned termination. This makes a vague future feel real.

It can also be helpful to review with supervisees themes that are commonly discussed during the termination phase, have them read articles and chapters on termination, and explore how they would like to conduct their final sessions. A recent study (Norcross et al. 2017) described eight pan-theoretical themes that are commonly discussed during the termination phase: talking about the feelings of patient *and* therapist (which includes attention to positive and negative feelings), discussing the patient's future coping and identifying risks for relapse, noting the option of returning for treatment, helping the patient use new skills beyond therapy, framing personal development as invariably unfinished, anticipating posttherapy growth and generalization, preparing explicitly for termination, and reflecting on patient gains and consolidation.

At the end of the termination of a mental health treatment relationship, supervisors should help supervisees appreciate what has been learned and felt to be good and healing. Supervisees should also be able to bear some degree of sadness, hopefully balanced by the satisfaction of being able to take a part in a patient's recovery and growth. The experience of a "good goodbye" fosters the ability to engage in continued social learning in an ever-changing social and cultural context (Fonagy et al. 2014).

Specific Challenges and Strategies

- **My supervisee is transferring his patient to another provider. Do I need him to go through a full termination with his patient?** Common in training, transfers from one provider to another are an end for the provider but not the patient. Nevertheless, the transfer needs to be treated as a relationship end even though it is not a treatment end. The supervisee should be attuned to the patient's helplessness about not having a choice and how that may stimulate them to reassert control, withdraw or displace anger. On the other hand, the supervisee may feel guilt, anxiety, sadness or relief as they face telling their patients they will be leaving the clinic. Supervisors should help supervisees notice, accept, and contain these feelings lest they delay telling the patient about the transfer. In year-long treatments, supervisees can be taught the routine of telling patients about the time limit at the beginning of the therapy, and reminding them 3–6 months before the end of treatment. The existing provider should help the patient anticipate the experience emotionally, describe the administrative process, and introduce the patient to the new provider. The new provider should be ready to tolerate that the patient might engage in comparison, feel troubled by having to start with someone new, or continue mourning the previous treatment. Offering supervisees the concept of "institutional transference" (Reider 1953) can help supervisees appreciate that a patient's attachment to the clinic or institution allows them to tolerate the coming and going of therapists. With this idea, the supervisee can work with some patients' surprisingly low levels of feeling about the impending end of the relationship due to a transfer. When the focus of treatment has been medication management, it is helpful to recognize that each patient attributes meaning and value to the medicine beyond its specific pharmacology. In good enough experiences with the psychiatrist, the medicine can be experienced as a transitional object, representing the psychiatrist and the therapeutic relationship. Continuing with the prescribed medicine can mitigate a sense of loss in a medication management transfer. But each patient attributes meaning to the medicine according to their own psychology (Hausner 1985–1986).

- **My supervisee's patient unexpectedly started the session by saying, "This is my last session."** Although this scenario is not uncommon, there is usually a prodrome that the provider may have missed. Supervisors should ask supervisees what their frank subjective response is as a means to help them regulate their emotional reaction to the surprise and commonly felt irritation and hurt. Supervisors can help normalize these subjective reactions and experiment in discussion and role play what the supervisee can usefully say in the patient's presence. The supervisor is key in helping the supervisee regain balance in these situations, optimally with the supervisee having gained confidence that the supervisor will be curious, not critical, if a case runs into trouble or ends abruptly. It can be helpful to role-play this scenario before it happens. In the role-play, the supervisor can encourage the supervisee to explore the patient's reasons for making the asserted changes, to clarify any misunderstandings or questions, and to discuss options, including continuing in treatment or offering alternative resources and referrals. The supervisor can help the supervisee find their genuine concern for the patient which can get swamped by surprise and irritation. By working on this in a role play, the supervisee will be better prepared to respond when this happens in the real world. When unexpected terminations occur, the supervisor's extensive experience can be referenced to help the supervisee realize that therapy does not work for everyone or at all points in a patient's life. When it is necessary to do so, a supervisor can lend the supervisee this kind of resilient humility and encourage the supervisee's explicit demonstration to the patient that their well-being comes first.

- **Just before our planned ending, the patient presents in a real crisis.** On the other hand, sometimes diligent preparation for an ending is not enough when just before a planned ending the patient is in crisis or voices serious reservations about stopping treatment. Usually there is warning about this, as when a patient has high dependent needs and low self-confidence. In supervision, a thoughtful assessment of reality, including severity of the crisis, available resources, and the vulnerabilities of the patient, needs to be done. A supervisor might role-play with the supervisee how to provide additional encouragement to the patient to give the posttermination phase a try before attempting to resume treatment. The supervisee may need to borrow the supervisor's conviction that this will not be harmful to the patient. And the supervisor can encourage supervisees to share relevant evidence which suggests that the gains of the treatment are likely to be sustained and may increase (Huber et al. 2012).

- **We prepared for our ending well in advance, but my patient has missed the final session!** There are also dismissive emotional responses to ending that can come in the form of missing the final sessions of treatment. Often there is reason to anticipate this kind of ending—such as a patient not acknowledging the ending phase and feelings about it, or his or her having a history of dealing with sad feelings by ignoring them. In this situation, the supervisee can consider the various ways to reach the patient such as phone or letter. The main point is to acknowledge the end and to protect the patient's confidence that future treatment is possible. When a patient does not have a last meeting, the supervisee and supervisor can have an ending in absentia, where they discuss the treatment and the good work the supervisee has done. It is also an opportunity to increase the supervisee's attention to the complex emotional terrain of treatment termination and how best to anticipate the ending from the beginning.

Questions for the Supervisee

■ How do you characteristically feel when a relationship ends?

■ How do you cope with experiences of loss and limitation?

■ What goals are you and your patient identifying, and how will you know when you've achieved them? What will this look like in behavioral and intrapsychic terms?

■ Given a patient's psychological style, how would you predict he or she will deal with the ending of treatment?

■ What feelings do you have about a specific patient's termination? What, if any, feelings are you prepared to share with the patient?

■ What challenges do you expect the patient will face post termination?

■ Can you describe what you see the patient as having achieved in this treatment?

Additional Resources

Hilsenroth M: An introduction to the special issue on psychotherapy termination. Psychotherapy 54(1):1–3, 2017

Marmarosh C, Thompson B, Hill C, et al: Providers-in-training experiences of working with transfer clients: one relationship terminates and another begins. Psychotherapy 54(1):102–113, 2017

Schen C, Raymond L, Notman M: Transfer of care of psychotherapy patients: implications for psychiatry training. Psychodynamic Psychiatry 41(4):575–595, 2013

Shedler J: Efficacy of psychodynamic psychotherapy. American Psychologist 65(2):98–109, 2010

References

Fonagy P, Luyten P, Campbell C, et al: Epistemic trust, psychopathology and the great psychotherapy debate. 2014. Available at: http://www.societyforpsychotherapy.org/epistemic-trust-psychopathology-and-the-great-psychotherapy-debate. Accessed August 20, 2018.

Hausner R: Medication and transitional phenomena. Int J Psychoanal Psychother 11:375–407, 1985–1986 4086185

Huber D, Zimmermann J, Henrich G, et al: Comparison of cognitive-behavioral therapy with psychoanalytic and psychodynamic therapy for depressed patients—a three-year follow-up study. Z Psychosom Med Psychother 58:299–316, 2012 22987495

Norcross JC, Zimmerman BE, Greenberg RP, et al: Do all therapists do that when saying goodbye? A study of commonalities in termination behaviors. Psychotherapy (Chic) 54(1):66–75, 2017 28263653

Novick J, Novick KK: Good Goodbyes, Knowing How to End in Psychotherapy and Psychoanalysis, Lanham, MD, Jason Aronson, 2006

Reider N: A type of transference to institutions. Bull Menninger Clin 17(2):58–63, 1953 13009385

Swift JK, Greenberg RP: Premature discontinuation in adult psychotherapy: a meta-analysis. J Consult Clin Psychol 80(4):547–559, 2012 22506792

Chapter 41 Supervising Cross-Cultural Topics in a Clinical Setting

Ripal Shah, M.D., M.P.H.

Megan Tan, M.D., M.S.

Belinda S. Bandstra, M.D., M.A.

Shifting trends in diversity in the United States are driving a need for multicultural competence in psychiatry and psychology training settings. According to the U.S. Census Bureau, in 2010, 16% of the population self-identified as Hispanic or Latino and 13% self-identified as black or African American, American Indian or Alaska Native, or Native Hawaiian or Pacific Islander (U.S. Census Bureau 2012). In contrast, only 10% of U.S. medical school graduates in 2013 self-identified as any of the above groups, considered underrepresented minorities in medicine (Association of American Medical Colleges 2017). Similar significant disparities are thought to exist between mental health providers and patients, as well as for other minority statuses, including gender identity, sexual orientation, and religion. Additionally, minority patients or patients of low socioeconomic status often have a more difficult time accessing mental health resources; a working-class black man calls, on average, 80 therapists before securing an appointment, whereas a middle-class white woman may have only needed to reach out to five therapists prior to entering a therapist's office (Kugelmass 2016).

Recent research studies investigating the persistence of disparities in mental health service utilization suggest that minorities' perceptions of differences in treatment and services play a greater role in lower rates of accessing mental health care than demand for those services or access-related factors such as insurance status (Smedley et al. 2003).

Within this context, there is an increasing awareness that effectively navigating the complexities and nuances of cross-cultural topics is an essential skill for any supervisor, in clinical settings and beyond. Studies suggest that persons of color terminate at a rate of greater than 50% after the first session, a factor that has been attributed to the biased nature of services and lack of appreciation for differences in experience across culture (Sue and Sue 1999). Conversely, providers with high levels of multicultural counseling competence often have patients who report greater improvement in well-being (Dillon et al. 2016).

Despite this recognition, the affective potency of cultural topics such as race, ethnicity, religion, sexual orientation, and national origin may at times lead to an avoidance of this discussion in the supervisory setting. Even among providers who aspire to directly confront issues of culture in supervision, there is little consensus about how to approach such topics on a practical level. Recognizing that talking about culture can often evoke strong reactions, we aim, in this chapter, to provide the reader with a practical set of tools for approaching issues of culture with supervisees.

Key Points

- It is essential for supervisors to foster a safe and productive learning climate for supervisees to discuss uncomfortable topics related to race, ethnicity, class, gender, sexual orientation, nationality, age, identity, and other categories of cultural belonging.

- Supervisors may work together with their supervisees to identify situations in which both the supervisee and the supervisor require a "cultural consultation" to best serve the patient, or where they might learn together through the use of case studies, "critical incidents," literary works, and film to explore the complex and nuanced nature of cultural formulation.

- Supervisors should explore their own inherent cultural biases and be willing and able to discuss explicit and implicit bias with supervisees.

- Supervisors may benefit from familiarizing themselves with strategies such as the ADDRESSING mnemonic and the DSM-5 Cultural Formulation and how to discuss these with supervisees, especially as pertains to cultural and historical features in the power relationship between the patient and the clinician.

Fostering a Productive Learning Climate

Creating a safe and productive learning climate for supervisees to think with supervisors about issues of culture is an active and ongoing process. Supervisors must be cognizant of the greater degree of power inherent in their role and set the tone for this conversation. Discussing evidence from the literature about the role that culture may play in the patient-provider dynamic, in diagnosis, or in health outcomes can normalize talking about this topic and ameliorate the vulnerability the supervisee may experience. Supervisors are in a position to model discourse that effectively communicates their commitment to this topic.

Supervisors can convey the value they place on mutual respect and trust in supervision, and their recognition that both supervisor and supervisee must actively learn from each other's unique contributions and experiences. As they openly recognize that this can go in both directions, the supervisee also feels welcome to teach the supervisor when appropriate, or to express discomfort or uncertainty. Emphasizing the importance of cultural humility for both supervisor and supervisee in these settings will enable both to more smoothly navigate asymmetries or uncertainties across complex issues such as culture, race, ethnicity, socioeconomic status, sexual identity, and religion. The supervisor must also recognize that the supervisee's own culture or understanding of culture may influence his or her willingness to contribute openly and candidly in discussions about culture, and may shape the relationship between the supervisor, supervisee, and patient (see Chapter 35, "Cultural Issues Within the Supervisory Relationship").

At times, a supervisor may have limited knowledge or experience in the cultural background of the patient or with a particular population. In such situations, the supervisor should consider seeking cultural consultation together with the supervisee to learn more. Reaching out to colleagues who have more experience with a particular cultural background is usually the simplest starting point. In the absence of a colleague with specific cultural knowledge, supervisors may also consider reviewing curated films, narrative works, and case reports in supervision with supervisees. Viewing and reading such resources together may help broaden both the supervisor and supervisee's understanding of the culture.

Beyond the question of experience, supervisors may also feel varying degrees of personal discomfort or uncertainty when working with patients from different cultural backgrounds. Rather than trying to hide the discomfort or lack of knowledge, the literature suggests that supervisors should proactively disclose the limits of their own cultural knowledge. Such disclosures are associated with greater perceived effectiveness of supervision (Ancis and Ladany 2001). Indeed, even if a supervisor attempts to hide his or her unease, it may nonetheless be detected by the supervisee. For example, a supervisee may notice the supervisor overmodifying speech in the room with the patient, spending less time with a minority patient as a result of the perceived discomfort, having difficulty building rapport, or avoiding frequent follow-ups of cases that involve complicating cultural factors. Recognizing that all individuals bring their own unique cultural perspectives and biases into treatment, supervisors must learn how to explore and navigate the subjectivity of their own and their supervisees' cultural assumptions. One valuable way for this dialogue to be opened up is for supervisors to acknowledge their own assumptions and limitations, their implicit biases, or even the fact that they may have outdated information.

Incorporating Cultural Considerations Into Assessment of Patients

Given the nuances and complexity of cultural topics, it may be helpful to introduce a structured approach to discussing culture in supervision. Informed by work with culturally diverse older patients, the ADDRESSING mnemonic solicits patients' Age and generational influences, Developmental and other Disabilities, Religion, Ethnicity, Social status, Sexual orientation, Indigenous heritage (Indigenous or other), National origin, and Gender (Hays 1996), and may be a useful approach to better appreciate the range of cultural factors that frame patient experiences. This approach increases providers' awareness of within-group diversity while discouraging typecast generalizations of patients based on one single description of identity.

The outline to the DSM-5 cultural formulation (American Psychiatric Association 2013) also provides a practical framework for approaching cultural issues through the exploration of four domains:

1. **Self-identification:** How does the patient self-identify culturally? Questions to consider include whether patients identify as mainstream versus other, and whether they view themselves as having a single or unitary culture versus having multiple, divergent identities. Salient features of the patient's family and cultural history, such as displacement, immigration, war, or other trauma, are also an important part of this arena.
2. **Cultural conceptualizations of distress:** How is distress expressed within the patient's culture? Specific attention may be paid to internalizing versus externalizing expressions of distress, and the ways in which the distress is manifested (or not manifested) in the context of the clinical encounter. The patient's explanatory models for his or her illness are also important in this regard, as they can frame alliance with the clinician, treatment expectations, and adherence.
3. **Cultural features of vulnerability and resilience:** What are sources of stress that are unique to the patient's cultural background? What are sources of strength and resilience? How can the clinical encounter modulate or utilize stressors or strengths to therapeutic benefit?
4. **Cultural features in the relationship between the patient and the clinician:** How is power distributed in this clinical relationship? Does the clinician hold most of the authority? Does the patient? Does another party? The power dynamic may be influenced by various factors, some that pertain to the patient's cultures specifically, and others that pertain to the historical and current relationships between the patient's and clinician's cultures. In the patient's cultures, traditional relationships to authority and the cultures' individualism versus collectivism may impact this variable. In the relationship between the cultural identifications of the patient and the clinician, historical and current trust, distance, oppression, and stereotyping may all have an effect.

While by no means exhaustive, this formulation outline may be used in a number of ways. In a clinical setting, a supervisee may be encouraged to talk through this formulation for each of a series of patients. One recommendation is to complete this exercise both for patients who feel culturally "diverse" and for those who feel culturally "mainstream," to underscore that every clinical encounter carries cultural components. In a classroom or small-group supervisory setting, it may also be a useful exercise for supervisees to complete cultural formulations on themselves, and to consider how their own cultural identifies inform their clinical work, their professional relationships and participation on teams, and their professional development more broadly.

A formulation is just a starting point, and supervisors may be mindful to encourage supervisees to contribute more broadly to the discussion of culture with their supervisors and other learners. Reading material and open discussions may enhance understanding in certain cases or patient demographics. Beyond considering the theoretical, supervisors should work with supervisees on tailoring therapeutic techniques in a manner that is sensitive to patients' cultural differences and experiences (Sue 2010).

Specific Challenges and Strategies

- **As a supervisor, I'm not accustomed to working with patients from this particular culture, so I feel like I can't help my supervisee in this regard.** In this case, a supervisor may benefit from working through a cultural formulation with the supervisee and encouraging the supervisee to use open-ended questions to elicit more information about the patient's life experiences. In the Cultural Formulation section of DSM-5, behind the outline is a Cultural Formulation Inventory (CFI) that lists useful and specific ways of asking patients about their varied cultural idioms and reactions to distress, as well as how they frame their own cultural narratives (American Psychiatric Association 2013). It is also important for supervisors to reflect on their own reactions to patients and acknowledge their limitations in a way that is both respectful and embracing of patient diversity. As mentioned above, cultural consultation may also be a useful tool in these contexts.
- **My supervisee's patient has expressed racist or sexist thoughts directly to the supervisee.** Unfortunately, situations in which a patient directly expresses racism or sexism to a supervisee are relatively common (i.e., the patient directly tells the provider, "I don't feel comfortable working with you," or the patient refuses to work with a particular supervisee, requests a provider of a different race, gender, religion, etc.). In this context, supervisors should encourage supervisees to maintain boundaries with the patient, and provide support. Supervisors should also confirm that all supervisees are qualified, and emphasize that both the supervisor and the supervisee are colleagues with a shared purpose of caring for the patient. It may be useful to name specific core principles of the institution's commitment to diversity and inclusion, including mutual respect for patients and providers, the importance of both common and divergent experiences, and the way in which these attributes contribute to the clinic's therapeutic space.
- **My supervisee is exhibiting implicit bias or microaggression or has limited experience in the cultural background of the patient.** When the supervisee exhibits harmful biases toward the patient, it is the supervisor's role first to create a safe learning climate for the supervisee and then to uncover and address the biases with the supervisee. For supervisees who may be uncomfortable with this discussion, the process may be aided by the supervisor drawing attention to the fact that unconscious biases are common in all people. One way to accomplish this is to use the Implicit Association Test (IAT; Greenwald et al. 1998) to make the supervisee's implicit bias explicit. In addition, supervisors may consider the use of peer/group supervision to enhance opportunities for the supervisee to receive non-hierarchical feedback, which may be better received by the supervisee. The supervisor may also probe for strong feelings associated with cultural difference, including fear, anxiety, guilt, and

shame. It can also be useful to identify factors that inhibit discussion of cultural differences: either lack of awareness that differences exist, or discomfort/fear about discussion.

Questions for the Supervisee

■ How might the patient's culture(s) overlap or differ from our own (both supervisor and supervisee)?

■ What implicit biases might we be bringing to our formulation and treatment plan? (How might your formulation and treatment plan be different if you changed certain demographic features?)

■ What do we actually know about the cultures that inform our patient? Can we complete a DSM-5 cultural formulation outline for our patient?

■ How might what we know about our patient's cultures properly inform our understanding of our formulation and treatment plan?

■ How might we be sensitive to issues of power in your relationship with the patient?

■ How might the patient's cultural concepts of distress be informing the presentation?

■ How might features of the patient's cultures be contributing to the presentation?

■ How might the patient's cultures serve as sources of strength and resilience for the patient in this context?

Additional Resources

Transcultural Psychiatry

McGill University Division of Social and Transcultural Psychiatry: www.mcgill.ca/tcpsych. Resource includes links to publications, online resources, and curated films for teaching transcultural psychiatry.

Transcultural Psychiatry: a peer reviewed journal with relevant articles on cultural psychiatry and mental health. https://www.ncbi.nlm.nih.gov/labs/journals/transcult-psychiatry

Psychoanalysis, Culture and Society: an international journal exploring the intersection between psychoanalysis and the social world. https://link.springer.com/journal/41282

Trusty J, Looby EJ, Sandhu DS (eds): Multicultural Counseling: Context, Theory and Practice, and Competence. Huntington, NY, Nova Publishers, 2002 (See Chapter 13: "Supervision from a Multicultural Perspective," in this volume.)

Cultural Formulation

American Psychiatric Association Diagnostic and Statistical Manual of Mental Disorders, 5th Edition. Arlington, VA, American Psychiatric Publishing, 2013, pp 749–759

Lewis-Fernandez R, Aggarwal NK, Hinton L, et al: DSM-5 Handbook on the Cultural Formulation Interview. Washington, DC, American Psychiatric Publishing, 2016. Provides detail on how a DSM-5 Cultural Formulation Interview can be conducted, and an interview worksheet is made available by the American Psychiatric Association at: https://www.psychiatry.org/File%20Library/Psychiatrists/Practice/DSM/APA_DSM5_Cultural-Formulation-Interview.pdf

Implicit Bias

Greenwald AG, McGhee DE, Schwartz JLK: Measuring individual differences in implicit cognition: the Implicit Association Test. Journal of Personality and Social Psychology 74(6):1464–1480, 1998

Fourteen publicly available tests retrievable at: http://www.implicit.harvard.edu

---

References

American Psychiatric Association: Cultural formulation, in Diagnostic and Statistical Manual of Mental Disorders, 5th Edition. Arlington, VA, American Psychiatric Association, 2013, pp 749–759

Ancis JRJ, Ladany N: A multicultural framework for counselor supervision, in Counselor Supervision: Principles, Process, and Practice. Edited by Bradley LJ, Ladany N. Philadelphia, PA, Brunner-Routledge, 2001, pp 63–90

Association of American Medical Colleges: Total U.S. medical school graduates by race/ethnicity and sex, 201–2013 through 2016–2017, 2017. Table B-4. November 21, 2017. Available at: https://www.aamc.org/data/facts/enrollmentgraduate/85956/bysexraceandethnicity.html. Accessed on August 20, 2018.

Dillon FR, Odera L, Fons-Scheyd A, et al: A dyadic study of multicultural counseling competence. J Couns Psychol 63(1):57–66, 2016 26436724

Greenwald AG, McGhee DE, Schwartz JLK: Measuring individual differences in implicit cognition: the implicit association test. J Pers Soc Psychol 74(6):1464–1480, 1998 9654756

Hays PA: Culturally responsive assessment with diverse older clients. Prof Psychol Res Pr 27(2):188–193, 1996

Kugelmass H: "Sorry, I'm not accepting new patients": an audit study of access to mental health care. J Health Soc Behav 57(2):168–183, 2016 27251890

Smedley BD, Smith AY, Nelson AR: Unequal Treatment: Confronting Racial and Ethnic Disparities in Health Care. Washington, DC, National Academies Press, 2003, p 764

Sue S: Cultural adaptations in treatment. Sci Rev Ment Health Pract 7:31–33, 2010

Sue DW, Sue D: Counseling the Culturally Diverse: Theory and Practice, 3rd Edition. New York, Wiley, 1999

U.S. Census Bureau: Population division, Table 1: Summary of modified race and census 2010 race distributions for the United States (US-MR2010–01), 2010. July 2012. Available at: https://www.census.gov/data/datasets/2010/demo/popest/modified-race-data-2010.html. Accessed on August 20, 2018.

Chapter 42   Integrating Measurement-Based Care Into Supervision

John M. Manring, M.D.

Zsuzsa Szombathyne Meszaros, M.D., Ph.D.

Joseph Biedrzycki, D.O.

Katherine Walia Cerio, M.D.

It is one thing to know something; it is another thing to turn what you know into behavior. Supervision is the process by which we help supervisees turn their knowledge into skills and techniques in treating patients. The ultimate goal of treating patients is the relief of their suffering. In medicine and surgery we have physical signs, laboratory tests, and diagnostic imaging to inform us of the sources of our patients' suffering and the relief of those sources of suffering. In psychiatry this suffering is most often an emotional suffering, a suffering on the inside. A fundamental challenge of supervision in psychiatry is that we often do not have clear markers for when we have relieved our patients' suffering. Without these markers, neither knowledge nor adherence to a technique guarantees relief of the patient's suffering (Dewan et al. 2017). To be most effective, one must be able to recognize when a patient has improved or has worsened. Outcome measures provide psychiatrists and other mental health providers with that direct feedback about patient suffering (Table 42–1); outcome measures become the "lab results" for psychiatric patients.

TABLE 42–1.   Commonly used questionnaires

Measure	What is it used for?	When would one use it?	Strengths	Limitations
Patient Health Question-naire–9 (PHQ-9; Löwe et al. 2004)	Depression	Screening and outcome monitoring	Free (public domain); widely available; brief and easily administered or incorpo-rated into EMR; patient-completed	Designed as diagnostic screening tool for DSM-IV MDE; tracks limited range of symptoms; little sensitivity to measures of health; limited norm group
General Anxiety Disorder–7 (GAD-7; Spitzer et al. 2006)	Anxiety	Screening and outcome monitoring	Free (public domain); widely available; brief and easily administered or incorpo-rated into EMR; patient-completed	Designed as diagnostic screening tool for DSM-IV GAD; tracks limited range of symptoms; little sensitivity to measures of health; limited norm group
World Health Organization Disability Assessment Schedule (WHODAS; American Psychiatric Association 2013, pp. 743–745)	Global mental health assessment	Initial evaluation then as outcome measure	Measures overall level of impairment; designed as outcome measure; widely available in DSM-5; patient-completed; broad tracking of symptoms; validated across many cultures	Cumbersome to administer and track; less sensitive to internal emotional state; relatively new; does not necessarily aid diagnosis
Beck Depression Inventory (BDI; Beck et al. 1996)	Measure depressive symptoms	Initial evaluation then as outcome measure	Designed as outcome measure; tracks internal symptoms of depression as well as signs; widely used in psychotherapy research; patient- completed	Proprietary measure (requires paying fee); limited to depressive symptoms

TABLE 42–1. Commonly used questionnaires *(continued)*

Measure	What is it used for?	When would one use it?	Strengths	Limitations
Outcome Questionaire–45 (OQ-45; Hawkins et al. 2004)	Global mental health assessment	Initial evaluation for level of distress then as outcome measure	Measures overall level of impairment; designed as outcome measure; patient-completed; broad tracking of symptoms; wide variety of platforms; informative readout of results; includes substance abuse queries; includes wellness measures; based on large norm group with measures of normal range	Proprietary measure (requires paying fee); does not necessarily aid diagnosis
Brief Psychiatric Rating Scale (BPRS; Faustman and Overall 1999)	Monitoring psychotic symptoms (in schizophrenia and bipolar disorder)	Initial assessment of severity of psychotic illness then to monitor improvement	Designed as outcome measure; used widely in research	Therapist-rated scale open to therapist bias

Note. EMR=electronic medical record; MDE=major depressive episode.

Nonmedical educational models emphasize planning any training by focusing on the results being sought and then working backward to the knowledge necessary to support acquisition of behaviors or techniques required to reach those results (Kirkpatrick and Kirkpatrick 1994). An emphasis on results becomes doubly important when we recognize that the therapist's role in negative outcomes with a patient is not found in gross errors of technique per se, but in the working alliance being damaged by frank or subtle rejections of the patient by the clinician (Lambert and Shimokawa 2011). As a result, improvement of the markers of patient suffering must be used as a measure of a supervisee's developing competence as a healer along with measures of adherence to technique (Dewan et al. 2017). In fact, these markers of patient suffering—these psychiatry "lab results"—are more directly accessible to the supervisee and more directly pertinent to treatment of an individual patient than are measures of adherence to technique; outcome measures allow immediate and continued self-learning.

Key Points

- Supervisors should develop a framework for supervisees to understand the strengths and limitations of using outcome measures at the start of supervisory work, whether for pharmacotherapy or psychotherapy.

- Measurement-based care includes the thoughtful choice and frequent administration of outcome measures shortly before or during a session allowing the supervisee to know the score during the session.

- Outcome measures must either be specific to the condition being treated or be a validated global rating scale, and when the patient's functioning allows it, measures completed by the patient trump those completed by the clinician.

- Scanning the changes in patients' outcome measure scores provides supervisors with direct, quantified guidance as to which patients require most attention in supervision.

- Developing protocols or policies for incorporating completion of outcome measures during or shortly before each contact with the clinician in the training clinic and/or the inpatient unit can reduce the external barriers to measurement-based outcomes.

Promoting the Rationale for Use of Measures

At present, regular administration of rating scales is used by only a minority of psychiatrists and psychologists in their clinical practice. Currently, less than one-fifth of psychiatrists and just over one-tenth psychologists in the United States regularly incorporate administration of rating scales into their clinical practice (Fortney et al. 2017). One corollary of this is the likelihood that few faculty supervisors have experience or are comfortable with the use of outcome measures. In supervision, providing a framework for why rating scales are used prior to seeing patients is as key for faculty as for trainees; resistance to incorporation of measurement-based care can be linked to concerns about utility (Fortney et al. 2017). Validated rating scales are used as a supplement to clinical judgment and not a substitute, much as laboratory tests and imaging are used in other medical specialties. Recognizing that a parallel process may have occurred in the supervisor's experience with rating scales, the supervisor may find it helpful to provide examples from his or her own experience. Additionally, it is valuable to educate supervisees regarding the role repeated outcome measures can take in facilitating a dialogue between the patient and the provider: changing scores can signal regression, impending rupture of the therapeutic alliance, or suboptimal gains during treatment or can reinforce work that is progressing, giving the clinician and patient real-world feedback.

Preparing for the First Session

At the first session, or when preparing for a new intake if possible, supervisors should discuss symptoms, differential diagnosis, and rating scales available prior to the first visit. Global measures are particularly useful at a first session, often validating for a patient the suffering he or she feels. Supervisors should have validated measures for the most common diagnoses available and review strengths and weaknesses of the chosen scales. These may be standardized within the institution as global measures or individualized based on the individual's presenting symptoms. It will be important to distinguish diagnostic screening scales from outcome measures; some scales (e.g., Patient Health Questionnaire–9 [PHQ-9; Löwe et al. 2004]) can serve in both capacities. The results of the scales should be revisited after the initial diagnostic interview to supplement the case formulation. In addition to the natural questions about a case that foster competence in pharmacological or therapeutic technique, discussing expected outcomes from treatment is critical. At the first and subsequent supervision sessions regarding a case, it is recommended that the supervisor either have automatic access to the supervisee's outcome measure scores or else ask for the session's rating scales. It is also helpful to note any change or stability of symptoms, the next interventions needed based on the supervisee's formulation of the patient, and the time expected prior to seeing the results of these interventions.

Using Outcome Measures During Supervision

Addressing outcome measure scores as the first order of business in each supervision session models as well as emphasizes the importance of acquiring the measures within the window of outcome measure utility when the scores can be used by the supervisee and the supervisor as "fresh data" during the session (Fortney et al. 2017). It also allows for discussion of some challenges of using repeated outcome measures such as how much does a score have to change to be clinically significant or ways in which patients may over- or underreport symptoms over time (although the effect is low for state-specific scores). Some authors have suggested that when a patient has been in treatment for more than eight sessions, one could consider reducing the frequency to once per month (Lambert and Hawkins 2004).

Specific Challenges and Strategies

- **My workflow doesn't accommodate completion of outcome measures.** While a motivated supervisee can find ways to effectively utilize outcome measures and to incorporate them routinely into supervision for all supervisees, it is crucial to develop a workflow in the clinic that facilitates the process by which patients complete their outcome measures in advance of the session. This can be done electronically through a patient portal, on an outcome measure website (a powerful argument for some proprietary measures like the Outcome Questionnaire–45 [OQ-45; Hawkins et al. 2004]), or in the waiting room on paper or at a computerized kiosk prior to the appointment. While serving to acculturate patients to completing measures, these arrangements reduce the amount of time needed to address results in the session and can tackle the resistance by patients as well as supervisees on a system level. Supervisees could use either paper or online rating scales; while paper scales can be easy to administer in the office, they require more time in the session to score and compare with prior results if at least part of this workflow is not completed by support staff or by the patient in the waiting room. When support staff is not available, the online completion of a measure the day prior to or on the morning of the visit, as in the case of the OQ-45, has allowed supervisees to easily access and share the results graphically during the session. Users of this method have cited moments when the scores helped to validate progress or challenge areas of poor engagement. An additional organizational step may be necessary to ensure electronically completed scores are readily available for comparison; this could be within the electronic medical record's patient portal or other tracking system, such as OQ-45's online platform.
- **My supervisee expresses resistance to rating scales, either verbally or behaviorally.** Invite exploration of their reasons for lack of completion while reinforcing the utility of rating scales in patient care. Try to address systems issues outside of the supervision process as well as the patient's or supervisee's own resistance.
- **My supervisee relies too heavily on the rating scale.** Supervisees sometimes utilize the scale without further discussion of the patient's current presentation, or most importantly the process of the therapeutic work. Use the supervisory space to explore reasons why the trainee may be using the scales as a distancing tool in the therapeutic relationship. Overreliance on scales may be a sign of countertransference that needs to be addressed, or it may be a sign that the trainee has misunderstood the role of scales in the larger treatment process.
- **The rating scales all show worsening of the patient over time.** As noted above, worsening (usually rising) scale scores can be a sign of deviation in technique or countertransference problems. This may reflect worsening of the therapeutic alliance, which can be further detailed through measures such as the Working Alliance Inventory (Horvath and Greenberg 1989) or the Barrett-Lennard Relationship Scale (Barrett-Lennard 1962; Simmons et al. 1995); or this may be due to nonadherence to technique, which can be assessed through the appropriate assessment tools, such as the Revised Cognitive Therapy Scale (Blackburn et al. 2001), IPT Quality and Adherence Scale (https://iptinstitute.com/ipt-training-materials/ipt-quality-adherence-scale), or Comparative Psychotherapy Process Scale (Hilsenroth et al. 2005), or, perhaps most effectively, through the review of video recordings of

patient sessions or direct observation of a session (Manring et al. 2011). For those providing medication management, this also becomes an opportunity to evaluate the medication regimen and compliance.

- **The supervisors in my system don't have any experience with outcome measures.** This may be one of the more frequent problems encountered in the training clinic. Most clinicians are wary of perceived intrusions into the clinical space, as much for themselves as for their patients. If there is no philosophical objection to use of rating scales, providing the same kind of system support for the supervisors' use of rating scales in their own practices as the supervisees receive and an attitude of "We're ALL new to this" can go a long way to allow them to gain experience. Providing grand rounds or didactic presentations to the supervisors is another way to help support this change. For those with philosophical objections, the administration can consider developing a QI study in which the objecting supervisor and/or his or her supervisees are in a "control group" of cases without use of measures versus another supervisor and supervisees with cases using outcome measures. Perhaps most important will be remembering that it takes 2–3 years to change a system or culture; these are changes for the long haul.

- **I've heard that there may be some drawbacks to using outcome measures in psychiatric treatment. How should I discuss this with my supervisees?** There is some emerging evidence that certain diagnostic categories can pose problems for patient-completed outcome measures. It may be useful to discuss current research with supervisees to help them think through these issues. For example, psychotic patients often report little distress about their emotional lives, leading to the greater utility of clinician-rated scales such as the BPRS or the PANSS. Patients with borderline personality disorder may have adverse reactions to the weekly administration of outcome measure questions (de Jong et al. 2018). A colleague who runs our High Risk Clinic has found that administering measures every 3 months mitigates some of this iatrogenic distress (Robert Gregory, M.D., personal communication, June 2018).

Questions for the Supervisee

- What is your experience of using measurements or rating scales in your work with patients?

- Do you have concerns about including questionnaires or rating scales in treatment?

- Which scale(s) would you choose to use given the patient's intake packet?

- How soon do you expect to see change in the scale after this intervention?

- Are you surprised by the results you see? If yes, why? If no, why not?

- What else (besides your therapy or the meds) may be contributing to the change in the score?

- Do you plan to share the results of the scales with your patient? If so, under what circumstances? If not, why not?

Additional Resources

Fortney JC, Unutzer J, Wrenn G, et al: A tipping point for measurement-based care. Psychiatr Serv 68(2):179–188, 2017

Norcross JC (ed): Psychotherapy Relationships That Work: Evidence Based Responsiveness, 2nd Edition. New York, Oxford University Press, 2011

Kirkpatrick DL, Kirkpatrick JD: Evaluating Training Programs. San Francisco, CA Barrett-Koehler Publishers 1994

References

American Psychiatric Association: Cultural formulation, in Diagnostic and Statistical Manual of Mental Disorders, 5th Edition. Arlington, VA, American Psychiatric Association, 2013, pp 749–759

Barrett-Lennard GT: Dimensions of therapist responses as causal factors in therapeutic change. Psychological Monographs 76(43, 562), 1962

Beck AT, Steer RA, Brown GK: Beck Depression Inventory–II. San Antonio, TX, Psychological Corporation, 1996

Blackburn IM, James IA, Milne DL, et al: The Revised Cognitive Therapy Scale (CTS-R); psychometric properties. Behavioral and Cognitive Psychotherapy 29:431–446, 2001

de Jong K, Segaar J, Ingenhoven T, et al: Adverse effects of outcome monitoring feedback in patients with personality disorders: a randomized controlled trial in day treatment and inpatient settings. J Pers Disord 32(3):393–413, 2018 28594629

Dewan M, Walia K, Meszaros ZS, et al: Using Meaningful Outcomes to Differentiate Change from Innovation in Medical Education. Acad Psychiatry 41(1):100–105, 2017 26976400

Faustman WO, Overall JE: Brief Psychiatric Rating Scale, in The Use of Psychological Testing for Treatment Planning and Outcomes Assessment. Edited by Maruish ME. Mahwah, NJ, Erlbaum, 1999, pp 791–830

Fortney JC, Unützer J, Wrenn G, et al: A tipping point for measurement-based care. Psychiatr Serv 68(2):179–188, 2017 27582237

Hawkins EJ, Lambert MJ, Vermeersch DA, et al: The therapeutic effects of providing patient progress information to therapists and patients. Psychother Res 14:308–327, 2004

Hilsenroth MJ, Bonge DR, Blagys MD, et al: Measuring psychodynamic-interpersonal and cognitive-behavioral techniques: development of the comparative psychotherapy process scale. Psychotherapy: Theory, Research, Practice, Training 42:340–356, 2005

Horvath AO, Greenberg LS: Development and validation of the Working Alliance Inventory. Journal of Counseling Psychology 36(2):223-233, 1989

Kirkpatrick DL, Kirkpatrick JD: Evaluating Training Programs. San Francisco, CA, Barrett-Koehler, 1994

Lambert M, Hawkins E: Measuring outcome in professional practice: considerations in selecting and using brief outcome instruments. Prof Psychol Res Pr 35(5):492–499, 2004

Lambert M, Shimokawa K: Collecting client feedback, in Psychotherapy Relationships That Work: Evidence-Based Responsiveness, 2nd Edition. Edited by Norcross JC. New York, Oxford University Press, 2011, pp 202–223

Löwe B, Kroenke K, Herzog W, et al: Measuring depression outcome with a brief self-report instrument: sensitivity to change of the Patient Health Questionnaire (PHQ-9). J Affect Disord 81(1):61–66, 2004 15183601

Manring J, Greenberg RP, Gregory R, et al: Learning psychotherapy in the digital age. Psychotherapy (Chic) 48(2):119–126, 2011 21639655

Simmons J, Roberge L, Kendrick SB Jr, Richards B: The interpersonal relationship in clinical practice. The Barrett-Lennard Relationship Inventory as an assessment instrument. Eval Health Prof 18(1):103–112, 1995 10140858

Spitzer RL, Kroenke K, Williams JB, et al: A brief measure for assessing generalized anxiety disorder: the GAD-7. Arch Intern Med 166(10):1092–1097, 2006 16717171

Chapter 43 Neuroscience in Clinical Supervision

Toward a Neurobiopsychosocial Approach

Kristin S. Raj, M.D.

Agnes Kalinowski, M.D., Ph.D.

Belinda S. Bandstra, M.D., M.A.

Historically, neurology and psychiatry were considered a single branch of medicine. In the twentieth century, a separation evolved whereby neurological conditions were "brain disorders" and psychiatric conditions were "mental disorders" (Baker et al. 2002). In several cases, once a specific brain lesion or cause was thought to be identified for a mental disorder, its classification was switched from psychiatric to neurological. With the advent of functional brain scans allowing us to visualize brain regions and circuits involved in psychiatric disorders, there has been a rapid progression of recognizing psychiatric "mental" conditions as "brain" conditions. For psychiatrists to remain at the forefront of evidence-based understanding, prevention, and treatment of psychiatric conditions, it is essential to incorporate clinical neuroscience into psychiatry training, especially in clinical supervision (Insel and Quirion 2005; Schildkrout et al. 2016). The future of our understanding of psychiatric conditions will include biomarkers, cognitive tasks, and neuroimaging, and psychiatrists need to be versed in these topics as diagnosis and treatments continue to evolve.

Key Points

- Psychiatrists need to learn neuroscience as the clinical applicability of the science continues to grow.

- Supervision can be a key learning space for teaching neuroscience due to the benefits of the individual or small-group learning environment and opportunities for case-based learning.

- Incorporation of neuroscience formulation as part of case conceptualization in supervision is an effective teaching strategy.

- Integrating neuroscience into supervision settings can serve three purposes: 1) enhance understanding of patient cases, 2) offer new ways to help patients make sense of what they are experiencing, and 3) inform treatment options.

Enhancing Understanding of a Patient Case

As neuroscience becomes increasingly clinically relevant, biopsychosocial formulations can be expanded into neurobiopsychosocial case conceptualizations (Silbersweig 2015). This parallels the field's movement toward utilizing neuropsychiatric domains in research, as reflected by the National Institute of Mental Health's Research Domain Criteria (RDoC) versus traditional DSM criteria (Insel 2014). The RDoC lists five higher-level domains of human behavior and functioning that are meant to capture the breadth of contemporary knowledge about major systems of emotion, cognition, motivation, and social behavior. Within each of these domains, RDoC identifies dimensional psychological concepts called *constructs*. Although developed for research purposes and not at present intended to guide diagnostic criteria, it can serve as a gateway to teaching a brain-based conceptualization. For example, a supervisor and supervisee might consider together how a patient's presenting symptoms map on to specific RDoC constructs (Ramage et al. 2018). This exercise may help supervisees find patterns among different groups of patients with the same diagnosis. It may also help supervisees recognize questions or concepts that they have not yet considered but would like to explore with their patients. For additional neuroscience formulations in the literature, see "Additional Resources."

Offering New Ways to Talk to Patients

One can also use supervision to discuss how a supervisee would talk to patients about the effect of their brain's functioning on their symptoms. Although it has yet to be formally studied, integrating neuroscience into discussions about diagnoses has been noted clinically to be useful and validating to certain patients, especially those who may worry or have been told that their symptoms are "made up" or "all in their heads." One strategy is to use supervision to role-play how this discussion could go. This can foster curiosity and engagement: As a patient, what questions about the brain are likely to arise? What would matter to a patient? It can also allow one to rehearse how to translate scientific knowledge to a patient in a relevant and accurate fashion.

Informing Treatment Options

Psychiatry is in the process of elucidating how to select neuroscience-informed treatment modalities for a specific patient (e.g., selection of psychotherapy vs. medication as first-line for a patient with depression, prediction of lithium response in a patient with bipolar disorder with the use of imaging). Supervisors and supervisees can review studies together to stay at the forefront of the field, as well as to foster excitement about neuroscience. One method is to consult accessible and manageable resources: review articles, books, and tools such as videos on the National Neuroscience Curriculum Initiative website (see "Additional Resources"). Another method is to collaborate with neuroscientists if possible: some may be as interested in a clinical perspective as clinicians are in a neuroscientific one. If experts are available, one can organize an interdisciplinary case conference that includes neurologists, neuropsychologists, radiologists, neuroscientists, and psychiatric geneticists (Benjamin et al. 2014).

Case Example

You are the supervising attending in a general psychiatry clinic, and your resident presents the following case:

> A 43-year-old woman with history of childhood trauma presents to clinic asking for help in gaining more control over episodes of binge eating. She reports using eating to cope with stress and feels badly about herself for this. She doesn't believe this is a "disorder," saying rather that she should just have more control, and that she only presented because her partner insisted she come to clinic.

How might you supervise a resident in integrating neuroscience in this case using the above approaches?

Enhancing Understanding of a Patient Case

A quick attempt to map this case onto RDoC domains and constructs yields a number of questions that the supervisor and supervisee could clarify to better understand the case. For example, in looking at the constructs Initial Responsiveness to Reward Attainment and Habit, one could further explore in supervision if the patient experiences a positive sensation when she eats, or if she eats more compulsively, without conscious awareness or oversight. This may be a helpful question to ask to tease out what kind of treatment she would most benefit from. Another area to further learn about is her cognition—in particular her Cognitive Control and ability to inhibit thoughts and responses or get tasks done; what is learned may impact her treatment significantly. Furthermore, the supervisor and supervisee could investigate Systems for Social Processes, or how much these episodes are affected by her brain's responses to interpersonal settings.

Offering New Ways to Talk to Patients

The patient doesn't believe this is a "disorder," and she gives herself a hard time around her difficulty controlling her eating. This might be a patient for whom the message that her behaviors are brain-mediated might be really powerful. The supervisor and supervisee could role-play how to discuss with the patient that the relationship (circuitry) between different parts of her brain may be overactive or underactive, leading to these behavioral patterns, and that treatment might help to regulate these circuits.

Informing Treatment Options

Finally, considering how neuroscience might inform the treatment planning would be important. The supervisor and supervisee might plan to take a quick look at the literature before the next visit with the patient to see if there are any studies about this. In the meantime, the supervisor and supervisee already know that the questions generated in their attempt at formulation will lead them to consider her evidence-based treatment options with a more complete appreciation of her experience.

Specific Challenges and Strategies

- **I feel hesitant about incorporating neuroscience into supervision because I'm not that familiar with what is clinically applicable in the field myself.** Do not fear—you and many psychiatrists are in the same boat! Psychiatrists who feel hesitant may find it helpful to begin by familiarizing themselves with the neuroscience that is most widely applicable to the patient population with whom they regularly work. For example, the reward circuit is a very relevant neuroscience topic for addiction specialists. Practice generating a brain-based question around each patient that supervisees see, and engage in real-time co-investigation into resources to answer questions together. Also consider social neuroscience, such as the neurobiology of social bonds, attachment, and resilience.
- **If we focus on neuroscience too much in psychiatry, I'm afraid that psychotherapy and the value of the therapeutic alliance will fall by the wayside in supervision.** Therapeutic alliance and a rich and multidimensional understanding of our patients' lives should continue to be a cornerstone of our field. Rather than detract from this, an understanding of an individual's brain can serve to further deepen an understanding of the individual. There is evidence that understanding more about an individual's brain and imaging biomarkers may help guide which treatment will be most beneficial (McGrath et al. 2013). Additionally, there may be some people for whom openly discussing their individual neuroscience will be particularly helpful in their treatment, as a means of destigmatization and self-conceptualization. For others, it may not be helpful, because they may feel such information is reductionistic or feel not fully understood. In this way, the alliance will prove continually necessary to provide individualized discussion and care.

Questions for the Supervisee

- What do we know (or what might we postulate) from the neuroscience literature that might be helpful in conceptualizing the case?

- Are there any RDoC domains in which your patient seems to have problems? Strengths? Does thinking about this add any dimension to our understanding of them that their diagnosis doesn't convey?

- Do you think that providing some education to your patient about this aspect of how their brain might be working would be helpful to them?

- Does the neuroscience support the use of a particular treatment?

Additional Resources

Center on the Developing Child: https://developingchild.harvard.edu/
   Presents summary of scientific findings related to neurobiology of brain development in format meant for a wide audience.
The Dana Foundation, The Dana Alliance for Brain Initiatives: www.dana.org
   A nonprofit organization committed to advancing public awareness about the progress and promise of brain research and to disseminating information on the brain in an understandable and accessible fashion.

Neuroscience Behind Various Disorders

Genes to Cognition: http://www.g2conline.org

Research Domain Criteria (RDoC)

National Institute of Mental Health's Research Domain Criteria (RDoC): https://www.nimh.nih.gov/research-priorities/rdoc/index.shtml

Social Neuroscience Resources

National Neuroscience Curriculum Initiative: www.NNCIonline.org
Nature.com: https://www.nature.com/subjects/social-neuroscience

Select Journals With Clinical Psychiatric Neuroscience Reviews

Trends in Neurosciences
Trends in Cognitive Sciences
Biological Psychiatry

Neuroscience Formulations: Examples of Clinical Cases

Ramage T, Bandstra BS, Williams L: RDoC: the card game. National Neuroscience Curriculum Initiative, 2018. Available at: http://www.nncionline.org/course/rdoc-the-card-game/. Accessed August 21, 2018.
Ross DA, Arbuckle MR, Travis MJ, et al: An integrated neuroscience perspective on formulation and treatment planning for posttraumatic stress disorder. JAMA Psychiatry 74(4):407, 2017

Torous J, Stern AP, Padmanabhan JL, et al: A proposed solution to integrating cognitive-affective neuroscience and neuropsychiatry in psychiatry residency training: the time is now. Asian Journal of Psychiatry 17:116–121, 2015

Vanden Bussche AB, Haug NA, Ball TM, et al: Utilizing a transdiagnostic neuroscience-informed approach to differentiate the components of a complex clinical presentation: a case report. Personalized Medicine in Psychiatry 3:30–37, 2017

Yager J, Feinstein RE: Potential applications of the national institute of mental health's research domain criteria (RDoC) to clinical psychiatric practice. J Clin Psychiatry 78(4):423–432, 2017

References

Baker MG, Kale R, Menken M: The wall between neurology and psychiatry. BMJ 324(7352):1468–1469, 2002 12077018

Benjamin S, Widge A, Shaw K: Neuropsychiatry and neuroscience milestones for general psychiatry trainees. Acad Psychiatry 38(3):275–282, 2014 24715675

Insel TR: The NIMH Research Domain Criteria (RDoC) Project: precision medicine for psychiatry. Am J Psychiatry 171(4):395–397, 2014 24687194

Insel TR, Quirion R: Psychiatry as a clinical neuroscience discipline. JAMA 294(17):2221–2224, 2005 16264165

McGrath CL, Kelley ME, Holtzheimer PE, et al: Toward a neuroimaging treatment selection biomarker for major depressive disorder. JAMA Psychiatry 70(8):821–829, 2013 23760393

Ramage T, Bandstra BS, Williams L: RDoC: the card game. National Neuroscience Curriculum Initiative, 2018. Available at: http://www.nncionline.org/course/rdoc-the-card-game/. Accessed August 21, 2018.

Schildkrout B, Benjamin S, Lauterbach MD: Integrating neuroscience knowledge and neuropsychiatric skills into psychiatry: the way forward. Acad Med 91(5):650–656, 2016 26630604

Silbersweig DA: Bridging the brain-mind divide in psychiatric education: The neuro-bio-psychosocial formulation. Asian J Psychiatr 17:122–123, 2015 26464238

Chapter 44 Suicide and Suicidal Behaviors

Supervising Adverse Outcomes

Deepak Prabhakar, M.D., M.P.H.

Lisa MacLean, M.D.

Esther Akinyemi, M.D.

From 1994 through 2014, there was a 24% rise in the U.S. national suicide rate; at 13 per 100,000, the suicide rate in 1994 was the highest it had been in the previous 30 years (Curtin et al. 2016). Even with the ongoing research, increased recognition of risk factors, and available treatments, the suicide rate increased across all age groups (ages 10–74 years) in the United States (Centers for Disease Control and Prevention 2014). The increase in the suicide rate brings attention to ongoing education and development of effective suicide prevention strategies (Swanson et al. 2015), so one must also take into account the impact of suicide on the lives of near and dear ones, including providers and especially those in training (Prabhakar et al. 2013). Providers experience myriad emotions following a patient's death by suicide; some may even experience stress comparable to that experienced with the loss of a parent (Chemtob et al. 1988). Further, the impact can be especially devastating to a less-experienced clinician, particularly supervisees (Fang et al. 2007). Supervisees often care for the most challenging patients and are prone to experiencing a sense of personal failure in the event of patient suicide (Brown 1987). Considering that many of the risk factors related to suicide can change during the course of treatment, effective supervision offers an opportunity to address questions and concerns related to patient suicide while helping nurture the career and growth of both supervisors and supervisees.

Key Points

- Supervisors are expected to assess for supervisee knowledge gaps and be aware of useful evidence-based strategies to mitigate the risk of suicide.

- If the supervisee is providing treatment to a patient at higher risk for suicide, the supervisor should consider more intensive and even daily or weekly supervision.

- The impact of patient suicide (or any adverse outcome) on supervisors and supervisees is often a neglected area of clinical medicine, and most institutions do not have specific curriculum to address the negative impact of this serious event.

- Supervisees are especially at increased risk of negative consequences related to patient suicide. This is particularly true of supervisees in the early years of training.

- Supervision offers a useful opportunity to address not only pertinent suicide-related issues for specific patients but also the emotional and educational needs of supervisees.

The Psychiatric Diagnosis

Most individuals who die by suicide have a psychiatric illness; many times, these conditions are underappreciated and left untreated. In patients with suicide-related behaviors, supervision must address the supervisee's knowledge base to clarify the patient's diagnosis and ensure that the management plan for the psychiatric condition is appropriate. Furthermore, supervisees should be knowledgeable about risk factors and warning signs that may help to adequately assess and treat the suicidal patient. The importance of corroborating factors such as substance abuse, life stressors, and medical illnesses should also be underscored when applicable. In the event a knowledge deficit is identified, the supervisor should teach to these gaps assigning readings as indicated.

Assessment of Suicidal Behavior and Suicide Risk

The supervisor should review with the supervisee the assessment of the patient's suicidal behavior, including not only the frequency, intensity, and duration but also the antecedents and consequences of these behaviors. The patient's degree of hopelessness, ability to tolerate negative emotions, and environment stressors should be assessed. A focus on reasons to survive versus reasons to end one's life can help the patient work toward finding effective risk mitigation strategies. The assessment should be treatment focused and reinforce alternatives the patient has to deal with his or her problems (Chiles et al. 2019). Additionally, the supervisor should review with the supervisee the creation of an effective safety plan to prevent suicide. This includes helping the patient to specify steps he or she can take when suicidal to soothe himself or herself, to identify important reasons to live, and to move toward focusing on positive thoughts when suicidal. Finally, the supervisor should ensure that the supervisee has educated the patient about who the patient can call or where he or she should go if these coping strategies do not work.

Chronically Suicidal Patients

Working with chronically suicidal patients is a challenge for any clinician and can be especially anxiety provoking for supervisees. These patients often experience long-term difficulty with emotional dysregulation and psychosocial functioning. Chronically suicidal patients often describe pervasive maladaptive responses that are persistent, resistant to change, and self-defeating. The supervisor must help the supervisee to focus on breaking patterns of dysfunctional behavior by helping the supervisee see the world through the eyes of the patient and to label these dysfunctional behaviors so that action can be taken to mitigate and reduce suicidal thinking. Effective treatment avoids confrontation and focuses on problem-solving skills. Though some may feel compelled to repeatedly hospitalize the patient, there is little evidence to support this as an effective strategy of care, and this should be adequately addressed in supervision. If inpatient hospitalization is needed, it should be for acute stabilization and involve a short stay with specific treatment goals (Chiles et al. 2019). Supervision should also address other potential knowledge gaps and clinical skills that may help address suicidal behaviors, including evidence-based suicide mitigation strategies, such as dialectical behavior therapy, cognitive-behavioral therapy, and medications with antisuicidal properties such as clozapine and lithium for specific conditions.

Suicidal Fantasy and Contagion

Supervisors should help supervisees explore patients' suicidal fantasies. Patients who express suicidal thinking may have powerful fantasies that their death will be better for those around them. They may feel they cannot measure up to their fantasies of self-perfection and believe that suicide is the only viable option (Smith and Eyman 1988). Working in supervision to process these unrealistic fantasies will help the supervisee to develop strategies to address these thoughts and help the patient to develop a more moderate expectation of self. Additionally, a suicidal patient may have a strong desire for revenge and have an intense wish to destroy the lives of others through his or her suicide. Or the patient may have reunion fantasies in which he or she hopes to be reunited with a loved one. The more these fantasies are explored, the more the patient may be able to see other possible alternatives to continue to live with his or her inner pain instead of dying by suicide (Gabbard 2014). Similarly, issues related to contagion of suicide or suicide-related behaviors should be addressed in supervision; even though the "copy-cat" phenomenon is well addressed in popular press, providers often miss an opportunity to discuss the impact of suicide on the community and their own patients.

Countertransference

Supervisors should help supervisees and other providers improve their skills in dealing with suicidality by helping them to explore their own individual emotional responses to these unpredictable patients. Emotional responses could include anger, hopelessness, wariness, resignation, passivity, powerlessness, and ambivalence. Helping the supervisee to continue to treat the patient and not react negatively is part of the supervisory process. Supervisees should also be encouraged to explore their moral, religious, and personal values, which could impact their ability to effectively treat a suicidal patient and interfere with a person's ability to pick the best evidence-based treatment strategy. Rescue fantasies are common among people who enter into helping professions. In their role as healers, supervisees may fail to see how their actions could lead them down a slippery slope. What starts out as ethical and caring could quickly become a professional boundary violation. The key to avoiding these transgressions is to recognize them early on and address them actively in supervision (Gabbard 2017).

Practical Strategies
Missed Appointments

Supervision should address the need to call a suicidal patient who misses an appointment and to document this telephone call in the patient's chart. If a message is left and the patient does not return the call, a letter should be sent. If a patient misses two consecutive appointments or this behavior becomes a pattern, it should be discussed with the patient. If the supervisee is concerned about the patient's safety, the supervisee with the support of the supervisor, could reach out to the patient's family or call the police and have them go to the person's home to check on him or her. The supervisee should always seek consultation with his or her supervisor to discuss therapeutic issues and to determine the continuation of treatment if the pattern of missing appointments persists (Gabbard 2017).

Suicide Contracts

Suicide contracts have not been shown to reduce suicide. Providers who use this method could falsely believe that they have reduced a patient's risk for suicide when they have not. Use of this prevention method may cause providers to be less vigilant despite increasing suicide risk. The use of suicide contracts should be discouraged in supervision (Rudd et al. 2006).

Safety Plan

A good safety plan is a collaborative strategic document developed by the provider and the patient. The plan addresses 1) warning signs that are generally identified as antecedents to suicidal behaviors, 2) internal positive coping strategies such as physical activity or relaxations techniques, 3) people and personal/professional contacts to whom the patient can reach out for support and care in times of crisis, and 4) suggestions (removing weapons, alcohol) for making the immediate environment safe. Supervision must also address specific practical strategies that may be used to decrease a person's social isolation, increase their physical activity, and help develop other coping skills (Chiles et al. 2019).

Supervision Considerations for Attempted Suicide

In the event of a suicide attempt, a supervisor needs to immediately reach out to a supervisee to assess both the clinical situation and the well-being of the supervisee. A suicide attempt can shake the confidence of a supervisee. The first goal will be to stabilize the patient and ensure his or her safety. Involving the patient's family and other support systems during this high-risk time can help to reduce patient's suicidal thinking. Once the patient is stabilized, supervisor and supervisee should explore their emotional reactions in the supervision encounter.

Supervision Considerations for Death by Suicide

The impact of a suicide on a treatment provider can be profound. Supervisees often experience feelings of anger, guilt, shame, bitterness and helplessness after a patient-suicide, coupled with loss of self-efficacy and knowledge gaps such as believing that suicide can be predicted, many consider a change in career after the death of a patient by suicide (Prabhakar et al. 2014). Initial reactions may be that of shock, numbing, sadness, dissociation, and experiencing intrusive thoughts (Prabhakar et al. 2014). Supervision must help explore a supervisees' concerns about continuing in the field and their fear about suicide in other patients, anger, confusion, guilt, helplessness, and loss of self-esteem. Some supervisees may immediately feel vulnerable and fear outside criticism or a lawsuit. Although some supervisees may see the suicide as a betrayal, others may identify with the death. Significant anxiety and feelings of horror have been described in the literature (Plakun and Tillman 2005). In some instances, a patient suicide may cause a supervisees to have a greater appreciation for their own limitations. They may grieve the loss of how they previously viewed themselves as a professional. Responses to a patient suicide are variable, with some supervisees building their suicide prevention skills and others refusing to treat high acuity and suicidal patients (Kleespies et al. 1993). Supervision should help address any of these concerns to help meet the needs of supervisees on either end of the emotional response spectrum, including thoughts of perceived failure (Figueroa and Dalack 2013; Prabhakar et al. 2013).

The loss of patient to suicide is devastating at any point in a person's career, but especially distressing when a person is still in training. Effective supervision offers an opportunity to help address some of these issues in order to mitigate the impact of patient suicide on supervisees. The supervisor should listen empathically without blame or judgment and not be quick to prematurely reassure the supervisee and thereby minimize the supervisee's distress or invalidate his or her feelings. The supervisor needs to encourage the supervisee, normalize the grief experience, and help him or her effectively address personal needs. There is opportunity to explore what the trainee learned from this experience. Ultimately, supervisors can contribute to promoting a culture of caring and support by helping their trainees to understand that in the psychiatric profession, exposure to suicide or suicide related behaviors is inevitable and a sequela of severe mental illness. Further, supervisors should address and encourage self-care by appropriately suggesting time away from clinical care, addressing grief, reducing isolation, and ultimately fostering resilience. See Table 44–1 for specific guidelines for supervisors and supervisees after a patient suicide.

Specific Challenges and Strategies

- **My supervisee is anxious about risk management in the event of a patient suicide.** Supervisors must pay attention to addressing any concerns related to this issue by emphasizing the productive and collaborative nature of the quality assurance process. It should be emphasized that the focus of risk management is on improving process and providing logistic support to the providers.
- **My supervisee has feelings of hopelessness about the patient.** Supervisors should pay attention to the unique countertransference reactions and address these in a timely manner. Supervisees may also benefit from learning specific therapeutic strategies addressing hopelessness in suicidal patients.
- **My supervisee has received threats of suicide from his patient.** It is not uncommon for supervisees to receive written or voice messages from patients threatening suicide. The supervisee should be encouraged to prospectively develop a team of concerned family members and friends with the patient's consent as a part of her safety plan. In these scenarios, if the patient is unreachable, the supervisee can reach out to the individuals who were identified by the patient earlier. In rare scenarios, in order to protect life, the local police department may be alerted.

Questions for the Supervisee

■ How did you learn about the patient suicide?

■ What are your concerns?

■ Are you worried about the documentation that was completed at the time of last visit?

■ Do you have a support system?

■ Is the training program supporting you and providing appropriate resources?

■ Do you have questions about condolence cards or attending the funeral service?

TABLE 44–1.	Patient suicide guidelines for supervision

For supervisees

A. Immediate

    a. Avoid isolation.

    b. Notify supervisor (if trainees, notify training director).

    c. Contact hospital attorney or insurance carrier.

    d. Consider contacting family.

        i. Plan in advance how you will manage the confidentiality boundary.

        ii. Consult with risk management to help think through unforeseen circumstances.

        iii. Offer a blame-free, nonjudgmental, nondefensive space to recognize and contain their grief and anger.

        iv. Offer your genuine condolences and state your sorrow without self-criticism.

    e. Consider attending funeral with family's permission.

B. Intermediate

    a. Take care of your need to mourn and seek help if needed.

    b. Consider time away from work.

    c. Address countertransference reaction in supervision.

    d. Do not second-guess treatment decisions. There is no evidence that suicide can be predicted.

    e. Seek support from supervisor, colleagues, and significant others.

C. Later

    a. Review the chart but never ever change anything.

    b. Consider writing a case summary for supervision.

    c. Participate in a psychological autopsy or case review, which should provide support and focus on understanding the events and examining the procedures with the goal of improving care.

    d. Attend to and address self-care needs. Be patient with yourself.

For institution and supervisors

A. Before the adverse event:

    a. Train faculty on supervisory issues pertaining to patient suicide.

    b. Schedule regularly occurring process groups to address adverse events.

    c. Educate all supervisees about adverse events.

    d. Educate all supervisees on self-care and burnout.

TABLE 44–1.   **Patient suicide guidelines for supervision** *(continued)*

For institution and supervisors *(continued)*

B. During the adverse event:

    a. Collect information on the adverse event.

    b. Support supervisees and providers in communicating with other members of the team.

    c. Validate immediate cognitive and emotional reaction.

    d. Ensure adequate and appropriate documentation.

    e. Ensure notification to appropriate individuals in the chain of command.

C. After the adverse event

    a. Maintain regular contact.

    b. Program directors should reach out to the trainee(s) involved in the adverse event.

    c. Provide opportunities for individual debriefing with trainee(s) involved in the adverse event.

    d. Provide opportunities for focus groups.

    e. Empower and train peers to be supportive.

Additional Resources

Collaborative Assessment and Management of Suicidality (CAMS): https://cams-care.com

American Foundation for Suicide Prevention (AFSP): https://afsp.org

Now Matters Now: https://www.nowmattersnow.org/skills

Zero Suicide: http://zerosuicide.sprc.org

References

Brown HN: The impact of suicide on therapists in training. Compr Psychiatry 28(2):101–112, 1987 3829653

Centers for Disease Control and Prevention: CDC National Health Report Highlights. Atlanta, GA, Centers for Disease Control and Prevention, 2014

Chemtob CM, Hamada RS, Bauer G, et al: Patients' suicides: frequency and impact on psychiatrists. Am J Psychiatry 145(2):224–228, 1988 3341466

Chiles JA, Strosahl KD, Roberts LW: Clinical Manual for Assessment and Treatment of Suicidal Patients, 2nd Edition. Washington, DC, American Psychiatric Association Publishing, 2019

Curtin SC, Warner M, Hedegaard H: Increase in Suicide in the United States, 1999–2014. NCHS Data Brief, No 241. Hyattsville, MD, National Center for Health Statistics, Centers for Disease Control and Prevention. 2016

Fang F, Kemp J, Jawandha A, et al: Encountering patient suicide: a resident's experience. Acad Psychiatry 31(5):340–344, 2007 17875615

Figueroa S, Dalack GW: Exploring the impact of suicide on clinicians: a multidisciplinary retreat model. J Psychiatr Pract 19(1):72–77, 2013 23334682

Gabbard GO: Psychodynamic Psychiatry in Clinical Practice, 5th Edition. Arlington, VA, American Psychiatric Publishing, 2014

Gabbard GO: Long-Term Psychodynamic Psychotherapy: A Basic Text, 3rd Edition. Washington, DC, American Psychiatric Association Publishing, 2017

Kleespies PM, Penk WE, Forsyth JP: The stress of patient suicidal behavior during clinical training: incidence, impact and recover. Prof Psychol Res Pr 24(3):293–303, 1993

Plakun EM, Tillman GG: Responding to clinicians after loss of a patient to suicide. Dir Psychiatry 25(26):301–310, 2005

Prabhakar D, Anzia JM, Balon R, et al: "Collateral damages": preparing residents for coping with patient suicide. Acad Psychiatry 37(6):429–430, 2013 23653109

Prabhakar D, Balon R, Anzia JM, et al: Helping psychiatry residents cope with patient suicide. Acad Psychiatry 38(5):593–597, 2014 24664605

Rudd MD, Mandrusiak M, Joiner TE Jr: The case against no-suicide contracts: the commitment to treatment statement as a practice alternative. J Clin Psychol 62(2):243–251, 2006 16342293

Smith K, Eyman J: Ego structure and object differentiation in suicidal patients, in Primitive Mental States of the Rorschach. Edit by Learner HD, Learner PM. Madison, CT, International Universities Press, 1988, pp 176–202

Swanson JW, Bonnie RJ, Appelbaum PS: Getting serious about reducing suicide: more "how" and less "why." JAMA 314(21):2229–2230, 2015 26524461

Chapter 45 Supervision in a Specialty Clinic

A New Frontier

Katherine E. Williams, M.D.

Thalia Robakis, M.D., Ph.D.

"Best practices" for supervision in specialty psychiatry clinics are a new frontier for academic psychiatry research. Over the past 20 years, one of the notable developments in psychiatry and psychology education has been the opportunity for advanced practicum work in many types of specialty clinics, such as women's mental health, eating disorders, obsessive-compulsive and related disorders, impulse disorders, and sports psychiatry and psychology.

To date, there is very little written to guide "best practices" for supervision in these specialty clinics. For some of the specialty clinics, educational objectives are shaped by established Accreditation Council for Graduate Medical Education (ACGME) fellowship criteria, such as those of addiction medicine or geriatric psychiatry (Accreditation Council for Graduate Medical Education 2017a, 2017b). However, most of the recently developed specialty clinic opportunities do not have an established ACGME curriculum, and historically, specialty clinic supervisors have developed their own educational objectives, materials, and supervision methods. Although patient populations and knowledge to be learned will vary from specialty clinic to specialty clinic, there are several shared challenges and opportunities for both supervisors and supervisees in this learning format.

Key Points

- A clear and consistent definition of specialty clinic patient populations is an integral responsibility of the supervisor in these clinics.

- There should be clearly articulated educational objectives that cover the content areas of the specialty and, when possible, be guided by the corresponding ACGME fellowship, or national specialty education committee, recommendations.

- Methods for assessing the attainment of specialized knowledge, such as examinations assessing mastery of fundamental concepts and skills in the specialty, should be used.

Developing Mastery

To facilitate the mastery of knowledge regarding the specialty, supervisors should provide clear educational objectives, as well as reading lists and representative articles.

Didactics

A separate group didactic session is an excellent method of facilitating this mastery and might ideally include lectures, case-based learning, and journal article reviews. A "flipped classroom" approach, in which trainees watch taped lectures from specialty clinic faculty prior to class and then work with instructors on representative cases, is a useful method (Prober and Heath 2012). The use of online "living" classrooms—learning management systems (LMS), where all PowerPoint slides, videos, and important articles can be easily accessed—is another very helpful method of encouraging mastery of core knowledge. Collaborative online case conferences including specialists from around the country are also a promising method of supervision (Lockhart et al. 2017). The use of pre- and posttests after lectures is yet another way to solidify core concepts and assess knowledge development.

Modeling

Refinement in evaluation of the specialty's patients is facilitated by modeling supervisor interview techniques. In some clinics, a one-way mirror is used, and the supervisor interviews the patient while trainees observe and take notes. Alternatively, the trainee may sit in the same room with the supervisor, and this method facilitates the patient's future work with the trainee, since the supervisor can explain to the patient that they will do the first part of the interview, and leave room for the resident—who will be their ongoing main physician—to complete the interview. For ongoing treatment in the specialty clinic, the supervisor and supervisee may make use of audiovisual techniques, as well as observations by the supervisor of the resident through the one-way mirror (see Chapter 9, "Video Recordings: Learning Through Facilitated Observation and Feedback," and Chapter 11, "Live Supervision: Behind the One-Way Mirror").

Patient Evaluation Methods

Supervisors should provide pertinent articles as well, to help the trainee understand the rationale for certain unique questions. Another important evaluation technique is the use of measures that are unique to the specialty clinic (see Chapter 42, "Integrating Measurement-Based Care Into Supervision"). Although most residents will enter their specialty clinic training with experience using the most common measures used in general psychiatry, such as the Patient Health Questionnaire–9 (PHQ-9) or the Generalized Anxiety Disorder–7 (GAD-7), many are unfamiliar with the measures used in individual specialty clinics, such as the Edinburgh Postnatal Depression Scale (EPDS), which is now recommended by multiple national medical organizations for screening depression in all perinatal women (Committee on Obstetric Practice 2015; Earls 2010; O'Connor et al. 2016).

Case Conferences

While weekly didactics are a key method of ensuring mastery of core knowledge in the specialty, an ideal learning format will also provide room for discussion of ongoing cases, and involvement of ancillary providers in the supervision in order for the trainees to learn about practice-based learning in the specialty. An important aspect of supervision in a specialty clinic is supervision around the unique role of the specialist within the greater health care delivery system. As a way of facilitating such supervision, nurses, social workers, and other medical specialists who interact regularly with the psychiatry specialist should be encouraged to attend group case conferences. Supervisors should observe trainees as they interact with these other health care providers and provide feedback to them about their interpersonal effectiveness.

Documentation

A very important aspect of practice-based learning in specialty clinics is the documentation of consultations. Specialty clinics vary in the types of communication generated. While it is expected that all of them generate a consultative report for referring clinicians, some of them also create written recommendations and reports for the patients. Consequently, a very important role of the supervisor in a specialty clinic is to create expectations for communications, review trainee write-ups, and provide direct feedback. Just as modeling interviews for trainees is recommended at the start of specialty rotations, providing sample write-ups is an excellent way to clarify best practices for communication within a specialty.

Keeping Abreast of the Literature

Some specialty clinics make generous use of references to recent research in their write-ups. Since the ability to analyze research in the field is an important core competency for specialty clinic training, supervisors should provide opportunities in the didactic sessions to review seminal articles in the field. Just as the supervisor should track the trainee's success in mastering core knowledge in the field, the supervisor should also track the trainee's success in mastering an understanding of what is not yet known in the field. What are the questions still to be answered by this specialty? What are the areas of research that need to be done?

Specific Challenges and Strategies

- **My resident is uncomfortable with "starting over" and is not interested in the unique specialty.** The specialty clinic rotation is usually an advanced rotation for psychiatry and psychology trainees, and some residents are very uncomfortable with "starting over" and learning a new subset of psychiatry. For many trainees, the specialty clinic is a desired elective; however, for some, it is a rotation that they have been assigned to, and they may have minimal interest in the unique patient population. To address these two challenges, faculty members should take extra care to create a supportive atmosphere where students feel free to ask even the most basic of questions. Starting the rotation with several opportunities for students to observe supervisors completing a model interview is a very useful method for helping students to feel more comfortable "starting over" and learning what specialized questions to ask. If a resident demonstrates disinterest in the specialty, the supervisor should help the trainee understand what the resistance is to the specialty, as this may help them become more engaged. This would be best done in individual supervision sessions, as it is important to create a sense of safety. Another method is to provide opportunities for directed reading on topics related to the specialty clinic that the student may be interested in that will enhance and deepen his or her overall experience. Another way to stimulate interest is to include guest speakers in the didactics that intersect with the specialty who can provide an example of the importance of the specialty to other fields.
- **My specialty clinic does not have an established curriculum.** Supervisors in specialty clinics without a well-developed national curriculum face the challenge of creating their own educational objectives, teaching materials and methods of student evaluation. One way to address this challenge is to partner with faculty in programs with similar specialty clinics. For instance, the National Task Force on Women's Reproductive Mental Health has created diverse educational materials (including videos and case-based learning exercises) for women's mental health clinics, in residency programs (Osborne et al. 2015).
- **There is too much to know and do; how can I also supervise?** Supervisors in specialty clinics are challenged by the constantly evolving fund of knowledge that they are expected to be experts in, and many are actively involved in ongoing research in their field. Furthermore, since they are specialists in the field, they are often taxed with providing care to some of the most challenging patients. One way to address this problem of overburdened supervisors is to encourage trainees to be responsible active learners. For instance, supervisors can share didactics with a trainee by providing them with PowerPoint presentations on a topic, and engaging them in updating the presentation with a literature review dated from the time of the last updated power point. The use of small private online courses is another method of leveraging "super specialists" within one's field. Another way to address this challenge of overextended faculty is to encourage the development of a fellowship program in the field at the residency, or an advanced specialty rotation so that students are teaching students.

Questions for the Supervisor

■ Has the trainee mastered the core fund of knowledge of the specialty?

■ Has the trainee demonstrated an appreciation for research methods used to determine this fund of knowledge?

■ Does the trainee know where to obtain ongoing "lifelong" learning in the specialty? Does he or she know the most relevant journals, societies, and committees?

■ Has the trainee demonstrated an ability to refine the clinical interview and use appropriate measures for this patient population?

■ Does the trainee demonstrate an appreciation for the role of other health care providers in this specialty area, and can he or she communicate effectively with them?

Additional Resources

Ross DA, Rohrbaugh R: Integrating neuroscience in the training of psychiatrists: a patient-centered didactic curriculum based on adult learning principles. Acad Psychiatry 38(2):154–62, 2014

Ross DA, Arbuckle M, Travis M: National Neuroscience Curriculum Initiative. Available at: http://www.nncionline.org.

References

Accreditation Council for Graduate Medical Education: ACGME program requirements for graduate medical education in geriatric psychiatry. July 1, 2017a. Available at: https://www.acgme.org/Portals/0/PFAssets/ProgramRequirements/407_geriatric_psych_2017-07-01.pdf. Accessed August 21, 2018.

Accreditation Council for Graduate Medical Education: ACGME program requirements for graduate medical education in addiction psychiatry. July 1, 2017b. Available at: https://www.acgme.org/Portals/0/PFAssets/ProgramRequirements/401_addiction_psych_2017-07-01.pdf?ver=2017-09-12-140227-900. Accessed August 21, 2018.

Committee on Obstetric Practice: The American College of Obstetricians and Gynecologists Committee Opinion No. 630. Screening for perinatal depression. Obstet Gynecol 125(5):1268–1271, 2015 25932866

Earls MF; Committee on Psychosocial Aspects of Child and Family Health American Academy of Pediatrics: Incorporating recognition and management of perinatal and postpartum depression into pediatric practice. Pediatrics 126(5):1032–1039, 2010 20974776

Lockhart BJ, Capurso NA, Chase I, et al: The use of a small private online course to allow educators to share teaching resources across diverse sites. The future of psychiatric case conferences? Acad Psychiatry 41(1):81–85, 2017 26620806

O'Connor E, Rossom RC, Henninger M, et al: Primary care screening for and treatment of depression in pregnant and postpartum women: evidence report and systematic review for the U.S. preventative task force. JAMA 315(4):388–406, 2016 26813212

Osborne LM, Hermann A, Burt V, et al; National Task Force on Women's Reproductive Mental Health: Reproductive psychiatry: the gap between clinical need and education. Am J Psychiatry 172(10):946–948, 2015 26423479

Prober CG, Heath C: Lecture halls without lectures—a proposal for medical education. N Engl J Med 366(18):1657–1659, 2012 22551125

Chapter 46

Supervision of Auxiliary Health Care Providers

Roles, Goals, and Learning Opportunities

Sheila Lahijani, M.D.

With a significant prevalence of mental health problems worldwide, enhanced methods of delivering care are needed to close the gap of psychiatric services by psychiatrists. In the United States alone, there is a shortage of psychiatrists and other mental health providers—particularly in rural regions, many urban neighborhoods, and community mental health centers (World Health Organization 2017). Psychiatric providers, including psychiatrists, advanced practice providers (nurse practitioners and physician assistants), social workers, and psychologists, will remain in demand in 2025, as projected by the National Council for Behavioral Health (National Council for Behavioral Health 2017) (Figure 46–1). As a result, psychiatrists play an important role in supervising expert auxiliary health care providers who often work closely with them. Implementing effective approaches for supervision and strategies to provide constructive feedback can facilitate these working relationships. Additionally, patient care can be optimized while providing opportunities for educational and professional development for all team members. In this chapter, I address salient points on how to cultivate both the relationships and the individual learning with the goal of utilizing the scope of expertise of all team members to provide comprehensive psychiatric care.

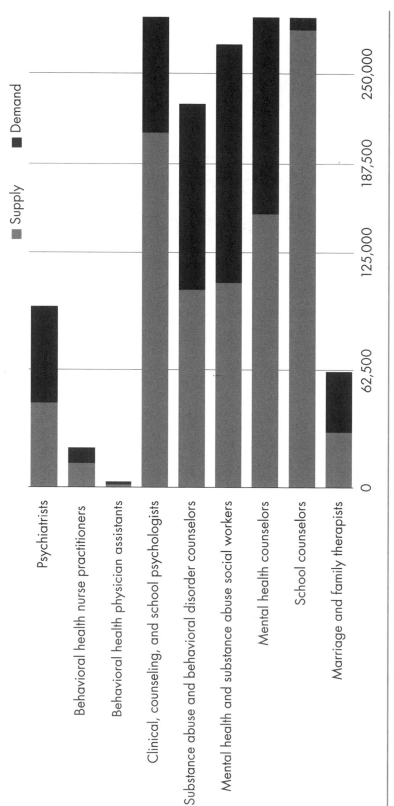

Figure 46–1. Projected surpluses and shortages of behavioral health practitioners full-time equivalents (FTEs) in 2025.

Source. Adapted from National Center for Health Workforce Analysis 2016.

Key Points

- Psychiatrists can play an important role in increasing access to care through supervising auxiliary health care providers.

- Auxiliary health care provider supervision is a function of the setting in which the care is delivered.

- Various approaches to supervision can be used to manage challenging clinical cases with multi-professional teams.

- Psychiatrists can benefit from specialized training programs to develop expertise for supervision of auxiliary providers.

The Scope of Supervision

Nonphysician psychiatric providers include a wide range of professionals, such as advanced practice providers, social workers, marriage and family therapists, and psychiatric and neurologic pharmacists, who have separate training, skill sets, certifications, clinical requirements, and memberships to national organizations. Furthermore, state medical boards determine the rules and regulations for these providers for their scope of practice. Depending on the setting, there may be one or more of these nonphysician clinicians working with a supervising provider, such as a psychiatrist.

Supervision of auxiliary health providers can help standardize diagnostic and therapeutic methods and serve to validate decisions in complex and challenging clinical situations, such as those found in acute medical settings like an emergency department, as well as improve liaison responsibilities of these providers who often interface with nonpsychiatric providers. Supervision in this context includes the monitoring, including providing guidance and feedback on, matters of personal, professional, and educational development in patient care. Assessment of strengths and weaknesses of the auxiliary care provider can not only identify areas for improvement but also promote patient safety (Woltmann et al. 2012).

Supervision of auxiliary care providers can also foster reflection on difficult encounters with patients and staff as well as provide opportunities for supporting the auxiliary provider's role. This is particularly germane to multiprofessional settings where the auxiliary care provider may communicate and collaborate with several providers at a time, serving as a liaison as well as a specialist. An example of this includes a psychiatric nurse practitioner who is a consultant to the cardiac surgery service in evaluating and managing a patient with schizophrenia hospitalized with an aortic dissection. In this setting, the psychiatric nurse practitioner is providing psychiatric services, including bedside supportive psychotherapy and offering of antipsychotic treatment, while simultaneously collaborating with cardiac surgery team members. This psychiatric nurse practitioner serves as the primary psychiatric provider to the surgical team while presenting the clinical data and making recommendations under the supervision of a psychiatrist who may not regularly collaborate with the consulting team. Supervision by the psychiatrist would offer guidance in therapeutic planning while also promoting the role of the psychiatric nurse practitioner as the primary psychiatric provider. Thus, understanding the ecosystem in which the auxiliary care provider is working can contribute to better clinical decision making while supporting the morale of team members and enhancing the quality of care for patients.

The Supervisor's Responsibility

Communication is of absolute importance to ensure that the medical, ethical, and legal responsibilities toward the patient are met (American Psychiatric Association 1980). Clinical supervision of auxiliary providers may have positive effects on outcomes, and the lack of supervision may subsequently result in negative outcomes for patients. Effective supervision is dependent on the relationship between the supervisor and the supervisee (Kilminster and Jolly 2000). A supervising psychiatrist therefore should undergo his or her own training, continued learning, self-assessment, and evaluation by the auxiliary providers to optimize his or her competence as a supervisor.

In a supervisory relationship of an auxiliary provider, the supervising provider is directly responsible for the patient's care and provides instruction and guidance that are congruent with the auxiliary care provider's training and expertise. For example, when a psychiatrist is supervising a clinical social worker, the psychiatrist may offer direction related to psychopharmacological regimens and recommend further diagnostic evaluation in the form of biomarkers and brain imaging; this augments the educational and experiential scope of the clinical social worker while supporting that auxiliary provider's own expertise and skill set. The supervising psychiatrist's responsibility extends throughout the duration of supervising the social worker. Implicit in this cross-disciplinary relationship is shared responsibility for the patient's care that is in accordance with the qualifications and limitations of the social worker. A patient may independently seek the services of a nonphysician clinician, at which point the psychiatrist would no longer have a supervisory role (American Psychiatric Association 1980).

The Structure of Supervision

Because of the wide range of training and competence among auxiliary care providers, determining the exact amount of supervision, consultation, or collaboration between the auxiliary care providers and supervising psychiatrists is difficult. Understanding the training, certification, and clinical experience of each auxiliary psychiatric provider by a supervisor is paramount for effective multiprofessional collaboration.

Supervision of auxiliary providers should have structure, which includes rules and learning objectives, while offering flexibility, given the competing responsibilities that the auxiliary providers have (e.g., calling for collateral information, writing notes, writing prescriptions, disposition planning). What is effective and suitable for one group of auxiliary providers may not be for another group (e.g., clinical social workers vs. physician's assistants). Therefore, it may be worthwhile to undertake trials of both individual supervision and team supervision to provide both separate attention to each auxiliary provider as well as group support and guidance. The system within which the supervision is provided must both create and enforce a setting that allows access to supervision, feedback, and support for the supervisor and the supervisee (Hore et al. 2009).

Rules that pertain to supervision of auxiliary psychiatric providers vary in different states. Therefore, the supervision of the auxiliary provider is dependent on the setting in which he or she practices. The delegation of medical tasks must be appropriate to the skill level and competence of each auxiliary provider (Table 46–1). A written doc-

TABLE 46–1. Examples of psychiatric auxiliary care providers and interprofessional roles

Auxiliary psychiatric provider supervisee	Nurse practitioner	Physician assistant	Clinical social worker	Marriage and family therapist	Psychiatric and neurologic pharmacist
Interprofessional roles	Assess, diagnose, and manage mental health problems and psychiatric disorders. Train and support peers, including nurses, and nonpsychiatric providers, and others. Provide teaching and interdisciplinary education, including medical education. Seek and acquire professional development activities within a respective institution and more broadly. Manage resources and participate in cost effective clinical decision making. Perform disposition planning.			Diagnose and treat mental health problems and disorders with psychotherapy within the contexts of marriage, couples, and family systems.	Work collaboratively with teams to optimize drug therapy. Provide direct patient care, including treatment assessment and medication management activities.

ument or a guide may be created to outline the scope of practice and interprofessional responsibilities for the auxiliary provider and identify the practice arrangement between the supervisor and the auxiliary care provider. The format of supervision should be included in this guide. For example, the timing and frequency of the supervision may vary in an emergency department setting versus an integrated care setting, such as at a cancer center. The process for evaluating the supervisee's performance should be established from the beginning of the relationship to create accountability and offer a regular stream of feedback and opportunities for professional growth. Scheduled meetings in a private, nurturing environment can foster discussions about performance, areas for improvement and goals for professional development. Documentation of the meetings can offer further accountability and create benchmarks in the dyadic relationship. This is particularly important for auxiliary care providers who may otherwise function more autonomously yet have chosen to hold a position that requires supervision. For this reason, the mutual respect between a supervisor and the auxiliary care provider is a sine qua non for a productive and healthy professional relationship.

Specific Challenges and Strategies

- **My supervisee, a well-respected and skilled clinical social worker who develops strong therapeutic alliances with patients, lacks skills in developing differential diagnoses.** To manage this deficiency of a core competency, first identify what the social worker's education and training has been with regard to understanding psychiatric diagnoses. There is a wide range of variability, and it is best not to make assumptions about his or her background. After you ask some basic questions, it is worthwhile to learn what the social worker's previous work experience has been and if this is a competency that has not been developed in the past or is not part of the training repetoire. It is necessary to know if he or she is aware of this deficiency and is motivated to improve it. Next, develop a formal plan that may involve continued education and/or on-site learning by the psychiatrist supervisor as well as others. Offer all of this in concert with supporting the extant role of the social worker, identifying the strengths and expertise that the social worker possesses, and emphasizing the importance of professional development for all health care providers.
- **My supervisee is a nurse practitioner who has worked independently in prior jobs and currently is expressing frustration having less autonomy in his new role, which is contributing to some interpersonal challenges.** From the beginning, define the supervisory roles, differentiate them, and document this accordingly to promote transparency and to create a mutual and shared understanding of the dyadic relationship. Given his previous work experience and the need to now adapt to a role requiring supervision, a useful technique is to inquire what was fulfilling about his previous role and how can that be applied to his current role. Another technique is to reframe his being supervised as an opportunity for professional growth and advancement. To deliver and handle negative feedback from the nurse practitioner about his current role as a supervisee, create an environment that fosters listening and provides adequate time for discussion.

- **The physician assistant ordered the wrong dose of an antipsychotic, causing a patient to get overly sedated and hypotensive.** To manage this patient safety issue, it is best to separate out any of the emotion related to your reaction as the supervisor, despite possibly having direct responsibility for the error. Understand the root of the error and determine how much the auxiliary care provider's error was intentional or poorly planned. Providing opportunities in real time to do a root cause analysis and to discuss methods for improvement allows for more effective supervision and prevents rupturing the relationship with the supervisee. It is also important to express empathy and offer opportunities for greater learning to prevent future errors.

Questions for the Supervisee

■ What is your training and background so that I can understand your skill set better and offer tailored supervision?

■ What are your goals for your current role and how can they be best achieved? through supervision?

■ What format of supervision has worked for you and in what environment? Do you prefer meeting separately or receiving supervision with your other peers?

■ Is supervision helping your learning and professional development as a nonphysician clinician? Is supervision helping you reduce burnout? If so, how? If not, what should be improved?

Additional Resources

Books

Davys A, Beddoe L: Best Practice in Professional Supervision: A Guide for the Helping Professions. London, Jessica Kingsley, 2010

Milne DL: Evidence-Based Clinical Supervision: Principles and Practice. New York, Wiley, 2009

Professional Organizations and Websites

Psychiatrists

American Psychiatric Association (APA): https://www.psychiatry.org

Harvard Business Review: https://hbr.org/topic/managing-people

California Department of Human Resources: http://www.calhr.ca.gov/Training/Pages/index-training-for-managers-and-supervisors.aspx

SAMHSA-HRSA Center for Integrated Health Solutions: https://www.integration.samhsa.gov/workforce/supervision

Nurse Practitioners

American Psychiatric Nurses Association (APNA): https://www.apna.org

NursingLicensure.org (nursing licensure requirements): https://www.nursinglicensure.org

Nurse Practitioner Scope of Practice Laws: https://www.bartonassociates.com/locum-tenens-resources/nurse-practitioner-scope-of-practice-laws

American Association of Nurse Practitioners (state practice environment): https://www.aanp.org/legislation-regulation/state-legislation/state-practice-environment

Physician Assistants

Association of Physician Assistants in Psychiatry (APAP): http://psychpa.com

PhysicianAssistantEDU.org (state-by-state requirements to become a physician assistant): https://www.physicianassistantedu.org/psychiatry-mental-health

Social Workers

National Association of Social Workers (includes American Association of Psychiatric Social Workers): https://www.socialworkers.org

SocialWorkLicensure.org: https://socialworklicensure.org/types-of-social-workers/psychiatric-social-worker

Marriage and Family Therapists

American Association for Marriage and Family Therapy: https://aamft.org

Pharmacists

College of Psychiatric & Neurologic Pharmacists: https://cpnp.org

---

References

American Psychiatric Association: Guidelines for psychiatrists in consultative, supervisory, or collaborative relationships with nonmedical therapists. Am J Psychiatry 137(11):1489–1491, 1980

Hore CT, Lancashire W, Fassett RG: Clinical supervision by consultants in teaching hospitals. Med J Aust 191(4):220–222, 2009 19705984

Kilminster SM, Jolly BC: Effective supervision in clinical practice settings: a literature review. Med Educ 34(10):827–840, 2000 11012933

National Center for Health Workforce Analysis:National projections of supply and demand for behavioral health practitioners: 2013–2025. Rockville, MD, Health Resources and Services Administration, U.S. Department of Health and Human Services: November 2016. Available at: https://bhw.hrsa.gov/sites/default/files/bhw/health-workforce-analysis/research/projections/behavioral-health2013-2025.pdf. Accessed August 22, 2018.

National Council for Behavioral Health: The psychiatric shortage: 2017. March 28, 2017. Available at: https://www.thenationalcouncil.org/wp-content/uploads/2017/03/Psychiatric-Shortage_National-Council-.pdf. Accessed August 22, 2018.

Woltmann E, Grogan-Kaylor A, Perron B, et al: Comparative effectiveness of collaborative chronic care models for mental health conditions across primary, specialty, and behavioral health care settings: systematic review and meta-analysis. Am J Psychiatry 169(8):790–804, 2012 22772364

World Health Organization: Mental health action plan 2013–2020. 2017. Available at: http://www.who.int/iris/handle/10665/89966. Accessed August 22, 2018.

Chapter 47 Clinical Consultation

How Consulting Differs From Supervising

Camilla N. Van Voorhees, M.D.

Consultation in psychiatry can be deeply helpful and meaningful for both consultee and consultant at any point in one's career. The underlying structures of clinical consultation and supervision hold some similarities, but they also differ in that consultation, which is arranged privately, is not part of a training program, whereas supervision typically is. This allows for much more freedom in how consultation may be used. One may seek psychiatric consultation on a wide variety of issues, including psychotherapy, psychopharmacology, administrative issues, and so on, although in this chapter the primary focus is on psychotherapy consultation.

Key Points

- There are differences between the role of a consultant and that of a supervisor; a consultant is responsible only to the consultee, whereas supervisors have split responsibilities to the supervisee, the training institution, and to the supervisee's patient.

- A consultant is generally not legally responsible for the consultee's patient, whereas a supervisor is both clinically and legally responsible for the supervisee's patient.

- Consultation can be used in a variety of formats to discuss a wide range of topics.

Differences Between Consultation and Supervision

Responsibility to an Institution

The consultant's responsibility lies solely with the consultee—not to the institution. In contrast, supervisors have responsibilities to the training institution, which require them to evaluate and report on the progress of their supervisees as they become increasingly proficient clinicians. Unlike consultants, supervisors are thus in a position of power relative to supervisees, and supervisees' knowledge that they are being evaluated is likely to impact their openness in a way that can hinder the work of supervision. Also, if the supervisors need to give the institution a negative evaluation of their supervisees, their allegiance to their supervisees comes into conflict with their duties to the training institution, and that can lead to feelings of betrayal in supervisees who have worked openly with their supervisors.

Degree of Confidentiality

Consultation is generally confidential, although it is not legally mandated to be so. In supervision, the supervisor is responsible for reporting on the progress of the supervisee— meaning the relationship cannot be entirely confidential—and thus is less safe for the supervisee. A rare exception to confidentiality in consultation would occur if the consultee engaged in a serious ethical or professional violation, in which case the consultant would be ethically obligated to report this to the consultee's overseeing clinical board.

Length of Consultation

Unlike in supervision, there is no predefined length to consultation. In supervision, the institution generally dictates the time of the relationship, for example, lasting for an academic year or until the end of the training period. In consultation, one may meet from one time to numerous times at any desired frequency over many years.

Legal and Clinical Responsibilities

Whereas consultation that is documented in a patient's chart may at times be clinically and legally important (e.g., when the clinician is faced with uncertain decisions regarding diagnosis and treatment; Clayton and Bongar 1994), consultants who provide private psychotherapy consultation, unlike supervisors, are generally neither clinically nor legally (Grennel and Frankel 2007) responsible for their consultees' patients. As a result, consultants are freed from the need to know in detail most or all aspects of how treatment is proceeding. This allows consultants and consultees to focus on whatever is most important to them.

The legal difference between psychotherapy consultation and supervision is that there is no doctor-patient or therapist-client relationship between the consultant and the consultee's patient. Unlike consultants, supervisors may be held liable for acts and omissions by their supervisees (Grennel and Frankel 2007; Saccuzzo 1997).

A consultant's legal responsibility for a patient *may* include 1) when a formal consultation on a specific, identified patient is requested and paid for; 2) when the consultant and consultee are both working for the same treating institution; 3) when the consultant reviews the chart and meets with the patient; and 4) when the treating physician or therapist is obligated (e.g., by the treating institution) to accept the consultant's advice. Also, the more specific the information concerning a particular patient that is provided, the closer the consultant is to being part of the care team (Chesanow 2017). In cases where the consultant is legally part of the care team, especially when consultant and consultee are not practicing in the same treating institution, consultees may need to have their patients sign informed consents, and consultants may want to consider a formal legal agreement with their consultees. But consultation in its purest form is a type of instruction, and generally courts have seen educational instruction as different from treatment and have been unwilling to interfere with the exchange of information between professionals (Grennel and Frankel 2007).

Consultation Formats

A clinician may obtain brief or long-term consultation. The format will depend on particular clinical or research skills the consultee seeks to develop and/or the topic he or she seeks to explore.

Brief Consultation

One might seek brief consultation in order to discuss questions concerning a particular new medication or procedure, an area of research, an issue with a patient (inpatient or outpatient), political or personality issues with colleagues, cultural issues, leadership issues, a paper the consultee has written, a case conference or other presentation for which the consultee is preparing, a specific psychotherapy question, and so on.

Long-Term Consultation

Since consultation does not have to be time-limited, a consultee-consultant pair may work together for many years, as seen most often in psychotherapy consultation. This allows the degree of comfort and safety to develop that is necessary for deep psychological work and allows for the development of important skills and attitudes and for the development of deeper understandings of various topics. This level of trust and safety is also enhanced because consultation is nonevaluative, confidential, and focused on the consultee's needs rather than divided between the needs of the supervisee, the patient, and the training institution. The consultant also provides an empathetic, caring, well-boundaried frame that further ensures the consultee's "freedom to think and dream and be alive to what is occurring" both in the therapeutic relationship and in the consultation relationship (Ogden 2005). In this setting the consultee may develop his or her therapeutic skills and attitudes, including self-awareness in the context of work with patients, and self-confidence and independence as a clinician. In other words, consultants ideally help their consultees to become more fully themselves as clinicians by helping to develop their own style, voice, theoretical stance (Purcell 2004); their own abilities to use their thoughts and feelings for their patients' benefit; and an awareness of when their own defenses may be interfering with their patients' growth. The last of these suggests that this is a time for consultees to return to consultation and/or their own therapy (Ogden 2005). It is hoped that this development as a psychotherapist, and as a human being, continues throughout one's career and is enhanced by consultation.

In a long-term consultation the deepening interpersonal safety between consultant and consultee over months and years also allows both parties to feel increasingly comfortable exploring a wide range of topics, from medication and research questions to issues about interacting with other people, whether they be patients, colleagues, friends, or family members. In other words, they explore the deepest, most pleasurable and disturbing aspects of human relating. This may include exploring one's needs to both feel and express one's most intense loves, hatreds, excitements, shames, griefs, and so on, in their most tender and fierce forms. It also may include exploring the extreme vulnerability and dependency of early childhood (Ogden 2014; Winnicott 1974) and the sometimes loud transference echoes of these in adult life; the needs of later childhood and adulthood; and the limits in life, including limits in time and limits in one's own capacities and the capacities of loved ones, losses associated with aging, and one's own mortality. These most challenging feelings and experiences are what patients and people in general are most desperate and most privileged to share with one another, including with our clinicians and with our consultants.

Specific Challenges and Strategies

- **As a consultant, I would like to avoid becoming legally responsible for my consultee's patient.** In addition to not working for the same treating institution, the consultant might ask the consultee to avoid being too specific about a particular, identified patient (Chesanow 2017; Grennel and Frankel 2007). For example, a consultant who comes to know a particular patient quite well by watching extensive videotapes of a consultee's work with the patient may increase the risk that a particular judge would find this consultant to be part of the care team and therefore legally responsible for the patient.
- **My consultee has a serious skill deficit or is defended against certain material, and this is impeding his patient's progress. What do I do?** Many patients need their therapist to develop further in a particular area before the patient can be helped with that issue (Ferro 2002). A common example of this in private consultation is with boundary setting, especially keeping financial and time boundaries, even though it is extensively discussed in supervision. In private practice, one imposes these boundaries for one's own benefit, not just to follow the requirements of one's training institution. As a result, many consultees fear that their patients will be angry or sad (Gabbard 2003) with them directly rather than at the training institution. The consultant can kindly point out the consultee's difficulty setting a given boundary in spite of theoretical knowledge from prior supervision about what to do, and can suggest that either the consultee explore his underlying fears in his own therapy and/

or with the consultant (Frawley-O'Dea 1998, 2003; and Ogden 2005). Eventually, if no progress is being made in the therapy, the consultant may have to recommend that the consultee refer the patient to another therapist, problematic as that is.

Questions for the Consultee

- How might consultation be useful to you after you're licensed in your field?

- In what ways can you optimize and deepen your use of consultation?

Additional Resources

Grennel G, Frankel A: Supervision vs. consultation: what you need to know. June 3, 2007. Available at: http://clinicallawyer.com/2007/07/supervision-vs-consultation-what-you-need-to-know/. Accessed August 22, 2018.
Ogden TH: Reclaiming Unlived Life: Experiences in Psychoanalysis. New York, Routledge, 2016

References

Chesanow N: When a curbside consult is a liability risk. Medscape, October 4, 2017. Available at: https://www.medscape.com/viewarticle/883538. Accessed August 22, 2018.
Clayton S, Bongar B: The use of consultation in psychological practice: ethical, legal, and clinical considerations. Ethics Behav 4(1):43–57, 1994 11652713
Ferro A: In the Analyst's Consulting Room. New York, Taylor & Francis, 2002
Frawley-O'Dea MG: Revisiting the "teach/treat" boundary in psychoanalytic supervision: when the supervisee is or is not in concurrent treatment. J Am Acad Psychoanal 26(4):513–527, 1998 10096051
Frawley-O'Dea MG: Supervision is a relationship too: a contemporary approach to psychoanalytic supervision. Psychoanal Dialogues 13(3):355–366, 2003
Gabbard GO: Miscarriages of psychoanalytic treatment with suicidal patients. Int J Psychoanal 84(Pt 2):249–261, 2003 12856351
Grennel G, Frankel A: Supervision vs. consultation: what you need to know. June 3, 2007. Available at: http://clinicallawyer.com/2007/07/supervision-vs-consultation-what-you-need-to-know/. Accessed August 22, 2018.
Ogden TH: On psychoanalytic supervision. Int J Psychoanal 86(Pt 5):1265–1280, 2005 16174607
Ogden TH: Fear of breakdown and the unlived life. Int J Psychoanal 95(2):205–223, 2014 24620827
Purcell SD: The analyst's theory: a third source of countertransference. Int J Psychoanal 85(Pt 3):635–652, 2004 15228701
Saccuzzo D: Liability for failure to supervise adequately mental health assistants, unlicensed practitioners and students. California Western Law Review 34(1), Article 10, 1997. Available at: http://scholarlycommons.law.cwsl.edu/cwlr/vol34/iss1/10. Accessed on August 16, 2018.
Winnicott DW: Fear of breakdown. Int Rev Psychoanal 1:103–107, 1974

Chapter 48 Enhancing Learning in Supervision

Priyanthy Weerasekera, M.D., M.Ed.

Clinical supervision is a major method of teaching in postgraduate medical education, psychology doctoral internships, and other related mental health disciplines. In psychiatric residency training, the supervisory relationship is essential to the development of resident competence and identity formation. There is, however, great variability in how supervision is carried out across programs, and even within training programs.

There are many opinion papers on what makes a good clinical supervisor or teacher; few are supported by research. Stenfors-Hayes et al. (2011) make a distinction between good teachers and good supervisors based on reports from medical students. These students describe good teachers as focusing on students' learning, responding to students' content requests, and conveying knowledge. Good clinical supervisors are described as stimulating students' growth, sharing information on what it is like to be a doctor, and showing how things are done. From these definitions it is clear that a clinical supervisor in psychiatry should be both a good teacher and supervisor, and that teaching and mentoring activities are intertwined. It is unclear, however, whether there is a relationship between students' perspectives on effective supervisor characteristics and resident competence—this question remains open to empirical investigation.

Medicine follows an apprenticeship model, with the supervisor playing the role of the expert, mentor, and teacher. Supervisors therefore carry a big responsibility in ensuring that the supervisee not only attains a level of competence with respect to knowledge, skills, and attitudes in psychiatry, but that the most effective methods of teaching are utilized to assist trainees in reaching their goals. How do training programs or supervisors make decisions on how to supervise trainees? For the most part, supervisors utilize supervision methods that are most familiar to them, usually originating from their own training experience rather than the empirical literature. Many training programs and supervisors are not cognizant of the most effective teaching methods, and even those programs that are struggle with incorporating these techniques across all supervisors.

The most recent review on supervision in psychiatry concludes that "it is little researched" (MacDonald and Ellis 2012). A more recent review over the past 5 years using the search term "supervision" and "psychiatry," and search engines PsychINFO, PubMed, and specific medical education journals (e.g., *Academic Psychiatry*, *Academic Medicine*) did not yield further empirical papers on the topic. The literature does include many opinion papers on clinical supervision in psychiatry and a review of evidence-based psychotherapy supervision (Weerasekera 2013).

Despite the lack of empirical papers in clinical supervision in psychiatry, the past 20 years have yielded important findings in the area of teaching and learning. Much of this literature originates from cognitive psychology, learning theories, medicine, and psychotherapy. Empirical data from these areas point to specific evidence-based teaching methods that can be incorporated into clinical supervision. These methods are not specific to teaching psychiatric residents but can be applied broadly in education to enhance students learning in the area of knowledge and skills.

The specific teaching methods covered in this literature include using modeling-rehearsal (practice), and feedback; incorporating direct observation; making an evaluation; focusing on patient outcomes; encouraging learning to teach (supervise); and enhancing knowledge acquisition though case-based and test-enhanced learning. Each of these areas will be discussed briefly, followed by suggestions for future research.

Using Modeling, Rehearsal (Practice), and Feedback

Modeling, rehearsal (practice) and feedback has been demonstrated to be the key method for learning skills (Peters et al. 1978). Modeling is essential in the initial conceptualization of any skill and can be used to break down the necessary components of a complicated set of skills so that they can be learned separately, and later integrated into complex behavioral chains (Rosenbaum et al. 2001). In addition to observing the supervisor model skills, learners can also benefit from observing peers receiving corrective feedback on their skills. This refinement in modeling increases learning and suggests an advantage for group supervision (Rohbanfard and Proteau 2011). Rehearsal and deliberate practice are essential for the development and consolidation of interviewing and psychotherapeutic skills. Without practice (and feedback) learning does not occur (Mazor et al. 2011). Research demonstrates that learners have few opportunities for observed practice; in most cases they function independently, even at junior levels of training (Hauer et al. 2011).

As discussed already, feedback is essential to learning (Mazor et al. 2011). It must be specific to behaviors and goal directed (Peters et al. 1978). Feedback that is not based on observation is not valued. Many reasons are given for why supervisors do not give feedback: not enough time, lack of understanding, concerns that the resident will get upset, concerns about negative evaluations, and the feelings that the system will not always support it (Bing-You and Trowbridge 2009). Research demonstrates several essential methods for giving effective feedback: establish a respectful environment, communicate goals and objectives for feedback, begin sessions with learner's self-assessment even though we know this will be inaccurate, base feedback on direct observation, make feedback timely and regular, and reinforce and correct observed behaviors (Ramani and Krackov 2012). Research also demonstrates an inverted U-curve relationship between feedback frequency and performance, with very low and very high feedback frequency leading to poor performance (Lam et al. 2011). Therefore, it is essential that a moderate frequency of feedback be given to ensure an optimal level of performance. See Chapter 8, "Modeling, Rehearsal, and Feedback: A Simple Approach to Teaching Complex Skills," for practical tips on this approach.

Incorporating Direct Observation

The Accreditation Council for Graduate Medical Education emphasizes direct observation of residents performing skills and considers this essential for the reliable and valid assessment of resident competence (Jardine et al. 2017). Despite these requirements, few faculty observe students with patients, and very few evaluations are based on direct observation (Hauer et al. 2011). This is concerning given that evaluations based on actual student performance are more reliable and valid in predicting competence (Hasnain et al. 2004), are considered more valid by students (Mazor et al. 2011) and are more likely to change students' behavior (Watling et al. 2008). These findings indicate that observation is essential, because it provides direct access to resident "performance" for more accurate assessment of skills, which leads to better identification of learner difficulties. In many cases training programs rely on resident self-assessment in the evaluation process. Although self-reflection and self-assessment are important in the maturation process of a psychiatry resident, the data from such measures are highly unreliable and inaccurate in providing an objective assessment of knowledge and skills (Hodges et al. 2001). Observation therefore is essential for evaluation and for providing the feedback necessary for learning.

Making an Evaluation

When an evaluation of performance is being made, it is important to first define the competencies being assessed, and as much as possible these should be operationally defined. If there are empirically validated tools to assess competencies, such as the therapeutic alliance or psychotherapy competencies, these can be used to increase the likelihood that specific skills will be evaluated (Hatcher and Gillaspy 2006; Vallis et al. 1986). Tools developed by institutions should be behaviorally anchored so that the learner is aware of which skills are being assessed. Reliable assessment of trainee competence includes both formative and summative assessments. Formative assessments increase learning because they provide the learner with timely ongoing feedback. This feedback can also lead to the development of further goals and objectives. Use of multiple assessments over time, carried out by different assessors, contributes to a more valid and useful assessment of performance (Hauer et al. 2011). Evaluations must be provided in a timely manner in order for it to be useful and meaningful to the learner.

Focusing on Patient Outcomes

Many educators advocate for a relationship between resident competence and patient outcomes; however, programs rarely evaluate resident competence from this perspective. One general skill set essential for all clinicians who are delivering different forms of treatment, including medical management, is the ability to form a *therapeutic alliance*. Numerous empirically validated instruments exist to assess the therapeutic alliance, and these can be given to patients early and late in treatment. Although mainly studied in psychotherapy, some of these scales have been used in medication management. A positive therapeutic alliance predicts a good outcome as early as the third treatment session and predicts compliance with medication (Hatcher and Gillaspy 2006). The Working Alliance Inventory (WAI; Hatcher and Gillaspy 2006) is perhaps one of the most commonly used instruments across a variety of therapeutic modalities, and it can be used in training programs. The WAI contains 12 items rated on a 5-point scale that assess the bond, goals, and tasks in any form of treatment. High scores on goals and tasks early in treatment predict a good outcome and increase the chance that the patient will remain in treatment. The alliance assesses the resident's ability to engage the patient in treatment, reach common goals, and convey understanding in a nonjudgmental fashion. Other instruments that assess symptoms such as depression and anxiety, as well as functional impairment (Beck 1988; Derogatis and Savitz 1999), can be used early and late in treatment to see if patients have made any gains through the treatment process. Therapy-specific and symptom-specific measures will inform us on whether the treatment has been effective. In some cases, despite all attempts to develop a good therapeutic alliance and deliver competently delivered treatment, patient outcome will be poor. Possible reasons for this could be patient variables such as perfectionism, severe personality disorder, and illness severity, which interfere with alliance formation (Ackerman and Hilsenroth 2003). It is therefore important to keep in mind that patient outcomes alone do not convey an accurate account of therapist competence, as multiple factors influence the patient's capacity to engage in treatment.

Encouraging Learners to Teach

Increasingly, more and more attention has been given to the "resident as teacher" role, with programs now requiring all residents to have teaching experiences during their residency training. Although these requirements contribute to early faculty development, encouraging residents to teach enhances their learning (Bargh and Schul 1980). Recent research shows that when two methods of studying are used to prepare for an exam, those individuals who prepared to teach the material, and those who went on to teach, showed a better understanding of the material than those who studied for exam preparation (Fiorella and Mayer 2013). Findings from cognitive psychology indicate that preparing to teach—and actually teaching—increases depth of processing, which increases understanding and recall of information. When teachers answer students' questions, this leads to further reorganization and deeper processing of information, which enhances learning. Therefore, supervisors should provide opportunities for residents to teach other learners. This does not have to be limited to a seminar, or teaching rounds, but can also be focused on helping other learners learn psychiatric skills. The evidence in this area is very compelling and should encourage programs and clinical supervisors to incorporate teaching opportunities for residents in clinical rotations.

Enhancing Knowledge Through Case-Based and Test-Enhanced Learning

Supervisors use many methods to ensure that residents develop a sound knowledge base. Trainees are frequently questioned on their knowledge, their diagnostic skills, and the treatment plans they develop for their patients. Frequently supervisors provide reference material and suggest that residents research the literature for topics relevant for patient care. Although these approaches are helpful, recent evidence suggests additional methods that could be incorporated in clinical supervision.

It is clear from the empirical literature that some methods of learning are superior to others. First, it is well known that mass studying carried out just prior to an exam does not lead to long-term recall (Fiorella and Mayer 2013). Case-based learning and problem-based learning both lead to enhanced learning of the material because the material is processed at a deeper level (Srinivasan et al. 2007). Of recent interest is that repeated test taking, or test-enhanced learning, leads to superior learning and longer-term recall than mass studying over the same period of time (Roediger and Karpicke 2006). It is possible that the superior recall effect seen with repeated testing is due to the continuous reorganization of the material, which leads to a deeper level of processing. The main issue in recall is that the material needs to be processed at a deeper level and connected to prior learning. Cognitive psychology demonstrates exciting new findings that need to be incorporated into how supervisors teach residents across all clinical placements.

Future Directions

A preliminary review of the literature on clinical supervision in psychiatry does not yield significant evidence-based recommendations. Of note, however, are the exciting findings from cognitive psychology, medical education, and psychotherapy training that have implications for teaching in the clinical supervisory relationship. Clinical supervisors must be active teachers, incorporate evidence-based teaching methods, and be connected to the current literature on best methods for teaching and learning. Training programs must be responsible for assisting clinical supervisors through faculty development programs so they can keep up to date with these effective teaching methods. Junior faculty should receive an orientation program on the most effective methods of teaching prior to beginning their faculty appointment as a department member.

With continued research in education, and the application of these findings to clinical supervision, we will no doubt provide the best learning environment for our residents.

Specific Challenges and Strategies

- **I don't have time to observe all the time.** Educators work in very busy clinical settings and have teaching and administrative responsibilities. They may also be teaching many learners. This makes it hard to observe learners on an ongoing basis. As a solution to this it may be helpful to sit down with the learner and ask him or her to identify what skills they find challenging. This way time can be used efficiently so observation becomes more focused and specific, as opposed to broader and more general.

- **I don't know how to help learners teach others.** It is difficult to help others to teach when you have not been taught how to do this yourself. Most teachers follow approaches that they observed when they were students, even if these approaches may not be successful. As an educator you can teach learners to teach using the modeling–rehearsal (practice)–feedback paradigm. Start with giving the learner an opportunity to observe you teach. Review the teaching approach and steps with the learner. Give the learner a chance to teach junior learners while you are in attendance. Ask the junior learners to provide feedback to the junior teacher. Review the process with the junior teacher paying attention to objective behaviors. If possible these sessions can be recorded for later playback and review.

Questions for the Supervisor

- Have I operationally defined the competencies that will be evaluated in this supervision?

- Have I incorporated objective tools to assess various competencies?

- Have I incorporated patient outcome instruments to assess patient progress?

- Have I ensured that case-based learning will take place throughout this rotation?

- Have I ensured opportunities for the learner to teach other learners?

References

Ackerman SJ, Hilsenroth MJ: A review of therapist characteristics and techniques positively impacting the therapeutic alliance. Clin Psychol Rev 23(1):1–33, 2003 12559992

Bargh JA, Schul Y: On the cognitive effects of teaching. J Educ Psychol 72:593–604, 1980

Beck AT: Psychometric properties of the Beck Depression Inventory: twenty-five years of evaluation. Clin Psychol Rev 8(1):77–100, 1988

Bing-You RG, Trowbridge RL: Why medical educators may be failing at feedback. JAMA 302(12):1330–1331, 2009 19773569

Derogatis LR, Savitz KL: The SCL-90-R, Brief Symptom Inventory, and matching clinical rating scales, in The Use of Psychological Testing for Treatment Planning and Outcomes Assessment. Edited by Maruish ME. Mahwah, NJ, Lawrence Erlbaum, 1999, pp 679–724

Fiorella L, Mayer RE: The relative benefits of learning by teaching and teaching expectancy. Contemp Educ Psychol 38:281–288, 2013

Hasnain M, Connell KJ, Downing SM, et al: Toward meaningful evaluation of clinical competence: the role of direct observation in clerkship ratings. Acad Med 79(10)(Suppl):S21–S24, 2004 15383380

Hatcher RL, Gillaspy JA: Development and validation of a revised short version of the Working Alliance Inventory. Psychother Res 16:12–25, 2006

Hauer KE, Holmboe ES, Kogan JR: Twelve tips for implementing tools for direct observation of medical trainees' clinical skills during patient encounters. Med Teach 33(1):27–33, 2011 20874011

Hodges B, Regehr G, Martin D: Difficulties in recognizing one's own incompetence: novice physicians who are unskilled and unaware of it. Acad Med 76(10)(Suppl):S87–S89, 2001 11597883

Jardine D, Deslauriers J, Kamran SC, et al: Milestone guidebook for the residents and fellows. Accreditation Council for Graduate Medical Education, June 2017. Available at: https://www.acgme.org/Portals/0/PDFs/Milestones/MilestonesGuidebookforResidentsFellows.pdf. Accessed August 16, 2018.

Lam CF, DeRue DS, Karam EP, et al: The impact of feedback frequency on learning and task performance: challenging the "more is better" assumption. Organ Behav Hum Decis Process 116:217–228, 2011

MacDonald J, Ellis PM: Supervision in psychiatry: terra incognita? Curr Opin Psychiatry 25(4):322–326, 2012 22569311

Mazor KM, Holtman MC, Shchukin Y, et al: The relationship between direct observation, knowledge, and feedback: results of a national survey. Acad Med 86(10)(Suppl):S63–S67, quiz S68, 2011 21955772

Peters GA, Cormier LS, Cormier WH: Effects of modeling, rehearsal, feedback, and remediation on acquisition of a counseling strategy. J Couns Psychol 25:231–237, 1978

Ramani S, Krackov SK: Twelve tips for giving feedback effectively in the clinical environment. Med Teach 34(10):787–791, 2012 22730899

Roediger HL, Karpicke JD: Test-enhanced learning: taking memory tests improves long-term retention. Psychol Sci 17(3):249–255, 2006 16507066

Rohbanfard H, Proteau L: Learning through observation: a combination of expert and novice models favors learning. Exp Brain Res 215(3–4):183–197, 2011 21986667

Rosenbaum DA, Carlson RA, Gilmore RO: Acquisition of intellectual and perceptual-motor skills. Annu Rev Psychol 52:453–470, 2001 11148313

Srinivasan M, Wilkes M, Stevenson F, et al: Comparing problem-based learning with case-based learning: effects of a major curricular shift at two institutions. Acad Med 82(1):74–82, 2007 17198294

Stenfors-Hayes T, Hult H, Dahlgren LO: What does it mean to be a good teacher and clinical supervisor in medical education? Adv Health Sci Educ Theory Pract 16(2):197–210, 2011 20978840

Vallis TM, Shaw BF, Dobson KS: The Cognitive Therapy Scale: psychometric properties. J Consult Clin Psychol 54(3):381–385, 1986 3722567

Watling CJ, Kenyon CF, Zibrowski EM, et al: Rules of engagement: residents' perceptions of the in-training evaluation process. Acad Med 83(10)(Suppl):S97–S100, 2008 18820513

Weerasekera P: The state of psychotherapy supervision: recommendations for future training. Int Rev Psychiatry 25(3):255–264, 2013 23859088

Part 7   Legal and Ethical Issues

Chapter 49 Ethical and Legal Considerations in Supervision

John M. Greene, M.D.

Education and training of residents, psychology students, and counselors are essential in establishing competence in therapy and counseling for prospective healthcare providers. During the education of trainees, however, their inexperience can expose them to making potential mistakes with patients they treat during their training. This inexperience places the trainee at risk of liability for harm to his or her patient, but it also places the supervisor at risk of liability as well. Therefore, supervisors must understand the potential legal and ethical risks of undertaking the education of trainees in psychiatric, psychological, and counseling settings. In this chapter, I attempt to address potential legal and ethical risks that supervisors face with supervision in regard to the treatment of patients, and how to manage these risks.

Key Points

- The concept of "negligence" on the part of the trainee places the supervisor at risk for malpractice.

- There are different principles of liability that the supervisor must be aware of that define a trainee's negligence.

- The most common types of trainee negligence that result in legal action toward the supervisor relate to sexual contact between trainee and patient, and suicide by the patient.

- The concepts of "negligence" and "ethics" are different and require the supervisor to understand and watch for both in supervision.

- Competence, confidentiality, welfare protection, and informed consent are factors that the supervisor must monitor to ensure ethical practice by the trainee.

Legal Considerations in Supervision

Negligence and the Civil Tort

To assess the potential legal issues that can arise in the role as a supervisor, the supervisor must understand the general legal principles in which the healthcare professional can potentially be exposed to legal action on the part of their patient. The Model Penal Code (American Law Institute 1962) defines four types of culpability, or legal parameters, that enable one to be held legally responsible for their actions: when the offender purposely, knowingly, recklessly, or negligently acts, causing harm to another. The first three definitions, "purposely," "knowingly," and "recklessly," relate to criminal actions and therefore generally do not define a potential action that the healthcare provider can commit. However, the fourth parameter, that of negligence, generally considered to be a noncriminal act, does pertain to the majority of the healthcare provider's potential action against their patient, and defines the arena to which the patient can find legal recourse against the provider.

An accusation of negligence on the part of the patient is handled in civil rather than criminal court; the accusation itself, in civil court, is called a "tort," or a "civil wrong." The tort of negligence, as it pertains to the healthcare provider, has itself four parameters that the complaining patient, or plaintiff, must show in order to prove that negligence on the part of the healthcare provider, or defendant, was present: the provider had a duty to the patient; there was a dereliction, or breach, of duty to the patient; the breach of duty resulted in a direct cause of damage to the patient; and the patient suffered from evidence of actual damage. Once these four elements have been proven in court, the healthcare provider is determined to have committed negligence against the patient, which is also defined as "malpractice."

To prove that the healthcare worker had a duty to the patient requires only that the patient show evidence that the healthcare worker instigated treatment to the patient; this aspect of negligence is generally easily shown, because any provider-patient relationship automatically defines a duty on the part of the provider to treat the patient. Malpractice claims, then, are mostly focused on an attempt by the plaintiff to prove the second factor of negligence, in that the provider breached his or her duty to the patient by practicing below a determined standard of care. Once this has been established, it must be proved that damages were present and that they were directly caused by the negligent action. All healthcare workers, then, must attempt to treat all patients in accordance with the standard of care as defined by their peers, professional organizations, and learning institutions, in order to minimize the liability for any of their patients to provide evidence that the provider's treatment represented a dereliction of duty or a breach of the standard of care.

Vicarious and Direct Liability

General Considerations

The healthcare worker minimizes risk against claims of negligence by focusing on his or her personal conduct and conforming to the standard of care that defines his or her scope of practice. When the healthcare worker becomes a supervisor, however, liability becomes a much broader issue, because it is necessary to focus on not only his or her behavior but also the behavior of the trainee. Liability applies whether the supervisory role is toward residents in training, psychology students, counselors and therapists out of formal training, and practicing psychologists and psychiatrists seeking additional supervision. In contrast, liability does not apply when the healthcare worker acts as a consultant, because the law recognizes consultation as exclusive of the therapist-client treatment relationship (Alban and Frankel 2007).

According to Saccuzzo (1997), supervisors are exposed to two general types of liability: vicarious liability and direct liability. *Vicarious liability* is defined as liability present when a supervisor, who could be considered to be the "master" of (and controlling the actions of) the trainee, is liable for the trainee's actions toward the patient, even though the supervisor may have no treatment connection to the patient. This theory, also known as *respondeat superior* ("let the master respond"), is based on the premise that the "master" is responsible for his or her subordinate's actions (Disney and Stephens 1994). After a trainee harms a client, if it can be shown that the supervisor had "authority and control" (Saccuzzo 1997) over the trainee prior to the harm the trainee caused, the supervisor can be held liable through vicarious liability.

Vicarious liability, however, generally requires that an employer-employee relationship also be present; in other words, the supervisor must also be shown to have hired the trainee and to have benefited, usually monetarily, from the trainee's presence (Saccuzzo 1997). Direct liability, in contrast, is a more encompassing liability than vicarious liability, because it relies on the belief that any supervisor, who is expected to have learned how to properly care for patients, is responsible for any trainee he or she supervises, who is assumed to be learning how to properly care for patients. Should the trainee fall below the standard of care in treating their client, then, the trainee's actions can be considered reflective of the supervisor falling below the standard of care in supervising their trainee (Saccuzzo 1997). Therefore, any dereliction of duty toward the patient by the trainee could therefore be the responsibility of the supervisor and lead to a direct-liability claim against the supervisor.

The case of *Jerrie Simmons v. United States* (1986) is a good example of both types of liability, as in this case, the negligent actions of a supervisee led to a finding of both vicarious liability and direct liability on the part of the supervisor/employer. In 1973, Jerrie Simmons sought counseling from a social worker, Ted Kammers, employed through the Indian Health Service. In October 1978, Mr. Kammers began a sexual relationship with Ms. Simmons; in 1980, Mr. Kammers' supervisor, Victor Sansalone, was notified of the sexual activity. Mr. Sansalone did not end the therapy between Mr. Kammers and Ms. Simmons and did not correct Mr. Kammers' actions. Ms. Simmons eventually filed a lawsuit alleging damages from Mr. Kammers' negligent treatment of her. The trial court found that the Indian Health Service, the employer of Mr. Kammers, was vicariously liable for Ms. Simmons' harm because it employed Mr. Kammers, and

Mr. Sansalone was found to be guilty of negligent supervision for allowing Mr. Kammers' behavior to continue and for not taking corrective action as a supervisor.

Common Liability Situations

Simmons v. United States also illustrates a common scenario resulting in the filing of torts against therapists, that of sexual contact between the therapist and client. A 2014 joint report by insurance companies CNA and HPSO revealed that claims against CNA-insured counselors between 2003 and 2012 mostly involved inappropriate sexual or romantic relationships with clients (CNA/HPSO 2014). This study further noted that the most common reason an action was taken against a counselor's license or certification to practice, a different claim than negligence of patient care, was sexual misconduct, in the form of having relationships with current or former clients. It logically follows that the supervisee also presents with potential risk of sexual contact with his or her patients, and managing this risk is an important endeavor for the supervisor.

Suicide is another common reason that brings litigation against therapists (Resnick 2012). Suicidality must then be assessed by the supervisor, in regard to the trainee's patient, in order to effectively manage this risk. The duty of therapists to protect third parties, in light of the 1976 *Tarasoff II* decision (Tarasoff v. Regents of University of California 1976), represents another risk that must be managed by the supervisor when guiding supervisees in their treatment of their patients. Much discussion in training programs is in regard to the *Tarasoff* case, because in that case, it was found that the therapist, Dr. Moore, knew that his patient, Prosenjit Poddar, was threatening to harm Ms. Tarasoff. Because Ms. Tarasoff was not "protected" from this threat by being informed of it, liability for the death of Ms. Tarasoff after Mr. Poddar subsequently killed her fell to the University of California, who employed Dr. Moore. The focus on this case usually relates to the need to understand how to protect third parties from potential harm; however, this case is also important to understand from the standpoint of supervision, as Dr. Powelson, the psychiatrist who was supervising Dr. Moore, was personally found to be negligently liable in his supervision of Dr. Moore (Recupero and Rainey 2007).

Psychiatrist supervision carries the additional need to manage risk of medication administration and potential bad outcomes related to medication management that can occur on the part of the supervisee. According to Professional Risk Management Services (PRMS) (2014), "patient suicides might trigger the most lawsuits," but "cases with the largest verdicts or settlements don't involve the death of a patient, but significant and permanent physical and neurological damage requiring lifelong care." PRMS highlights renal failure from lithium toxicity and severe Stevens-Johnson syndrome as frequent causes for lawsuits. In 2014, CPH and Associates (2014) noted that the number-one liability risk for psychiatrists is psychopharmacology, with overdose and lithium toxicity given as common reasons for litigation. These data underscore the need for the supervising psychiatrist to closely monitor the supervisee's actions, if the supervisee is prescribing medication to his or her clients.

Recupero and Rainey (2007) highlight additional situations that could lead the supervisor to a claim of negligence while providing supervision. They note that evidence regarding a failure to provide oversight of the resident, of showing carelessness in monitoring the resident's work, of failing to maintain administrative requirements as defined by the Accreditation Council for Graduate Medical Education, or of failing to enforce established hospital or clinic policy could connect the supervisor to negligent supervision, should the trainee harm his or her patient. They consider that negligent supervision could apply when the trainee has physically or emotionally harmed the patient, particularly if evidence shows that any risk factors for this behavior by the trainee were identified by the supervisor but not addressed. Close monitoring of the trainee, early identification of risk factors, and careful assessment are essential factors of supervision, then, in order to manage these risks and minimize any potential bad outcomes of actions by the trainee.

Ethical Considerations in Supervision

Much as supervisors have an incentive to address risk factors for negligence in their own practice and that of their supervisees, supervisors must also act in an ethical manner toward their patients and supervisees, and must ensure that their supervisees also behave ethically. Although there can be an overlap between actions on the part of the healthcare professional as both unethical and negligent in regard to treatment of the patient, the two concepts are not equivalent. Should a healthcare provider be found to conduct behavior that is unethical but not negligent, their action could lead to a reprimand or loss of licensure by his or her governing board but would not lead to legal action against them in civil court.

Beauchamp and Childress (2012) describe four moral principles that provide a framework for defining ethical behavior: respect for patient autonomy, actions of beneficence toward the patient, actions of nonmaleficence toward the patient, and justice in administration of care to the patient. These concepts are considered and expanded on in American Psychiatric Association's Commentary on Ethics in Practice (American Psychiatric Association 2015), in which it is noted that professionally competent care, avoidance of dual agency and overlapping roles, confidentiality, honesty and integrity, informed consent, and therapeutic boundary keeping are essential in maintaining an ethical practice. Establishing good ethical practice of supervisees is noted to require "not only clinical expertise but also a high standard of professional ethics" on the part of supervisors, as well as acknowledgement of the "asymmetry in power between themselves and their trainees, with a resulting responsibility on teachers" to avoid dual-agency roles (American Psychiatric Association 2015, p. 8).

According to Saccuzzo (1997), case law and ethical codes have determined five ethical principles necessary in making sure the supervisor and supervisee act ethically in the care of the supervisee's patient. The supervisor must first be aware of his or her own competence in their ability to supervise, must be able to assess and direct the competence of the supervisee in patient care during the supervisory process, and must act on issues with trainee competence to ensure proper patient care. Confidentiality must be addressed by ensuring that the patient is aware of confidentiality limitations and that exchange of information between supervisor and supervisee occur under the understood confidentiality requirements. Protection of the welfare of the patient must be present at all times of supervision, by ensuring that monitoring and intervention occur on a regular basis by the supervisor. Informed consent must be addressed comprehensively, including disclosure to the patient of the role of the supervisor and supervisee in their care, as well as disclosure to the trainee of the type of supervision, expectations and goals of supervision.

Lastly, Saccuzzo (1997) highlights that case law and ethical codes dictate that the supervisor must avoid dual-agency roles, as has been described by the American Psychiatric Association in its Commentary on Ethics in Practice (American Psychiatric Association 2015). The major example of dual agency is that of sexual contact between supervisors and their trainees. The concern of this is reflected in Hall et al. (2007), summarizing that surveys conducted by the American Psychiatric Association and American Psychological Association from 1979 to 1988 revealed that 5%–17% of respondents polled reported having sexual relationships with trainees or supervisors. The frequency of the occurrence of sexual relationships by this evidence is troubling and underscores the importance of addressing and managing this potential ethics violation between the supervisor and their trainee. Other dual-agency roles between the supervisor and trainee include social relationships, financial agreements outside of patient treatment, and the supervisor acting as both therapist and supervisor to the trainee. Since all of these situations reflect a potential dual-agency, they potentially can be ethics violations and should be avoided.

Ways to Minimize Legal and Ethical Risk

The several legal and ethical situations described in this chapter suggest that becoming a supervisor could be intimidating; this conclusion could be reached when considering that there are more potential legal and ethical concerns not covered in this chapter that may be presented to the supervisor. However, if the supervisor follows general principles in supervision, covering potential legal and ethical risks can be managed as effectively as therapists managing the potential legal and ethical issues in their own practices. Recupero and Rainey (2007) provide risk management suggestions for psychotherapy supervision that serve as good general guidelines in supervision, providing steps to assess and document issues present for supervision. Saccuzzo (1997) provides a comprehensive informed consent document that can be used between the supervisor and his trainee to set the parameters of therapy. The California Board of Psychology (State of California Department of Consumer Affairs 2017) provides a list of steps taken to address potential legal and ethical issues in supervision that could be used as a framework for initiating and continuing supervision in therapy situations. By being conscious of these issues, the supervisor can conduct supervision in an ethical manner, while managing legal risks, and be effective instructors to their trainees and effective agents of patient care in the supervision setting.

Specific Challenges and Strategies

- **I feel uncomfortable that my supervisee is not communicating important therapeutic issues to me, and I worry this is placing me at risk for litigation.** In order to avoid this type of situation from developing, it is important to discuss all parameters of supervision with the supervisee prior to the onset of therapy, and to define how to proceed for potentially difficult situations, such as confidentiality limits, suicidal thinking or behavior by the patient, side effects to medication, and exacerbation of symptoms and how to address them. Defining what potential situations require additional intervention and communication on the part of the supervisee to the supervisor will assist in beginning supervision with greater protection against risk, and will assist with enabling the supervisor to feel comfortable about the relationship that emerges between supervisor, supervisee, and patient. The additional resources listed in this chapter provide several examples of how to organize a discussion with the supervisee prior to the onset of supervision, to encourage mutual understanding of handling difficult topics. After therapy has begun, it is beneficial for the supervisor to periodically check in with the supervisee in regard to the potentially difficult situations to make sure they are not present, and document that this was performed. Should unanticipated issues arise after therapy begins, reviewing the issue with the supervisee, determining how to minimize risk in the situation, and altering treatment to reflect that the issue has been addressed are necessary.

- **I suspect that my supervisee is getting too emotionally close to his patient.** It is understandable that supervisees will have emotional connections to their pa-tients; one aspect of supervision is determining how the supervisee expresses this connection to the patient and whether the expression is reasonable, or whether it represents either an unethical or an illegal action. Regular monitoring of how the supervisee is interacting with the patient is necessary, both in regard to what transpires in therapy and in regard to the type of communication, if any, that occurs out-side of therapy. Any actions that could potentially develop in dual-agency roles on the part of the supervisee, such as exchange of gifts or money, or any potential or actual interaction in a social environment, must be addressed and discussed as a part of the supervision process. Should any potential issue arise, documentation that the discussion has occurred, that the potential action has been addressed, and that the supervisee has altered their communication or behavior in regard to the patient is necessary.

Questions for the Supervisor

- Have you provided broad communication to your supervisee about the expectations of supervision, and have received confirmation that the supervisee under-stands?

- Do you feel you have set a plan in place for times when the supervisee doubts how to proceed, and how this will be addressed?

- Do you understand the limitations of your supervisee, and can you identify potential issues in those limitations?

- Have you described the issues that your supervisee is to call you about urgently, less urgently, routinely?

Additional Resources

General Legal Information for Psychiatrists and Supervision

American Academy of Psychiatry and the Law: aapl.org

Information for Psychologists and Therapists

American Psychiatric Association: psychiatry.org

State of California Department of Consumer Affairs: California board of psychology supervision checklist. 2017. Available at: http://www.psychology.ca.gov/applicants/sup_checklist.pdf.

Managing Supervision Risk

Recupero P, Rainey S: Liability and risk management in outpatient psychotherapy supervision. J Am Acad Psychiatry Law 35(2):188–195, 2007 (See appendix on risk management suggestions for psychotherapy supervision.)

Informed Consent Example

Saccuzzo DP: Liability for failure to supervise adequately mental health assistants, unlicensed practitioners, and students. California Western Law Review Vol 34, No 1, Article 10, 1997 (Appendix A contains sample informed consent for supervisees.)

References

Alban A, Frankel AS: Supervision vs. consultation: what you need to know. June 3, 2007. Available at: https://www.clinicallawyer.com/2007/07/supervision-vs-consultation-what-you-need-to-know/. Accessed August 23, 2018.

American Law Institute: Model penal code. 1962. Available at: https://www.ali.org/publications/show/model-penal-code. Accessed August 23, 2018.

American Psychiatric Association: APA commentary on ethics in practice. 2015. Available at: https://www.psychiatry.org/psychiatrists/practice/ethics. Accessed August 23, 2018.

Beauchamp T, Childress J: Principles of Biomedical Ethics, 7th Edition. New York, Oxford University Press, 2012

CNA/Healthcare Providers Service Organization: Understanding counselor liability risk. 2014. Available at: http://www.hpso.com/Documents/pdfs/CNA_-CLS_COUNS_022814p_CF_PROD_ASIZE_online_SEC.pdf. Accessed August 23, 2018.

CPH and Associates: Top liability risks for psychiatrists. 2014. Available at: https://www.cphins.com/top-liability-risks-for-psychiatrists. Accessed August 23, 2018.

Disney M, Stephens A: Legal Issues in Clinical Supervision (The ACA Legal Series, Vol 10). Alexandria, VA, American Counseling Association Publishing, 1994

Hall RC, Macvaugh GS 3rd, Merideth P, et al: Commentary: delving further into liability for psychotherapy supervision. J Am Acad Psychiatry Law 35(2):196–199, 2007 17592165

Professional Risk Management Services: Two top liability risks for psychiatrist: patients with suicidal behavior and psychopharmacology. 2014. Available at: https://www.prms.com/news/2010-top-risks.html. Accessed August 23, 2018.

Recupero PR, Rainey SE: Liability and risk management in outpatient psychotherapy supervision. J Am Acad Psychiatry Law 35(2):188–195, 2007 17592164

Resnick P: Psychiatric malpractice. Presentation at annual meeting of American Academy of Psychiatry and the Law Forensic Psychiatry Review Course, Montreal, Canada, October 2012

Saccuzzo DP: Liability for failure to supervise adequately mental health assistants, unlicensed practitioners and students. Calif West Law Rev 34(1):10, 1997

Simmons v. United States, 805 F.2d 1363 (9th Cir 1986). Available at: http://law.justia.com/cases/federal/appellate-courts/F2/805/1363/170932. Accessed August 23, 2018.

State of California Department of Consumer Affairs: California board of psychology supervision checklist. 2017. Available at: http://www.psychology.ca.gov/applicants/sup_checklist.pdf. Accessed August 23, 2018.

Tarasoff v. Regents of University of California, 17 Cal.3d 425 (1976). Available at: http://law.justia.com/cases/california/supreme-court/3d/17/425.html. Accessed August 23, 2018.

Part 8   Professional Development

Chapter 50 Professional Development

Strategies for Supervision and Growth of Supervisors

Jesse David Markman, M.D., M.B.A.

Deborah Suzanne Cowley, M.D.

Clinical supervision is central to psychiatric education. However, few clinical supervisors receive formal preparation for this role. Instead, most learn to supervise through their own personal experience of supervision. Previous chapters in this book have provided practical approaches for supervisors in a variety of different psychiatric practice settings. In this chapter, we address professional development for clinical supervisors, and specifically how one might design a program to prepare new supervisors, build skills around the approaches and topics discussed in previous chapters, and enhance clinical supervision skills for supervisors at any stage of their careers.

Clinical supervision is understudied, and there is even less literature regarding professional development programs for psychiatry supervisors. For this reason, we look broadly at literature examining professional development programs across medical education and across mental health fields. From this review of the relevant literature, we propose guiding principles and practical strategies for providing professional development around clinical supervision in psychiatry.

Key Points

- Professional development programs for clinical supervisors should utilize a combination of didactic education and experiential learning.

- A model of supervision for supervisors provides longitudinal, experience-based learning with the opportunity for direct observation and feedback.

- More rigorous studies using outcomes beyond participant self-report are needed to identify the most effective approaches to professional development.

Review of the Relevant Literature

There is scant published literature within psychiatry regarding professional development programs for clinical supervisors. There is, however, more extensive literature on topics such as teaching psychiatry residents to teach and supervise medical students, encouraging faculty development to address teaching and supervision skills across medical specialties, and teaching psychotherapy supervision skills to psychologists. In what follows, we review this literature and its limitations, as well as highlight some suggested best practices for designing professional development programs.

Professional Development Programs for Psychiatry Supervisors

Riess and Herman (2008) described an eight-session course for current and prospective psychodynamic psychotherapy supervisors. Core educational methods were class participation and discussion of case examples. Topics included the history of supervision in psychodynamic psychotherapy; the opening phase of supervision, including forming an alliance with the supervisee and establishing a frame and goals; assessment of learning; boundaries; the differences between supervision and psychotherapy; evaluation and feedback; legal, ethical, and cross-cultural issues in supervision; supervising intense affect; and characteristics of excellent supervisors. Participant ratings of this course were high (3.70–4.00 on a 4-point scale, with 4 being "excellent"). The authors suggested possible future directions of showing video examples of effective and ineffective supervision, providing video feedback to supervisors, and peer supervision of supervisors.

Teaching Psychiatry Residents to Teach

Several authors have reported on programs teaching psychiatry residents to teach, in both classroom and clinical settings. An editorial summarizing such studies (Polan and Riba 2010) noted the wide variety of programs (ranging from 1.5 hours to multiyear clinician-educator residency tracks), skills taught (including teaching clinical skills such as interviewing, mental status examination, and case formulation; giving, eliciting, and using feedback; the one-minute preceptor model; and how to be an oral examiner), and teaching methods (e.g., didactics, supervision, mentoring, direct observation and feedback). The editorial authors also highlighted the importance of evaluating such professional development programs using assessments of learner performance and observed standardized teaching evaluations, not merely participant self-report.

One early experimental study of a program training psychiatry residents to teach interviewing skills to medical students (Naji et al.1986) emphasized the importance of experiential learning in professional development for clinical supervisors. Twenty-four psychiatry residents were randomly assigned to one of four training conditions to learn how to teach interviewing skills: experiential supervised (ES), experiential unsupervised (EU), didactic supervised (DS), and didactic unsupervised (DU). Didactic instruction included receiving a handout about areas to cover and a rating scale to use in assessing students' interviewing skills. Residents then viewed and discussed a videotape demonstrating the interviewing skills to be taught. Twelve of the residents (ES and EU groups) also received experiential training, including self-assessment and group discussion of their own patient interviews and interviewing skills. Supervised residents (ES and DS groups) additionally received supervision and feedback about their first four teaching sessions with medical students. Two hundred eighty-seven medical students on their psychiatry clerkship participated in this study. Compared with a control group of students who received no training, medical students receiving training showed significantly greater improvements in interviewing skills. Medical students taught by residents who themselves received experiential training (ES and EU groups) performed significantly better in interviewing patients than those taught by residents trained in a solely didactic manner. Neither supervision nor the residents' own interviewing skills had a significant effect on medical student performance.

Professional Development Programs to Enhance Teaching Effectiveness in Medicine

Across medical specialties, most faculty development programs to improve teaching effectiveness, including clinical supervision, take the form of workshops or longitudinal programs such as teaching scholar programs or degree or certificate programs. For example, in reviewing 111 studies of such faculty development programs published between 2002 and 2012, Steinert and colleagues (2016) found that 29% described workshops and 36% longitudinal programs. Other, less common, interventions included seminars, short courses, or "other" (e.g., observed teaching, Objective Structured Teaching Encounters, coaching programs). Only 32% of the interventions were based on an underlying conceptual framework or theory of learning, and most emphasized skill acquisition rather than participants' motivation for teaching, values, or professional identities.

One area of professional development that appears to be gaining more momentum in the literature in recent years is the use of peer observation. Observation and feedback constitute one of the cornerstones of experience-based medical education, and learners value direct observation by teachers. It is not surprising, then, that observation and feedback would be useful in the development of supervisor skills. Mookherjee and colleagues (2014) designed a faculty development program based on direct observation and feedback of clinical teaching skills in hospitalists. Their program utilized the SFDP-26, a 26-item teaching evaluation from the Stanford Faculty Development Program framework for optimal clinical teaching. The study selected 10 items from this

26-item scale as the observable behaviors for evaluation. Participants were trained for 2 hours on optimal teaching skills, and then paired up to have their teaching observed and evaluated, based on those 10 items, by a peer, at least twice over the next year. The observed participant then received both written and verbal feedback from their observer. Most participants of the program rated the program highly and described improvement in their teaching skills. Although this study measured only self-assessed outcomes and was uncontrolled, it does demonstrate how peer observation and feedback can be implemented in a teaching faculty group without significant training requirements.

The use of objective structured teaching exercises (OSTEs) is another vehicle for introducing peer observation and feedback into professional development. OSTEs consist of simulated teaching scenarios in which an actor plays a learner and presents a scenario for a teacher to react to. The teacher can then receive real-time feedback on his or her performance once the scenario is complete (Boillat et al. 2012). Julian et al. (2012) evaluated the impact of using OSTEs on faculty clinical teaching skills. They demonstrated that their faculty group from across multiple specialties rated OSTEs very highly in improving self-assessed teaching skills. Comparing faculty teaching evaluations pre and 6 months post intervention did not demonstrate significant change, however. The authors hypothesized that this result was due to the very highly rated teaching evaluations at both time points for all participants.

Another example of peer observation of teaching is the co-teaching model described by Orlander et al. (2000). In this model, junior and senior faculty members are paired for teaching experiences. The model consists of an initial orientation and then phases of teaching, debriefing, and planning for the next teaching experience. Co-teachers develop a set of shared goals for both the teaching encounter and the exercise itself (i.e., goals the teachers have for the learners and goals the teachers have for themselves). This model lends itself well to learning and skill development on multiple levels. Senior and junior faculty can model skills for one another, observe one another practice skills, reflect on experiences together, and self-reflect on shared experiences. Evaluation of this model by the model authors, though limited, reflected that participants reported high levels of satisfaction and self-assessed skill development.

Increasingly, the faculty development literature within medicine also has examined the context in which professional development programs occur (O'Sullivan and Irby 2011; Steinert 2010; Steinert et al. 2016). O'Sullivan and Irby (2011) postulate that there are actually two major communities in faculty development, the faculty development community (i.e., those who participate in a training together) and the workplace in which faculty work (i.e., where learning is put into practice). They assert that both environments should be studied, as should the interaction between them. The context in which skills would be used must be considered and likely determines, to some degree, the effectiveness of the development methods used to teach a skill. Workplace-based professional development programs also allow participants to acquire new knowledge and skills directly relevant to their work environment, with their peers, thus forming a community of practice (Steinert et al. 2016). This approach is convenient for busy clinicians and supervisors and can include activities such as lunchtime professional development sessions, peer mentoring, coaching, reflection, and the peer observation and feedback approaches discussed above.

Professional Development for Psychology Supervisors

Clinical supervision skills in psychiatry are similar to those in other mental health professions, such as psychology, especially in the area of psychotherapy supervision. Thus, published reports of professional development for psychotherapy supervisors across mental health disciplines are relevant for psychiatrists. This literature increasingly has focused on the evidence base for supervision and for training supervisors. For example, Milne et al. (2011) reviewed 11 studies of professional development programs for supervisors. The most frequently covered topic was giving feedback, included in all 11 programs. Program outcomes were evaluated using reactions of supervisors to training, supervisor and supervisee development, and, in two studies, effects on patients. Outcomes were positive across studies, providing empirical support for supervisor training. The authors noted the marked overlap between methods used in supervision itself and in training supervisors, especially giving feedback, educational role-plays, modeling, and video demonstrations.

Milne (2010) described a trainer's manual for teaching professional development programs for psychotherapy supervisors and tested it in 10 workshops involving 25 trainers and 256 psychologist supervisors. The manual provided PowerPoint slides, supervision guideline handouts, video examples of supervision, and instructions for facilitating experiential learning exercises incorporating feedback, discussion, and action planning. Workshops included six sessions covering orientation to supervision, goal setting, facilitated learning, the supervisory relationship, evaluation and feedback, and the supervision system. Some trainers also received consultation regarding their teaching of the sessions. Trainers rated the manual and consultation highly. Participating supervisors reviewed the workshops positively and rated the instructors who received additional consultation more highly than instructors who used the manual alone. Supervisor participants also valued most the experiential part of their training.

Watkins (2012) conducted a comprehensive review of the literature and concluded that ideally, education of psychotherapy supervisors is made up of a combination of didactic material and experiential learning. This is consistent with much of the literature cited above and with findings in the medical and dental literature that continuing education practices are most effective when provided as a combination of didactic and experiential practices (Forsetlund et al. 2009; Hendricson et al. 2007). Watkins (2012) described the didactic component of educating supervisors as supplying information on the goals, frame, structure, and function of supervision, while the experiential component consists of "supervision of the supervision process." In this "supervision of supervision," the trainee supervisor brings evidence of or is observed doing supervision and then receives feedback and supervision regarding his or her supervision efforts.

Increasingly, psychology and other health professions have adopted a competency-based approach to training supervisors. For example, the American Psychological Association (2014) has outlined a set of seven competencies for clinical supervisors: 1) the supervisor's own clinical and professional competence; 2) knowledge regarding diversity; 3) ability to establish and maintain an effective supervisory relationship, including forming an alliance and managing the power differential inherent in supervision; 4) professionalism; 5) the ability to assess supervisee strengths and areas for improvement, provide effective feedback and formative and summative evaluation, foster self-assessment in the supervisee, and elicit feedback regarding the supervision process; 6) the ability to identify, address, and work to remediate performance problems in supervisees; and 7) knowledge of ethical, legal, and regulatory considerations, including establishing a supervision contract. This framework of competencies has been proposed as a guide for designing didactic and experiential components of professional development programs for psychology supervisors and self-assessment tools have been developed to guide supervisor development (see, e.g., Falender et al. 2014).

Limitations of the Professional Development Literature

There is some evidence that supervisor training is beneficial (e.g., Milne et al. 2011; Steinert et al. 2016; Watkins 2012). However, most studies of professional development programs use participant satisfaction as the major outcome measure. Although participant satisfaction rates tend to be high, such ratings provide limited information about the effectiveness of these programs in improving supervisors' actual skills and performance. Other commonly employed program outcome measures include increases in participant knowledge, confidence, and enthusiasm and increases in their self-reported skills and behaviors. Few studies assess observed changes in supervisors' behavior and very few examine changes in satisfaction or performance of their supervisees or in patient care outcomes.

Other weaknesses of the professional development literature regarding teaching and supervision include the relative lack of qualitative research to help understand how or why faculty development interventions are effective for particular participants, the limited use of control groups or randomized trials, and the paucity of direct comparisons of different interventions.

Best Practices for Faculty Development Programs

Despite the limitations of the literature on professional development for clinical teaching and supervisory skills, the data do suggest some best practices for successful programs. These include using an evidence-based educational design grounded in theory, providing content relevant to the context of the learner and based on desired supervisor competencies, incorporating experiential learning mixed with didactic education, and providing opportunities for practical application. In addition, there appears to be educational benefit to longitudinal programs that spread learning over time. Longitudinal programs provide greater opportunities for some of the aforementioned practices (i.e., experiential learning and practical application of skills) and also allow for greater community building, which supports and sustains educational gains at institutions. Workplace-based professional development also fosters community building and is convenient and accessible. Finally, institutional support is a clear asset to a successful program. This support extends beyond simple support of the education itself to the environment in which new knowledge and skills are to be used. If a faculty development program focuses on a particular skill or application, but then participants are unable to practice those skills in their clinical environments because of administrative or logistical constraints, how useful can the development program be?

Recommendations for Designing a Professional Development Program for Supervisors

Content

Particular supervision types and venues require specialized content knowledge. However, based on the literature and on desired supervisor competencies, we propose nine core content areas for professional development programs: 1) orientation to the role of supervisor and discussion of the theoretical model underpinning the particular type of supervision; 2) establishing a supervisory alliance; 3) setting goals and expectations; 4) educational methods for supervision; 5) assessment, feedback, and evaluation; 6) cultivating self-assessment and lifelong learning, both in supervisors and their supervisees; 7) ethical and legal issues in supervision; 8) cross-cultural and diversity issues in supervision, or how to supervise someone with a background and perspective different from one's own; and 9) addressing problems in supervision, including identifying a poor "fit" between the supervisor and supervisee, supervisee attendance or performance issues, and need for remediation. Specific content in each of these areas is included elsewhere in this book.

Program Structure

On the basis of the literature, we recommend that a professional development program for supervisors include both didactic and experiential components. Suggested content of the didactic material is detailed above and would also depend on the learning needs of participants. A longitudinal learning format would allow the program to capitalize on repeated skill demonstration and practice, internalization of learning over time, and building of a community among program participants.

Central to our recommended program would be supervision for the training supervisor, or "supervision of supervision" (Watkins 2012). This could include direct observation of the supervision itself, viewing of video recordings of past supervision, discussion of process notes, or some combination of these options. Such supervision would allow for observation and feedback as well as reflection for the training supervisor on the process of supervision from both sides. The training supervisor has the experience of being the supervisor with trainees and then being a supervisee with his or her supervisor. This dual experience should provide a rich environment for skill development and integration. An illustration of this program structure is provided in Figure 50–1.

Experiential training for the psychiatry supervisor could also follow a co-teaching model as described by Orlander and colleagues (2000). This would provide built-in supervision for the junior faculty member and encourage planning, reflection, and continuous assessment on the part of both parties. Integrating supervision of the supervisor into a longitudinal program either through a co-teaching model or via a more traditional supervision model would provide robust experiential learning. Individual supervision or co-teaching sessions could be linked with prescribed didactic topics to ensure that participants focused on relevant content areas.

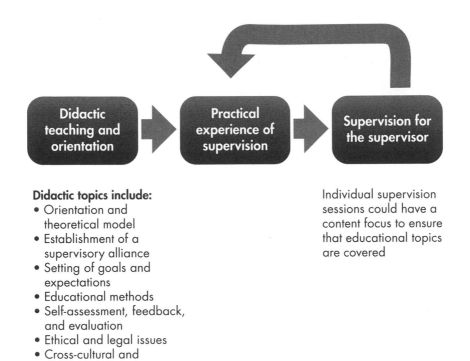

FIGURE 50–1.   Professional development program structure: an example.

Context

Professional development programs traditionally occur outside the supervisor's workplace and in fact could be accomplished from a distance, with didactic education online or via off-site workshops and supervision for the supervisor conducted remotely. However, there appear to be a number of benefits to integrating the program into the workplace as much as possible. Taking advantage of the workplace context for experience-based learning maximizes the relevance and practical application of learning. The process of either co-teaching or supervision for the supervisor is likely to create a collegial bond between the pair, which is likely to benefit the overall faculty culture and offer possible future mentorship opportunities. Finally, workplace-based professional development supports the local culture around faculty development and teaching skill improvement, fostering a continued, local impetus for quality improvement in supervision.

Assessing Outcomes

Determining whether professional development meaningfully enhances supervisors' performance requires measuring program outcomes beyond participant satisfaction or self-assessed improvement in knowledge and skills. Methods such as direct observation of supervision, OSTEs, co-teaching, and examining supervisee and patient outcomes would provide more robust measures of the effectiveness of a professional development program.

Specific Challenges and Strategies

- **There are no experts available in our area.** Many institutions and departments lack experts who are ready, willing, and able to provide high-quality professional development in all of the didactic content areas described in this chapter. Likely, departments will need to consider a combination of drawing on existing in-house resources within their own and other departments, bringing in national experts or programs, and using offsite training, for example, at national conferences or career development programs. Online and/or teleconferenced professional development would be an option providing a national peer group and exposure to topics and experts not locally available.

- **There is a lack of resources and/or support for our professional development program.** Professional development requires resources and support, not only in terms of direct program costs but also in terms of protected time for supervisors to participate. The clinical environment in which supervision exists may not support an optimal supervision technique or process that a professional development initiative may want to foster. Achieving support from department chairs and clinical leaders is important before starting a professional development program. Potential benefits include building a community of supervisors and increasing faculty and supervisor job satisfaction, well-being, and retention, as well as the possibility of improving supervision, training program quality, trainee satisfaction and recruitment, and patient outcomes. However, in the face of scarce resources, competing priorities, or lack of interest, it may not be possible to start with an ideal, fully formed professional development program. A pragmatic approach, beginning with a smaller intervention and demonstrating positive results, may allow progressive program development and the creation of a lasting and successful program.

Questions for Development Programs, Departments, and Institutions

■ What are the professional development needs of our faculty?

■ How could a faculty development program at our institution be best structured to meet the educational needs of the faculty?

■ What local resources can be drawn on to meet this need?

■ What partners will we need to support this development program?

■ How can our faculty development program support the needs or mission of our department?

Additional Resources

Online Resources

MedEdPORTAL: www.mededportal.org

An open -access, online, peer-reviewed repository of hundreds of resources related to faculty development and supervision to provide examples and support to educators developing their own programs and workshops.
Stanford Faculty Development Center for Medical Teachers: http://sfdc.stanford.edu/
Yale Supervision Program: www.supervision.yale.edu

Manual

Milne DL, Reiser RP: A Manual for Evidence-Based CBT Supervision. Hoboken, NJ, Wiley, 2017
Includes tools to evaluate supervisors and recommended readings regarding supervision and supervisor training.

References

American Psychological Association: Guidelines for clinical supervision in health service psychology. 2014. Available at: https://www.apa.org/about/policy/guidelines-supervision.pdf. Accessed August 23, 2018.

Boillat M, Bethune C, Ohle E, et al: Twelve tips for using the objective structured teaching exercise for faculty development. Med Teach 34(4):269–273, 2012 22455695

Falender CA, Shafranske EP, Ofek A: Competent clinical supervision: emerging effective practices. Couns Psychol Q 27:393–408, 2014

Forsetlund L, Bjørndal A, Rashidian A, et al: Continuing education meetings and workshops: effects on professional practice and health care outcomes. Cochrane Database Syst Rev (2):CD003030, 2009 19370580

Hendricson WD, Anderson E, Andrieu SC, et al: Does faculty development enhance teaching effectiveness? J Dent Educ 71(12):1513–1533, 2007 18096877

Julian K, Appelle N, O'Sullivan P, et al: The impact of an objective structured teaching evaluation on faculty teaching skills. Teach Learn Med 24(1):3–7, 2012 22250929

Milne D: Can we enhance the training of clinical supervisors? A national pilot study of an evidence-based approach. Clin Psychol Psychother 17(4):321–328, 2010 19911431

Milne DL, Sheikh AI, Pattison S, et al: Evidence-based training for clinical supervisors: a systematic review of 11 controlled studies. Clin Supervisor 30:53–71, 2011

Mookherjee S, Monash B, Wentworth KL, et al: Faculty development for hospitalists: structured peer observation of teaching. J Hosp Med 9(4):244–250, 2014 24446215

Naji SA, Maguire GP, Fairbairn SA, et al: Training clinical teachers in psychiatry to teach interviewing skills to medical students. Med Educ 20(2):140–147, 1986 3959930

O'Sullivan PS, Irby DM: Reframing research on faculty development. Acad Med 86(4):421–428, 2011 21346505

Orlander JD, Gupta M, Fincke BG, et al: Co-teaching: a faculty development strategy. Med Educ 34(4):257–265, 2000 10733721

Polan HJ, Riba M: Creative solutions to psychiatry's increasing reliance on residents as teachers. Acad Psychiatry 34(4):245–247, 2010 20576979

Riess H, Herman JB: Teaching the teachers: a model course for psychodynamic psychotherapy supervisors. Acad Psychiatry 32(3):259–264, 2008 18467486

Steinert Y: Becoming a better teacher: from intuition to intent, in Theory and Practice of Teaching Medicine. Edited by Ende T. Philadelphia, PA, American College of Physicians, 2010, pp 73–93

Steinert Y, Mann K, Anderson B, et al: A systematic review of faculty development initiatives designed to enhance teaching effectiveness: a 10-year update: BEME Guide No. 40. Med Teach 38(8):769–786, 2016 27420193

Watkins CE Jr: Educating psychotherapy supervisors. Am J Psychother 66(3):279–307, 2012 23091887

Index

Page numbers printed in **boldface** type refer to tables or figures.